PRACTICAL PATHOLOGY

This book is approved for the course of undergraduate and postgraduate Medical students and Laboratory technologists

PRACTICAL PATHOLOGY

including

MORBID ANATOMY AND HISTOPATHOLOGY WITH SPECIAL STAINS, EXFOLIATIVE CYTOLOGY, CLINICAL PATHOLOGY, CHEMICAL PATHOLOGY INCLUDING THE PRINCIPLES OF PHOTOELECTRIC COLORIMETER AND FLAME PHOTOMETER, EXPERIMENTAL PATHOLOGY AND POSTMORTEM STUDIES; IN ADDITION TO HAEMATOLOGY AND APPLICATION OF AUTOMATED INSTRUMENTS; DIAGRAMS OF RELEVANT INSTRUMENTS AND MUSEUM SPECIMENS ARE PRESENTED

N C Dey
BSc, MD, FDS, FRSM [London], DBact [Manchester], FISD [New York]

T K Dey
MD, DBact [Manchester], FISD [New York], FRSM [London], etc.

D Sinha, PhD

New Central Book Agency (P) Ltd

Co-Published by

Bijay Publications

E-mail : bijaypublications@gmail.com

Exclusively Distributed by

Bijay Pustak Bhandar (P) Ltd

90/6A M. G. Road, Bhawani Dutta Lane, Kolkata-700007

✆ : (033) 4605-7856, 8777898576, 8274916104

E-mail : bijaypustakbhandar@gmail.com

NCBA

REGD OFFICE
8/1 Chintamoni Das Lane, Kolkata 700 009, India
email: ncbakolkata@gmail.com

OVERSEAS
NCBA (UK) Ltd, 149 Park Avenue North, Northampton, NN3 2HY, UK
email: ncbauk@yahoo.com

CORPORATE OFFICE
12 Shahpur Jat, New Delhi 110 049
email: ncbaexports@ncbapvtltd.com

BIJAY PUBLICATIONS
90/6A M. G. Road, Bhawani Dutta Lane, Kolkata-7
E-mail : bijaypublications@gmail.com

BIJAY PUSTAK BHANDAR (P) LTD
90/6A M. G. Road, Bhawani Dutta Lane, Kolkata-7
E-mail : bijaypustakbhandar@gmail.com

PRACTICAL PATHOLOGY • N C Dey, T K Dey, M Dey, D Sinha

First Published: 1998
Reprinted: 1999, 2003, 2004, 2007, 2010, 2012, 2013, 2015
Thoroughly Revised and Updated Second Edition: 2017
Reprinted: 2018, 2019, 2021, 2022, 2023

PUBLISHER • TYPESETTER • PRINTER
New Central Book Agency (P) Ltd
8/1 Chintamoni Das Lane, Kolkata 700 009

CO-PUBLISHED BY
Bijay Publications
90/6A M G Road, Bhawani Dutta Lane, Kolkata 700007

TECHNICAL EDITORS
Dr Mita Sen, MBBS and Dipan Roy

PROJECT TEAM
Ashit Ghosh, Prodip Baidya and Pradip Biswas

ISBN: 978 93 5255 015 9

Price ₹ 595.00

Dedicated
to
the students of
Pathology

Contents

Preface to the Second Edition

This book titled **Practical Pathology** does not need any introduction as it is one of the most popular books on the subject vis-á-vis its merit. The book offers basic knowledge as regards the "up to date" techniques in different aspects of practical pathology.

The content of the book starts with the design of a microscope and its techniques including the focal length and magnifications of objectives and eye piece. Regarding staining techniques, the routine and the selective special stains of common usage have been explained including the directive formularies.

Various topics on general and special pathology have been discussed "chapter by chapter" including the special and selective points for diagnostic histopathology.

The book contains a chapter on Exfoliative Cytology with special reference to specialised stains, like PAP stain and the secret of success in accomplishment of Methyl green and Pyronin stain plus Unna-Papenheim stain.

Most of the diagrams of histological, hematological, biochemical and museum specimens are coloured with detailed histories of patients and the total number of diagrams is 193 in this book of 304 pages.

A good number of tests are laid down in Chapters 9, 10 and 11. The subjects include detailed examinations of A. Sputum, B. CSF, C. Urine, D. Gastric juice analyses, E. Liver function tests, F. Renal function tests, G. Thyroid function tests, H. Pregnancy tests, I. Seminal fluid analysis, etc. along with other immunological tests.

In Chapter 12 (Hematology) topics on blood collection and examinations have been discussed with incorporation of 23 blood charts with histories of the patients.

Chapter on Chemical Pathology includes various ways and the basic methods of chemical and biochemical tests including a number of parameters (non-enzymic, enzymic and others).

Chapters on A. **Automated and semi-automated methods** in pathology, B. **Preliminary experimental pathology** and C. **Autopsy pathology** are well documented.

Museum specimens are well-reproduced in Chapter 17. Appendix includes preparation of important buffers.

Last but not least, a complete and elaborate index has been incorporated for finding out the topics at a glance.

The book is designed for the undergraduate and postgraduate medical students, and advanced level learners of Chemistry, Biochemistry and Pathology. It will also cater to the needs of the 'Laboratory Assistants' working in pathological laboratories.

We would congratulate the readers who would be bestowed upon with exclusive and sumptuous knowledge in Practical Pathology reading the text.

N C DEY
T K DEY
M DEY
D SINHA

1st February 2017
Kolkata

Preface to the First Edition

This particular title is based on the existing book under the Title "Practical Pathology and Microbiology" by N C Dey and T K Dey in accord with the combined syllabus.

Since the subjects are upgraded, it has been necessary to upgrade the two parts of the book into Practical Pathology and Practical Microbiology, separately in the form of two separate books under new syllabus. The matters in these books are thoroughly rewritten and has been upgraded with newer additions as per the syllabus.

The book has been thoroughly revised, many additions made and its scope of utility is enlarged. It includes Morbid Anatomy and Histopathology, Clinical Pathology and Chemical Pathology including the principles of Photoelectric colorimeter and Flame photometer. Common routine microchemical techniques for biochemical estimations have been incorporated. Also included are Preliminary Experimental Pathology and Postmortem Techniques and proforma to make the book more useful for student and laboratory workers.

In addition, the important Museum Specimens, and the Instruments and Charts which are given and asked in the examinations have been serially incorporated for the benefit of the students during examination who can recapitulate them at a glance.

In publishing this edition, due care has been taken to review the various chapters thoroughly and to incorporate an index and uptodate developments wherever necessary. The text includes 'BIOPSY' and its classification in this edition lucidly, as the term is not clearly written in any of the common books on the subject.

The outstanding feature of this volume lies in the 23 charts of Hematological diseases, questions on which a student is likely to face during viva voice tests. A large number of important tests regarding urine examination have also been embodied in this volume, which are rarely available in other books on the subject.

The instruments have been incorporated in this edition of the book with their individual diagrams in addition to museum specimens of morbid anatomy which would be absolutely and necessarily helpful to the student of M.B.B.S. course. They have been meticulously checked with the syllabus in consultation with the examiners.

Hence a student will be well-advised to go through this volume more meticulously to enable him to build up a good standing in his medical career in the long term.

We take this opportunity of offering our sincere thanks to New Central Book Agency (P) Ltd., and Dr. Mita Sen without whose active co-operation and help it would have been impossible for us to make the progress of this edition upto the publishing stage within such a short time.

N C DEY
T K DEY
M DEY
D SINHA

25th December 1997
Kolkata

I. For Junior Class

The book is intended to be presented to the University During Practical Examination of Pathology

Students's Name ....

Roll No...................... Class..................... Batch.................... Session.....................

Remarks on Practical Works:

Complete/Incomplete:

....

Asst./Associate Professor/Reader Professor

Date .... Date ....

University Roll .... No......................... Year...............................

Examiner's Signature ....

Date ....

II. For Senior Class

The book is intended to be presented to the University During Practical Examination of Pathology

---

Students's Name ....

Roll No..................... Class.................. Batch..................... Session....................

Remarks on Practical Works:

Complete/Incomplete:

....

Asst./Associate Professor/Reader Professor

Date .... Date ....

University Roll .... No..................... Year...............................

Examiner's Signature ....

Date ....

General Instructions for the Students

Students must observe the following instructions strictly while working in the laboratory:

1. Every student must reach the practical class in time and should maintain discipline.
2. Students must carry their own apron, lead pencil and H & E pencils, Practical Note Book and handkerchief in Practical Class.
3. Microscope, slide and other articles needed for practical exercises will be provided by the Laboratory Assistant at the beginning of the class and they must be returned to the same person before leaving the laboratory.
4. Students should draw the diagrams and write down their observations during the practical period.
5. Reagent bottles and other articles must be kept in proper places after use.
6. Students should clean the microscope lenses every day after use with the aid of kerchief moistened with solvent and rotate the objective to low power before returning them, and put off the microscope light at their respective seats before leaving the laboratory.
7. Keep your trays and table clean before leaving the laboratory.
8. Students should not hesitate to express their difficulties to the staff.
9. Students will be responsible for any damage caused by themselves.

CARE OF MICROSCOPE

Remember that the microscope is a delicate and costly instrument, which must be handled with care. It is your responsibility to see that it is maintained properly.

1. Never carry the microscope with one hand. Use both hands one under the foot and the other holding the limb.
2. Never leave the microscope without the Eyepiece or Objectives in place.
3. Never put the microscope away with Immersion Oil Objective in focus.
4. Never touch the lenses of the Objectives or Eyepieces with your fingers.
5. Never use ordinary paper, fluffy or rough cloth or cotton wool to clean lenses. Clean the lenses with soft cloth.
6. Never clean the body of the microscope with Xylene.

USE OF MICROSCOPE

Set up the microscope at a convenient position facing the source of light. Place the object on the stage and adjust the mirror to the light source. Never tilt the stage of the microscope if examining any fluid specimen. Adjust the microscope as follows:

For Unstained Preparation

1. Lower the condenser.
2. Partially close the iris diaphragm.
3. Use a concave mirror.
4. Focus under low power and then turn on dry high power.

For Stained Preparation

1. Lower the condenser.
2. Use a concave mirror.
3. Adjust the iris diaphragm to give an even illumination of the microscopic field.

For Oil Immersion Examination

1. Raise up the condenser completely.
2. Open the iris diaphragm.

3. Use a plane mirror.
4. Study the object under low power first and then place a drop of cedar wood oil (paraffin oil is an accepted substitute) on the object and turn on the oil immersion lense. Rack the objective down until the tip of objective dips in the oil. Then examine the object (using the fine adjustment).
5. After use remove oil from the objective and clear the object with a cloth dipped in Xylol.
6. Turn the nosepiece until low power objective is in position.

HISTOPATHOLOGY SLIDES FOR STUDENTS

1–1 Acute apendicitis
1–2 Tuberculous lymph node
1–3 Chronic cholecystitis
1–4 Squamous papilloma
1–5 Squamous cell carcinoma (SCC)
1–6 Basal cell carcinoma (BCC)
1–7 Adenocarcinoma
1–8 Fibroma
1–9 Lipoma
1–10 Liposarcoma
1–11 Chronic venous congestion-spleen
1–12 Chronic venous congestion-lung
1–13 Infarction of spleen
1–14 Hodgkin's lymphoma
1–15 Amyloidosis of spleen
1–16 Amyloidosis-kidney
1–17 Myocardial infarction
1–18 Medial calcification of artery
1–19 Thromboangitis obliterans
1–20 Heamangioma
1–21 Lobar pneumonia
1–22 Bronchopneumonia
1–23 Bronchiectasis of lung
1–24 Frabrocasseous tuberculosis-lung
1–25 Bronchogenic carcinoma.

PART ONE

Histopathology and General Pathology

A. BASIC METHODS AND GENERAL PATHOLOGY

CHAPTER 1

HISTOPATHOLOGY

FIXATIVES AND STAINING

Fixation (For Fixative see Page 2):

Fixation is a complex series of chemical events. Fixation differs for different groups of chemical substances present in tissues.

Reactions of Fixatives with Proteins

Fixatives that **stabilize the proteins** are most important. **Fixatives forming cross links between proteins lead to formation of a "gel". Soluble proteins are fixed to structural proteins and render proteins insoluble**. Such insoluble substance **offers more mechanical strength** that **protects the tissue (substance)**. Fixation usually takes place in aqueous solution but occasionally "vapour" is used.

A. Primary Fixatives

I. ALDEHYDES:

Kinds of Formaldehyde Fixatives

1. **Formaldehyde Gas (Vapc ur)**

Formaldehyde vapour can b dissolved in water upto 35% to 40% to its **saturation**. :0% formaldehyde vapour is dissolved in water; this is called **formalin**. 10% of the formalin (i.e., 4% forma dehyde vapour) is dissolved in 90 ml. of saline, and this is called 10% formal saline or 4% formaldehyd vapour in NaCl solution (N/saline). **Ten percent formalin fixative is used** as a fixative for all the tissues in general; but **for fixing brains, 15% formalin is required**. Suitably a buffered (in phosphate buffer) formalin with addition of phenol formalin (0.5% phenol) is used for immunoperoxidase and electron microscopic studies.

2. **Formaldehyde (40%)** i.e., Formalin

Formaldehyde that reacts with amino acids and proteins is a "time honoured" ideal fixative. This forms the basis of fixation with other aldehydes as well. Cross links are formed between protein molecule; the reaction occurs **between the fixative and "lysine"** (the basic amino acids), the residues remain on exterior of protein molecule. With formaldehyde mostly the **fixation reaction is reversible (in excess of water)**.

3. **Glutaraldehyde**

With glutaraldehyde the fixation reaction is rapid and irreversible. The reaction between aldehydes and proteins is dependent on pH; **rapidity of reaction** occurs **with increase in pH** (towards the **alkaline side**).

Fixation denatures 10% to 30% protein, yet it is **easy and convenient for routine work, enzyme biochemica', and immunohistochemical work**, as well **as for electron microscopy**. Glutaraldehyde causes **30% loss of tissue specificity** by denaturation of protein, but the total property, tissue specificity, morphological preservation, and the biochemical activities are well-retained. **Osmic acid treatment following glutaraldehyde fixation** causes complete denaturation of protein but the total properties of tissue specificities are best maintained.

II. OXIDIZING AGENTS:

They are: (a) Osmium tetroxide, (b) Potassium dichromate and (c) Potassium permanganate

Osmium tetroxide breaks down protein into small subunits (reacting with **epidermal keratin**).

B. Secondary Fixatives

They are **postfixation fixatives.**

MERCURIC CHLORIDE (Secondary fixative)

This is used as a secondary fixative where amino acid residues (of proteins) are present, e.g., (a) **Thiol group, (b) Amino group, (c) Imidazole group, (d) Hydroxyl and (e) Phosphate groups react with mercuric chloride.**

Carboxyl groups of proteins do not react with mercuric chloride.

The secondary fixation, i.e., postfixation with mercuric chloride is satisfactory with the (i) **trichrome methods,** and (ii) **immunoperoxidase techniques.**

Most of the fixatives are for primary fixation that alone is enough to fix tissues. Sometimes tissues fixed with primary fixatives, e.g., aldehyde fixative which may not be stable enough, and in that case they **require secondary fixation** (or **post-fixation**).

Primarily fixed (e.g., tissue containing) catecholamine (monoamine oxide) requires **secondary fixation or post-fixation** (i.e., chromation) by **potassium dichromate solution** for showing the **chromaffin tissue** for the **demonstration of mitochondria clearly**.

Similarly tissues fixed in the **primary fixative,** like **glutaraldehyde** usually requires **post- (or secondary) fixation in Osmium tetroxide.** The **aldehyde-fixed tissues are not stabilized** (alpha-helix of proteins is completely lost) when it is **post-fixed by osmium tetroxide** that makes the membranes permeable, and hence percolation and retention of stains and dyes persists and renders them stained positively.

For study of other fixatives and section making and staining procedure in detail see page 5.

Tissue processing and section making procedures

Fixation:

Fixative: A fixative is an agent which penetrates and fixes the tissue to prevent autolysis.

Common fixative: Formal saline......

Formalin (commercial 40%)	— 10 ml
Water or normal saline	— 90 ml.

The **amount of fixative should be 20 times** the volume of tissue.

Dehydration, Clearing and Impregnation:

Fixed tissue is cut into sizes of about 1 cm^2, and a thickness of about 5 mm.

(a) Dehydrate by passing through ascending grades of alcohol for each tissue piece in 70%, 80%, 90% and 95% alcohol and **two changes in absolute alcohol.**

(b) Clear by two changes in xylol or chloroform: 1 hr. and 2 hrs. respectively.

(c) Put in saturated solution of paraffin (**melting points 54° to 56°C or celsius**).

Embedding:

Blocks are made in 2 "L" moulds. The surface to be cut is put downwards; pour molten paraffin (54-56°C).

Cool in cold water rapidly or by application of ice.

Section cutting:

Sections are cut in rotary microtome (razor, should be sharp and even); thickness of sections 3 μm to 5 μm is preferable.

Receive sections with a brush or lifter and float on **water bath (50°C).**

Receive the section **from water bath in albumin coated slides.**

Staining—Hematoxylin and Eosin method:

(a) Rehydration—pass through **descending grades of alcohol (90%, 70%, 50%)** each for five minutes and then bring down to water.

(b) Stain with hematoxylin solution for 3–5 mins. Wash in running water till **blue color** develops.

(c) Differentiate with acid-alcohol (1 ml of HCL + 99 ml of 70% alcohol).

(d) Counterstain with 1% aqueous solution of eosin for 1 minute.

(e) For study of other fixatives and section making and staining procedure in detail see page 5.

Mounting:

Mounting is done with DPX mountant and the section is ready for examination.

Method of Examination of Tissue section

(a) Hold the slide against light, examine the section in naked eye or by hand lens or by **inversed eye piece** of the microscope. Note the differences between normal and abnormal procedures.

(b) Examine the entire section with the low power objective. Observe the normal and abnormal sections.

(c) Change to high power objective to study the nature of cells; their size, shape and the staining character of the cytoplasm and nuclei.

METHODS AND TECHNICS

LABORATORY MANNERS AND METHODS

1. Do not be in a hurry to get the materials for the day's work and do not **overcrowd** the table where the materials are kept.

2. See that you are not on the **way of light** of anybody's microscope.

3. Do not **hesitate** to express your difficulties. The staff will always try to help you in every possible way.

4. Keep your **lenses** clean (*see—care of the microscope*).

5. **Draw sketches** of the preparation as seen under high and low power objectives.

6. **Keep** your **trays** and **table clean**; clean the watch glasses after use and wipe them dry. Wash your hands and use antiseptics, if required.

7. Do not lift the jar specimen. **Bend yourself to the level of the jar to examine the morbid anatomy** specimens.

8. Always put on **white apron** (coat) while working in the practical class room.

9. Always **make a habit to check** the gas taps, water taps and electric switches on entering, and before leaving the class room.

THE MICROSCOPE

Draw diagram of a microscope and label the parts.

Parts of a microscope

(a) Horse-shoe stand (**base**).

(b) **Body with coarse rack and pinion** adjustment, and a micrometer for fine adjustment. "Draw tube" is to be fixed at 160 mm.

(c) A revolving **triple nosepiece** containing three objectives:

1. 16 mm ($^2/_3$ inch) × 10 L.P: **low power**
2. 4 mm ($^1/_6$ inch) × 45 H.P: high power **(dry H.P)**
3. 2 mm ($^1/_{12}$ inch) × 90 or 100 oil-immersion **(immersion H.P)**.

(d) **Oculars** "6×" and "10×" Huygenian eye piece (eye piece)

(e) A mechanical stage to move the slide to and fro. In absence of a mechanical stage, the slide is moved with hand to obtain the view of different fields.

(f) A substage Abbe-condenser with rack and pinion (or swing out) is fitted with an **iris diaphragm** to regulate the entrance of light for clear definition of the object.

(g) A reversible plane and **concave mirror** to reflect light.

Magnification = $^T/_F$ × E.

T is tube length; F is the focal legth of the objective; E is the magnification of the ocular **(eye piece)**.

Magnification at 160 mm = initial magnification of the objective multiplied by the magnification of the eyepiece.

USE OF A MICROSCOPE

Put the slide on the stage and focus under low power and then under high power (dry H.P) or oil-immersion (immersion H.P) as the case may be.

Focussing

At first use the coarse adjustment and then the **fine (micrometer) adjustment**. When examining a slide under low or high power, lower the condenser to allow only **critical (optimum density of light)** and work with the concave mirror. In case of an unstained specimen, **close the iris diaphragm** for better definition of the object. The diaphragm and the condenser should be manipulated each time for critical illumination of the object to be examined.

The use of the oil-immersion (immersion H.P) ***objective.*** Find out the field to be examined under low power. Raise the condenser up, use the plane mirror and focus with the $^1/_{12}$" oil-immersion objective after putting a drop of cedar-wood oil or liquid paraffin on the slide.

Lower the $^1/_{12}$" objective into the oil cautiously till the objective nearly touches the surface of the slide;

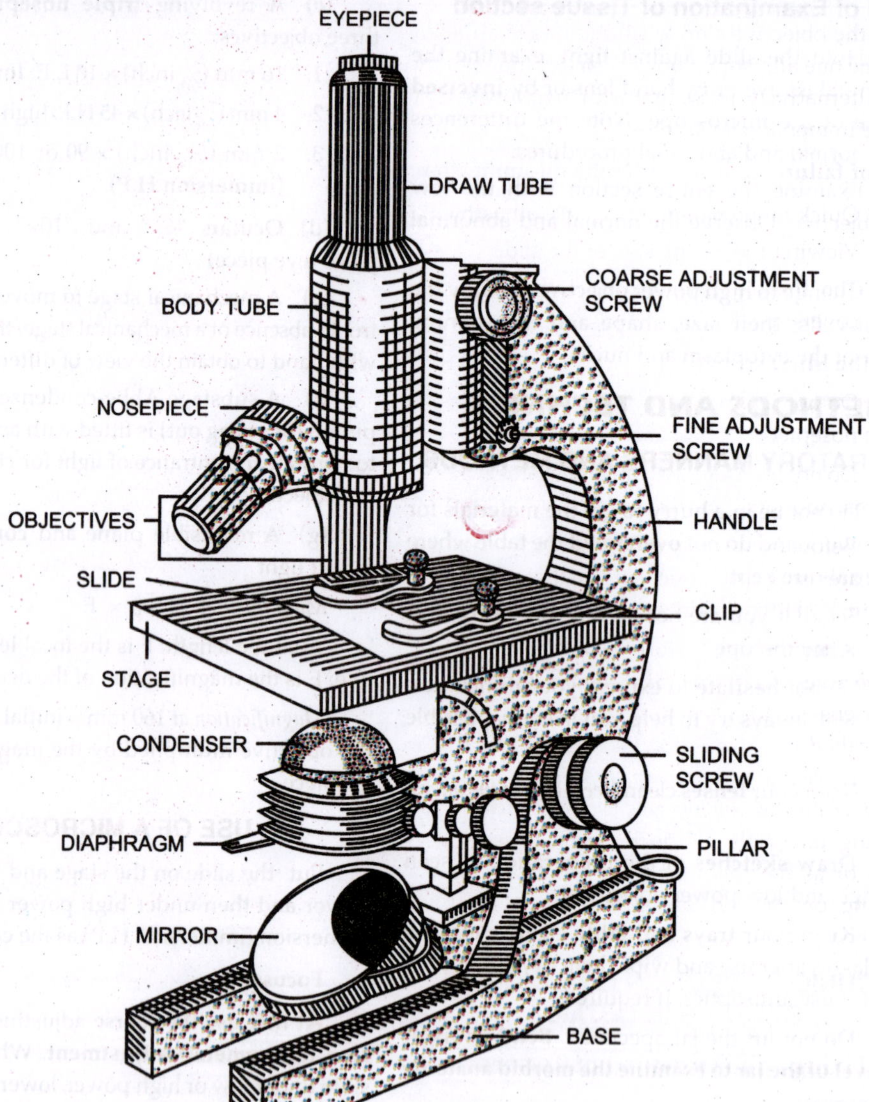

Fig. 1.1: A compound microscope

Table 1.1: Showing focal length of objectives and magnification of the microscope lenses

Objective (Focal length)	Magnification of the (i) Objective	(ii) Eyepieces (1 = 6 X; 2 = 10 X)		Total magnifications of object, i.e., Power of objective × Power of eyepieces	
$\frac{2}{3}$″ or 16 mm	X 10	1 = 6 X	2 = 10 X	1 = 60	2 = 100
$\frac{1}{6}$″ or 4 mm	X 45	1 = 6 X	2 = 10 X	1 = 270	2 = 450
$\frac{1}{12}$″ or 2 mm	X 90 or 100	1 = 6 X	2 = 10 X	1 = 540 or 1 = 600	2 = 900 or 1000

rack up the objective slowly till the image appears. Adjust the fine adjustment for a clear definition of the object. Alternatively, focus first with low power, then place the immersion lens.

Causes of failure to focus under the oil-immersion:

1. Quick movement of the coarse adjustment.
2. Viewing the wrong side of the slide.
3. Too thick a coverslip (always use a thin coverslip—No. 0).

Care of the Microscope

1. Do not remove the eyepiece, and the lenses from the nosepiece.

2. Do not interfere with any mechanical part of the microscope.

3. Before examining under the microscope, see that you are using the correct lens, so that oil may not spoil your $\frac{1}{6}$" H.P objective.

4. After the day's work, clean the oil immersion objective. First wipe off the oil with a piece of **silk**, or lens- or tissue-paper; clean again with the same, soaked in a drop of xylol. *Never use alcohol in any part of the microscope specially to clean the lenses, unless it is directed by the microscope company.* The cementing materials of the lenses is dissolved in alcohol, or as the manufacturer would advise. Oil remaining on the lens dries and spoils it, if left uncleaned.

TECHNIC OF SECTION CUTTING AND STAINING IN DETAIL

Fixing and Hardening of Tissues

FIXATIVES

Fixatives are substances which would maintain the cellular structure and tissue arrangements in vitro (outside the body) as it is present in vivo (inside the body).

A fixative is an agent which penetrates and fixes the tissue and prevents autolysis. It causes cell death but not necrosis.

Small pieces of fresh tissue should be put in 20 parts by volume in one of the following fixatives.

1. ***Alcohol* (Primary Fixative)/Absolute**

Fix in 95 to 100% alcohol for 24 hours. Put the tissue in water overnight before cutting on a (freezing) microtome.

2. ***Formal solution*** (1 : 10)

Formalin (commercial 40% formaldehyde solution) .... 10 ml

Water or normal saline .... 90 ml

It fixes tissues in a few hours to 24 hours depending on the thickness. It is not an ideal fixative but can be used for routine work.

Formal sublimate (1 : 10 $HgCl_2$)

Saturated soln. of mercuric chloride .... 9 parts

Formalin (commercial 40%) .... 1 part

It is a better fixative and less destructive than mercuric chloride. Fix for 8 to 18 hours. Wash for 2 hours. It may be used for routine work.

Zenker's fluid

Pot. bichromate ..... 25 g

Hydrarg perchloride ..... 5.0 g

Water to ..... 100 ml

Just before use add 5 ml of glacial acetic acid. It is a good general fixative and gives excellent details; 5 ml of formol saline instead of acetic acid makes **Zenker's formol**.

Fix tissue for 3-12 hours; wash in running water overnight to remove bichromate and then put in 70% alcohol containing sufficient **iodine** to keep the solution **brown**.

3. ***Carnoy's Fixative* (Primary Fixative)**

Carnoy, J. B. (1887). *La Cellule* 3, 276

It is a **rapid nuclear fixative**. This preserves glycogen and the **Nissl substance**. It has rapid **penetrating and dehydrating power**. This is often used for fixing biopsy specimens for urgent diagnosis. It is a good fixative for cytology as well, where H and E staining has to be done, e.g., **cytology of virus-infected monolayer cell culture.**

Solution:

Acetic acid, glacial ..... 10 ml

Chloroform ..... 30 ml

Ethyl alcohol, absolute ..... 60 ml

Mode of preparation

Combine the ingredients, mix well and label. Put in a well fitted screw-capped bottle to prevent evaporation.

Mode of use

Dissect small pieces of tissue and fix for 30 minutes to 2 hours.

4. *Bouin's Fixatives* (Primary Fixative)

Bouin, P. (1897). In Phenomenes Cytologique Anormaux dans 1' Histogenese. ***Nancy*, 1897.**

A **micro-anatomical fixative** which may also be used for **detailed nuclear study** and the **preservation of glycogen.**

***Solution*:**

1.	Acetic acid, glacial	.....	5 ml
2.	Concentrated formal-dehyde solution (40%)	.....	25 ml
3.	Picric acid, saturated aqueous solution	.....	75 ml

Mode of preparation

Add acetic acid and concentrated formaldehyde solution to the picric acid solution. Mix well and label.

Mode of use

Dissect small blocks of tissue (preferably not exceeding 1 cm in thickness) and fix for 3 to 24 hours, according to the size and consistency of the particular piece of tissue fixed.

For better preservation of glycogen, formaldehyde solution is replaced by 25 ml of absolute ethanol (Dey, 1974). This is called alcoholic, fixative, or **Alcoholic Bouin's** fixative.

5. *Alcoholic Bouin's Fluid* (Primary Fixative)

Ethyl alcohol	....	1 part
Bouin's fixative	....	1 part

It is a special fixative for endometrium (true glycogen vacuole gets prominent).

6. Bouin-Hollande Fluid (Primary Fixative)

Hartz, P. H. (1947). *Am. J. clin. Path.* 17, 750

It is a micro-anatomical fixative recommended by Hartz for fixation and gross demonstration of areas of **calcification**. Tissues for **von Kossa** staining may be fixed in this solution.

***Solution*:**

Copper acetate	....	2.5 g
Picric acid	....	4.0 g
Acetic acid, glacial	....	1.5 ml
Concentrated formaldehyde solution (40%)	....	10.0 ml
Distilled water	....	100.0 ml

Mode of preparation

Dissolve the copper acetate and picric acid in the distilled water at room temperature. Add the concentrated formaldehyde solution and the acetic acid. Mix well and label.

Mode of use

Fix tissues for 1 to 7 days.

7. *Zenker's fluid* (Secondary Fixative)

Pot. bichromate	....	25 g
Hydrarg. perchloride	....	5 g
Water upto	....	100 ml

Just before use add 5 ml of glacial acetic acid. It is a good **general fixative and gives excellent details;** 5 ml of formal saline instead of acetic acid makes **Zenker's formal.**

Fix tissue for 3-12 hours; wash in running water overnight to remove bichromate and then put in 70% alcohol containing sufficient iodine to keep the solution brown.

MORDANT: Mordant is an agent (substance) that stabilizes the dye (stain) during the staining procedure.

FOR BONY AND CALCIFIED TISSUE (DECALCIFICATION)

(a) Saw the bone into small discs of 3 to 5 mm thickness.

(b) The tissue should be fixed in 5% buffered formal-saline.

(c) **Then it should be decalcified in the following solution till the calcareous matter is dissolved. Keep the tissue hanging in a large volume of the following solution.**

Formal Nitric Acid

Formalin (commercial 40%)	....	5 ml
Nitric acid (Inorganic acid)	....	5 to 10 ml
Water	....	80 to 85 ml

Change the solution once or twice daily. Treat till the bone is soft and decalcified; it requires 4 days or more (sometimes 15 days) for decalcification. **When decalcified, it can be easily punctured by a needle.** Wash in running water and **harden in 70% alcohol.**

TISSUE DEHYDRATION, CLEARING AND IMPREGNATION

Tissues usually fixed in **formal-saline**, or in special cases in **Zenker's fluid**, are cut into sizes of about 1 cm square with thickness of about 5 mm. Zenker-fixed tissue is washed overnight under running tap water.

(a) Dehydrate by passing through ascending grades of alcohol for 12 to 24 hours in each of 70% and 90% alcohol and then 2 changes in absolute alcohol—2 hours each.

(b) Clear by two changes in xylol or **chloroform** (first change 1 hour, second change 2 hours, or till it is clear).

(c) Put in saturated solution of paraffin (melting point **54°C–56°C**), or in xylol, or **chloroform**.

EMBEDDING

(a) Embed in paraffin (melting point 54°C–56°C) in constant temperature (thermostatic)—paraffin-bath at 56°C (one change in 8 hours). Thorough and uniform impregnation is necessary. To ensure impregnation, use of a **vacuum embedding bath** which is necessary.

(b) Block in moulds—the **surface to be cut being placed downwards**; cool in cold water rapidly by application of ice as soon as the scum forms.

PARAFFIN SECTION

(a) Cut with a rocking or a rotary microtome; razor should be sharp with even edge. Thickness of 3–5 μ is preferable. The cuts are done at 1 μ with expert hands (**THIN CUTS**).

(b) Receive sections with a brush or a lifter and float on a warm thermostatic water-bath (50°C), with rounded margin, care to be taken to put the glossy surface downwards.

(c) Receive the section in albumen-coated slides. For this, collect the white of an egg, filter it and then add equal part of **pure glycerine** to it. Mix them thoroughly and preserve the mixture with a crystal of **thymol** in a glass-stoppered wide-mouthed bottle. Put a drop of this mixture and spread it on the slide.

(d) When the floated sections spread well on the surface of warm water, they are taken on **albuminated (albumin-coated) slides** with the help of a soft painting brush. If necessary, **cut the ribbon** with the warm blade of a knife.

(e) The slides with the sections are dried in the incubator overnight. But this is often not necessary.

FROZEN SECTION

Use :

For fat staining, for rapid diagnosis (2 hours), etc.

Solution:

(a) *Cane sugar*—450 g. Water—300 ml. Dissolve and filter.

(b) *Gum acacia*—120 g. Water—150 ml. Dissolve and filter.

Mix three parts of (a) and five parts of (b) and add a few crystals of **thymol as preservative.**

Fix small pieces of tissue in 10% formal-saline (for ordinary work) and (for special work 12.5% formalin), for 12 to 24 hours, but for rapid work fix the tissue at 37°C for 10 minutes. Wash as usual.

(a) Transfer in gum solution, and

(b) Leave in it for at least ½ hour or more in a warm oven.

(c) Freeze the tissue in gum solution on the microtome platform by **passing CO_2 gas over it**.

(d) Wait a little-while and cut sections quickly when the snow is just thawing (in 5 to 10 minutes preferably).

(e) Transfer the section with a soft camel hair brush to a watch glass containing distilled water; transfer to 70% alcohol, and stain with routine stain or any special stain.

BIOPSY

It is the small piece of tissue taken out from a living body for histopathological or cytopathological study for investigational purpose (DIAGNOSTIC BIOPSY), or for irradication of a lesion (EXCISIONAL BIOPSY).

TYPES OF BIOPSIES

(1) **Diagnostic Biopsy** (Conservative Biopsy). Biopsy is done for diagnostic purposes.

(2) **Fine Needle Aspiration Biopsy (FNAB) or Fine Needle Aspiration Cytology (FNAC)**

In this, a fine needle of No. 21 or 22 gauge is introduced into the tissue (even into the liver, lung or spleen also) for aspirating the minimum quantity of healthy or necrosed tissue causing minimum trauma. This tissue is used for diagnostic purposes.

(3) **Endoscopic Biopsy**

In this, an endoscope (Bronchoscope, Urethroscope or Cystoscope, Esophagoscope, Proctoscope or Colonoscope, Laryngoscope, Gastroscope, Laparoscope, etc.) is introduced to see the lesion and to take out the tissue either by the endoscope or withdrawing the endoscope, and then washing up the exfoliated cellular material (generated as a result of endoscopy) following its collection by a tubing system and finally submitting the material for Histopathology (**cell block**) or Exfoliative Cytology and FNAC smears.

(4) **Therapeutic or Excisional Biopsy**

It is the total excision of a small lesion which has the possibility to cure the patient radically.

Biopsy is the surgical procedure of taking out the tissue; while biopsy material examination is the job of a pathologist.

STAINING OF SECTIONS

Hematoxylin & Eosin Routine Method (H & E)

One of the following Hematoxylin solutions are used for hematoxylin-eosin (H & E) stain.

Delafield's Hematoxylin (mostly used)

Hematoxylin	.....	4 g
Absolute alcohol	.....	25 ml
Saturated solution of ammon. alum (2 : 13)	.....	400 ml

Expose to light and air in a stoppered bottle for **one month to complete oxidation**; filter. To the filtrate add 100 ml each of glycerine and **methyl alcohol**. **Ripen** the solution till it is dark purple in color. If necessary, keep it in an incubator at 37°C for quick **ripening (15 days). For use, dilute 1 in 4 in water.**

Harris' Hematoxylin

Hematoxylin	....	5 g
Ammon. alum	....	100 g
Ethyl alcohol	....	50 ml
$HgCl_2$ or HgO	....	2.5 mg
Water	....	1000 ml
Variant (Glacial Acetic acid)	....	40 ml

Dissolve hematoxylin in alcohol; heat to boiling for a few minutes till a purple color develops. Cool quickly and filter before use. Stain improves on addition of acetic acid. Mix other ingredients.

Ehrlich's Hematoxylin (acidic)

Hematoxylin	....	2 g
Absolute alcohol	....	100 ml
Glycerine	....	100 ml
Distilled water	....	100 ml
Glacial acetic acid	....	10 ml

Pot. alum in excess is used to saturate and make the solution blue. Ripen as for Delafield's.

> **N.B.** The solution will keep indefinitely. It does not usually overstain since the stain contains acetic acid. This is why a longer time is required to make the section **blue** in running water by removing the acid.

Preliminary treatment for staining

Paraffin sections are treated as follows:

1. Warm the slide just to melt the paraffin and dip in xylol. Two changes in xylol for 5 minutes each.
2. Remove xylol by putting in **absolute alcohol**; 2 changes for 5 minutes each.
3. Pass through **descending grades of alcohol** (90%, 70%, 50%) for 5 minutes each, and then to **water**.
4. In case of tissue fixed in Zenker's fluid or formal sublimate, treat the section with 70% alcohol containing iodine (to remove corrosive sublimate from the section) for 10 minutes and pass through **descending grades of alcohol** down to water.
5. Wash in water (5 minutes); and then put in 0.5% watery solution of sodium hyposulphite—10 minutes.
6. Finally wash under tap water for 10 minutes, before staining.

Staining with Hematoxylin and Eosin

1. Take the section down to water as above.
2. Stain with hematoxylin—3 to 5 mins.: wash in running water till a blue color develops (10 min).
3. Examine under the low power and **differentiate** with **acid alcohol (1 ml of HCl in 99 ml of 70% alcohol)** for a few seconds and soak in water. Continue differentiation with a check under the microscope till the maximum nuclear details are available.
4. **Leave in running water** till the section is blue (10 minutes to 30 minutes).

5. **Counterstain** with **1% aqueous** solution of eosin for a minute.

6. Pass through **ascending grades of alcohol** and **finally absolute alcohol**.

7. **Dehydrate** in dehydrated alcohol; clear in xylol and mount in neutral mountant **Canada balsam.***

Result: A well-stained preparation should show: Nuclei—**Blue**; Acidophilic nuclei—**Red**; Basophilic nuclei—**Blue**; Muscle, Collagen and Fibrils—**Pink**; Red cells—**Pink**; Eosinophilic granules—**Red**; Basophilic granules—**Blue**; and in general cytoplasm—**Blue**.

STAINING BY SPECIAL STAINS

WEIGERT'S IRON HEMATOXYLIN STAIN

This is specially useful for materials fixed in **Zenker's fluid** when ordinary hematoxylin stains may be inadequate.

Sol. A:

Hematoxylin	....	1 g
Absolute alcohol	....	100 ml

Sol. B:

Liq. Ferri perchlor—30% (aqueous)	....	4 ml
Hydrochloric acid (conc. 11N).	....	1 ml
Distilled water	....	100 ml

Filter and stock the solutions separately. For use, **equal parts of A and B are mixed** before use. Stain for 3 minutes; wash in tap water till blue.

If the section is deeply stained, differentiate with **acid alcohol (1 ml HCl in 99 ml 70% alcohol)**; wash in running water for 10 minutes to develop a light blue color. Proper staining is judged under the microscope by the appearance of the nuclei, which should show the nuclear details.

Counterstain with 1% aqueous solution of eosin for 1 minute. Dehydrate in absolute alcohol, and then in dehydrated alcohol. Clear in xylol and mount in DPX mountant.

FAT STAINING

Solution: Saturated solution of **Sudan IV**, or **Scharlach R** in a mixture of equal parts of 70% alcohol and acetone. It stains **Orange** and **Scarlet Red** respectively. Other stains are **Oil Red stains reddish to orange; Osmic acid stains black. Osmic acid** (osmium tetroxide) **is both a fixative and a stain**. Filter the solution before use.

Frozen section must be done (For details, see above). Otherwise **fat is dissolved in organic solvents** during processing.

Method

1. Put the *frozen section* in 70% alcohol in a staining jar.**

2. Transfer it to another staining jar containing freshly filtered **Sudan IV** or **Scharlach R solution**. Stain for 20 minutes, but maximum staining is obtained in 2 hours. Evaporation is avoided by covering the jar with a glass slab.

3. Rinse quickly in 50% ethyl or propyl alcohol (Isopropanol) and transfer to water.

4. Counterstain the nuclei in hematoxylin for 5 minutes, and wash in water till blue; dry with filter paper.

5. Receive on an albumen-slide and mount in **Apathy's medium or Kaiser's glycerine jelly**.

Apathy's medium: (Refractive index—1.524)

Pure gum arabic	....	50 g
Pure cane-sugar	....	50 g
Distilled water	....	50 ml
Thymol	....	0.05 g

Kaiser's Glycerine Jelly (Refractive index—1.47)

Gelatin	....	10 g
Distilled water	....	60 ml
Glycerine (pure)	....	70 ml
Phenol (crystal)	....	0.25 g

Dissolve gelatin in a beaker of water placing in a water bath (56 °C). When dissolved add glycerine and phenol. Keep in a balsam bottle. Melt in a warm bath before use.

Result: Nuclei are **blue, fat appears Orange** with **Sudan IV, Scarlet red** with **Scharlach R** and **Oil red**.

Fine fat droplets may become dissolved in 70% alcohol. In these cases, use 50% alcohol instead of 70%.

* Canada balsam should be neutral, otherwise the stain fades away after a time. Synthetic mounting medium like D.P.X. or Supermount (Pasteur Laboratory, Calcutta) is satisfactory.

** A coplin jar with a lid is preferable.

Sudan IV or Scharlach R are not specific for neutral fat; other lipids may stain also, though the staining is less deep.

VAN GIESON'S STAIN

(A **differential** Stain for **Fibrous Tissue** and **Muscle Tissue**)

Mix stock solutions:

A.	1% solution of **Acid Fuchsin**	5 to 10 ml
B.	Saturated aqueous solution of **Picric Acid**	90 to 95 ml

Procedure

1. Take the section down to water.
2. Stain deeply with Weigert's Iron hematoxylin for 5 minutes (See before).
3. Wash in water till blue.
4. Blot out and stain with **van Gieson's stain** or its substitute—3 to 5 minutes.
5. Rinse rapidly for a few seconds only.
6. Control the 'degree of staining' under the microscope.
7. Dehydrate, clear and mount in Canada balsam or supermount or DPX.

Results

Fibrous tissue (**collagen**) is stained **Red**, and

Muscle tissue **Yellow**.

For types of collagen see at the end of this chapter.

MASSON'S TRICHROME STAIN

A general purpose connective tissue stain ***Regaud's Iron-Hematoxylin***, (Sol. 1, 2 & 3).

Solution (1)—use working sol. at 45°C

Iron alum	....	5 g
Distilled water	....	100 ml

Mix and label.

Solution (2)

Hematoxylin	....	1 g
Ethyl alcohol, 95%	....	10 ml
Glycerol	....	10 ml
Distilled water	....	80 ml

Solution (3)

Picric acid, saturated alcoholic soln.

(approx. 7 g per 100 ml)	.....	2 volumes
Ethyl alcohol, 95%	.....	1 volume

***Solution (4) — see below**

Ponceau de xylidene	....	0.7 g
Acid fuchsin	....	0.3 g
Distilled water	....	100 ml
Acetic acid, glacial	....	1 ml

Solution (5)

Phosphomolybdic acid, 1% aqueous solution. Label and put date.

***Solution (6) — see below**

Aniline blue	....	2.5 g
Distilled water	....	100 ml
Acetic acid, glacial	....	2 ml

Solution (7)

Acetic acid, 1% aqueous solution

***Mode of preparations:**

Solution (4)

Dissolve acid fuchsin and **ponceau de xylidene** in distilled water and add acetic acid. Mix well and label.

Solution (6)

Dissolve aniline blue in distilled water and add acetic acid. Mix well and label.

Procedure

1. Bring sections to water.
2. Mordant in solution (1), previously heated to 45°C for 5 minutes.
3. Wash in tap water.
4. Stain in solution (2) for 5 minutes.
5. Rinse in 95% alcohol.
6. Differentiate in solution (3). Check the degree of differentiation repeatedly under a microscope.
7. Wash in running tap water for 5 to 10 minutes to remove traces of iron-alum.
8. Stain in solution (4) for 5 minutes.

9. Differentiate and mordant in solution **(5)** for 5 minutes.
10. Transfer to solution **(6)** for 5 minutes.
11. Rinse in distilled water.
12. Return to solution **(5)** for 5 minutes.
13. Transfer to solution **(7)** for 5 minutes.
14. Dehydrate, clear and mount.

Results

Cell nuclei — **Black;**

Cytoplasm, Neuroglia fibres and Muscle fibres—**red;** Collagen and mucus — **Blue.**

PER-IODIC ACID SCHIFF (PAS) REACTION AND STAINING (After McManus)

For demonstration of **glycogen and mucin** *and PAS positive substances*

Solution (1)

Per-iodic acid	....	1	g
Distilled water	....	100	ml

Mix and label

Solution (2) de Tomasi:

Basic fuchsin	....	1	g
Sodium metabisulphite ($Na_2S_2O_5$)	....	1	g
Activated charcoal	....	2	g
Distilled water	....	200	ml
Hydrochloric acid, (1N solution)	....	20	ml

Solution (3)

Potassium metabisulphite, 10% aqueous solution	....	5	ml
Hydrochloric acid, (1N solution)	....	5	ml
Distilled water	....	90	ml

Mix. Always prepare reagents freshly.

Solution (4) (Mayer's acid-hematoxylin):

Ammonium alum	....	50	g
Chloral hydrate	....	50	g
Hematoxylin	....	1	g
Citric acid	....	1	g
Sodium iodate	....	0.2	g
Distilled water	....	1000	ml

Mode of preparation

Solution (2)

Boil distilled water in a litre flask and add basic fuchsin gradually and cautiously. Remove from heating. Shake for 5 minutes. Cool to 50°C. Filter, add hydrochloric acid slowly. Further, cool to 25°C. Now add sodium metabisulphite. Keep the solution undisturbed in dark for 12 to 24 hours. Add activated charcoal. Shake for 1 minute to clarify. Filter, write batch and label. Store at 4°C in dark. For use, bring the solution to room temperature first.

Solution (4)

Dissolve the hematoxylin in (distilled) water by gentle heating and **add sodium iodate and alum,** shaking at intervals to affect solution of the alum. Dissolve the citric acid and chloral hydrate. Record date and label. The hematoxylin solution, which turns reddish-violet in color is ready for immediate use. No further ripening being necessary owing to the inclusion of sodium iodate. The solution remains stable for several months.

Procedure

1. Bring sections to water.
2. Oxidize in solution **(1)** for 5-10 minutes.
3. Wash in running water for 5 minutes, and rinse in distilled water.
4. Treat with solution **(2)** for 10-30 minutes.
5. Transfer to three baths of solution (3), (1), (2), for 2 minutes each, respectively.
6. Wash in running tap water for 10 minutes.
7. Stain with solution **(4)**.
8. Dehydrate, clear and mount.

Results:

Cell nuclei—**Blue;**

PAS-positive substances—**Bright Red** or **Light Magenta.**

PER-IODIC ACID SCHIFF REACTION AND STAINING (After Hotchkiss)

For demonstration of glycogen

Solution (1)

Per-iodic acid	....	0.4	g
Ethyl alcohol, absolute	....	35	ml
Distilled water	....	10	ml
Sodium acetate, 5M solution	...	5	ml

Solution (2)

Potassium iodide	....	1	g
Sodium thiosulphate, ($Na_2S_2O_3$, $5H_2O$)	....	1	g

Ethyl alcohol, absolute	....	30 ml
Distilled water	....	20 ml
Hydrochloric acid, 1N solution	....	0.5 ml

Solution (3)—Prepare as in **McManus' PAS** stain; solution (2):

Basic fuchsin	....	1 g
Sodium metabisulphite ($Na_2S_2O_5$)	....	1 g
Activated charcoal	....	2 g
Distilled water	....	200 ml
Hydrochloric acid, 1N solution	....	20 ml

Solution (4)—Prepare as in **McManus' PAS** stain; solution (4):

Ammonium alum	....	50 g
Chloral hydrate	....	50 g
Hematoxylin	....	1 g
Citric acid	....	1 g
Sodium iodate	....	0.2 g
Distilled water	....	1000 ml

Mode of preparation

Solution (1)

Dissolve **per-iodic acid** in **alcohol**. Add **sodium acetate solution** and distilled water. Mix well, make batch and label.

Solution (2)

Combine **alcohol** and **distilled water**. Dissolve **potassium iodide** and **sodium thiosulphate**. Add **hydrochloric acid** and mix. Make batch and label.

Procedure

1. Bring sections to water.
2. Rinse in 70% alcohol.
3. Oxidize with **solution (1)** for 5–10 minutes.
4. Rinse in 70% alcohol.
5. Treat with **solution (2)** for 1 minute.
6. Rinse in 70% alcohol.
7. Wash in running water for 10 minutes.
8. Treat with **solution (3)** for 20 minutes.
9. Wash in running tap water for 10 minutes.
10. **Stain with solution (4).**
11. Dehydrate with dehydrated alcohol. Clear in xylol, and mount.

Results:

Cell nuclei — **Blue;**

PAS-positive substances — **Bright Red.**

ALCIAN BLUE-PERIODIC ACID SCHIFF METHOD

For demonstration of acidic groups and **1–2 glycols of carbohydrates (glycogen).**

Solution (1):

Alcian blue (0.1%), in 3% acetic acid. Mix and label.

Solution (2):

Per-iodic acid, 0.5% aqueous solution. Mix and label.

***Solution (3): (See below)**

(a) ***Modification of Lillie's "Cold Schiff"***

Distilled water	.....	192 ml
Hydrochloric acid (sp. gr. 1.19)	.....	8 ml
Sodium sulphite	.....	5 g
Basic fuchsin	.....	2 g
Activated carbon (charcoal)	.....	1 g

Or

(b) ***Coleman's Feulgen reagent***

Basic fuchsin	.....	1 g
Potassium metabisulphite	.....	2 g
Distilled water	.....	200 ml
Hydrochloric acid, 1N solution	.....	10 ml
Activated carbon (Norit)	.....	0.5 g

***Solution (4): (See below)**

Reducing solution for a rinse:

Sodium acid sulphite, 10.4 g% in water (aqueous solution)	.....	1 volume
Distilled water	.....	20 volumes

***Solution (5) (See below)**

Weigert-Lillie alum-hematoxylin

Hematoxylin, 1% alcoholic soln.	.....	100 ml
Distilled water	.....	288 ml
Ferric chloride (29.1 g% in water)	.....	4 ml
Hydrochloric acid (sp. gr. 1.19)	.....	8 ml
Ferrous sulphate	.....	4.44 g

Mode of preparation

***Solution (3)**

(a) Measure the **distilled water** into a 500-ml flask. Add hydrochloric acid and dissolve **sodium sulphite** and **basic fuchsin**. Shake at intervals until the mixture is clear brown to brownish-red. Incorporate the activated carbon and shake for 2 minutes. Filter, and store in a suitable bottle at 4 °C. Record date and label. The final solution should be colorless.

(b) Measure distilled water into a 500-ml boiling flask; bring to the boil and dissolve the **basic fuchsin**. Cool to 50°C and add **potassium metabisulphite**. Add **hydrochloric acid**. Transfer to a brown bottle and allow to stand for 24 hours. Incorporate the carbon. Shake for 1 minute; filter through coarse paper until the dye becomes colorless. Record date, label and store at 4 °C.

***Solution (4)**

Add sodium acid sulphite solution to distilled water. Prepare immediately before use.

***Solution (5)**

Combine the ingredients in the order listed. Record date and label. The solution remains stable for 2-3 weeks.

Procedure

1. Bring sections to water.
2. Stain with solution (1) for 30 minutes.
3. Wash in running tap water for 2 minutes.
4. Rinse in distilled water.
5. **Oxidize** in solution (2) for 10 minutes.
6. Wash in running tap water for 5 minutes.
7. Rinse in distilled water.
8. Treat with solution (3) for 10 minutes.
9. Place in solution (4) and give 3 baths of 2 minutes each.
10. Wash in running tap water for 5 minutes.
11. Stain with solution (5) for 5 minutes.
12. Wash in running tap water for 2 minutes.
13. Dehydrate, clear and mount.

Results:

Exclusively acid substance — **Blue;**

Neutral polysaccharides — **Light Magenta;**

Epithelial mucins and ground substance of cartilage — varying shades of **Purple** to **Deep Blue;**

Cell bodies of fungi — **Red to Purple;**

White mucoid capsules — **Blue;**

Cell nuclei — **Blue.**

MUCIHEMATIN STAIN

(After Laskey, 1950)

For demonstration of mucin (epithelial and connective tissue)

Hematoxylin	.....	1	g
Aluminium chloride	.....	0.5	g
Sodium iodate, 1% aqueous soln.,	.....	5	ml
Ethyl alcohol, 70% v/v	to	500	ml

Mode of preparation

Dissolve hematoxylin in 100 ml of alcohol. Dissolve **aluminium chloride**. Add sodium iodate solution and make up the volume to 500 ml with 70 per cent alcohol. Record date and label.

Procedure

1. Bring sections to water and wash thoroughly in several changes of distilled water.
2. Stain with **mucihematin** for 5–10 minutes.
3. Wash in three changes of distilled water for 5 minutes in each.
4. Dehydrate, clear and mount.

Results:

Epithelial mucin—**Deep Blue** to **Violet**; connective tissue mucin and matrix of cartilage—**Light Violet**.

SOUTHGATE'S MUCICARMINE

(After Carleton and Drury, 1957)

For demonstration of Epithelial Mucin

Solution (1)

Mayer's acid-alum-hematoxylin:

Ammonium alum	.....	50	g
Chloral hydrate	.....	50	g
Hematoxylin	.....	1	g
Citric acid	.....	1	g
Sodium iodate	.....	0.2	g
Distilled water	.....	1000	ml

Mix and label; put date (for method see before)

***Solution (2) (See below)**

Carmine	.....	1 g
Aluminium hydroxide	.....	1 g
Aluminium chloride (anhydrous)	.....	0.5 g
Ethyl alcohol, 50%	.....	100 ml

Mode of preparation

***Solution (2)**

Weigh **carmine and aluminium hydroxide** into a 500 ml flask and then add alcohol. Shake well and add aluminium chloride during shaking. Place in a boiling bath for exactly 2 ½ minutes. Cool, filter, record date and label.

Procedure

1. Bring sections to water.
2. Stain with solution (1); for method see before.
3. Stain with solution (2) for 30-45 minutes.
4. Rinse in distilled water.
5. Dehydrate, clear and mount.

Results:

Cell nuclei — **Blue**

Epithelial mucin — **Red.**

BEST'S CARMINE STAIN FOR GLYCOGEN

For demonstration of glycogen

***Stock Carmine solution (See below)**

Potassium chloride	.....	5 g
Carmine	.....	2 g
Potassium carbonate	.....	1 g
Distilled water	.....	60 ml
Ammonia (sp. gr. 0.880)	.....	20 ml

Solution (1)

Ammonium or potassium alum.	.....	15 g
Hematoxylin	.....	2 g
Ethyl alcohol, 95%	.....	100 ml
Glycerol	.....	100 ml
Distilled water	.....	100 ml
Acetic acid, glacial	.....	10 ml

***Solution (2) (See below)**

Stock carmine solution	.....	20 ml
Ammonia (sp. gr. 0.880)	.....	30 ml
Methyl alcohol	.....	30 ml

Best's Differentiator

***Solution (3) (See below)**

Distilled water	.....	100 ml
Methyl alcohol	.....	80 ml
Ethyl alcohol	.....	40 ml

Mode of preparation

***Stock Carmine solution:**

Add dye components and salts to distilled water in a 250 ml boiling flask, and bring to the boil. Keep for 6 minutes, or until the color darkens. Cool; add ammonia and store in a tightly stoppered bottle at 4°–5°C. Record date, and label.

***Solution (2)**

Mix the carmine solution with the alcohol, add the ammonia and label.

***Solution (3)**

Add the **methyl alcohol** and ethyl alcohol to the distilled water and label.

Procedure

1. Prepare paraffin sections from tissue fixed in **Carnoy's, Bouin's, or Gendre's fluid.**
2. Bring sections to absolute alcohol.
3. Coat with 1% celloidin.
4. Harden in 80% alcohol.
5. Wash in water.
6. Stain with **solution (1)** for 5 minutes. Wash in water.
7. Stain with **solution (2)** for 5-30 minutes.
8. Differentiate in **solution (3)** for 1–5 minutes.
9. Dehydrate, **remove celloidin** with ether-alcohol mixture; clear and mount.

Results:

Cell nuclei — **Blue**

Glycogen — **Red.**

CONGO RED

(After Freudenthal)

For demonstration of **Amyloid**

Solution (1) [Formal saline]

Concentrated formaldehyde solution (40%)	.....	100 ml
Distilled water	.....	900 ml

Solution (2) [Alkaline Congo Red soln.]

Congo Red	.....	1 g
Sodium carbonate	.....	5 g
Distilled water	.....	100 ml

Solution (3) Ehrlich' Hematoxylin:

Ammonium or potassium alum	.....	15 g
Hematoxylin	.....	2 g
Ethyl alcohol, 95%	.....	100 ml
Glycerol	.....	100 ml
Distilled water	.....	100 ml
Acetic acid, glacial	.....	10 ml

Procedure

1. Bring sections to water.
2. Transfer to solution (1) for 15 minutes.
3. Stain with solution (2) for 15 minutes.
4. Wash in distilled water.
5. Counterstain nuclei in solution (3).
6. Dehydrate, clear and mount.

Results:

Cell nuclei — **Blue**

Amyloid — **Orange-Pink.**

FEULGEN REACTION FOR DNA

For demonstration of nucleoproteins, especially deoxy type.

Solution (1) (cold solution)

Hydrochloric acid, 1N solution (HCl 9.1 ml + distilled water 0.9 ml)

Solution (2) Schiff reagent *de Tomasi (See below)

Basic fuchsin	.....	1 g
Sodium metabisulphite ($Na_2S_2O_5$)	.....	1 g
Activated charcoal	.....	2 g
Distilled water	.....	200 ml
Hydrochloric acid, 1N solution	.....	20 ml

Or

Barger and de Lamater:

Basic fuchsin	.....	1 g
Activated charcoal	.....	2 g
Distilled water	.....	400 ml
Thionyl chloride ($SOCl_2$)	.....	1 ml

Or

Cold Schiff:

Basic fuchsin	.....	1 g
Sodium metabisulphite ($Na_2S_2O_5$)	.....	1.9 g
Hydrochloric acid, 0.15N solution	.....	100 ml
Activated charcoal	.....	0.5 g

Sulphite rinse

***Solution (3)**

Potassium metabisulphite, 10% aqueous	.....	5 ml
Hydrochloric acid, 1N solution	.....	5 ml
Distilled water	.....	90 ml

Mode of Preparation of *Solution (2)

Schiff reagent *de Tomasi*

Bring distilled water to the boil in a 1-litre boiling flask and add basic fuchsin. Shake for 5 minutes. Cool to 50°C, filter and add hydrochloric acid. Cool further to 25°C and **add sodium metabisulphite**. Keep the solution in the dark for 12–14 hours. Add activated charcoal, shake for 1 minute to clear, and filter. Bottle, record date and label. Store in a refrigerator at 4°C, but allow the solution to reach room temperature before use.

Or

Barger and de Lamater:

Bring the distilled water to the boil in a 1-litre boiling flask and add the basic fuchsin. Cool to 50°C and filter. Incorporate the thionyl chloride and stand the mixture in the dark for 12 hours. Add the activated charcoal, shake for 1 minute to clear, and filter. Bottle, record date and label. Store in a refrigerator at 4°C, but allow the solution to reach room temperature before use.

Or

Cold Schiff:

Using a 500-ml flask, dissolve basic fuchsin and sodium metabisulphite in hydrochloric acid. Shake the solution at intervals for over a period of 2 hours (a mechanical shaker is recommended). Add activated charcoal and shake for further 2 minutes to clear. Filter into a graduated cylinder and make up the filtrate to the original volume by washing the residue thoroughly with a little distilled water. Bottle, record date and label. Store in a refrigerator at 4°C. Allow the solution to reach room temperature before use.

***Solution (3)**

Add potassium metabisulphite solution and hydrochloric acid to distilled water. Prepare reagent immediately before use.

Procedure

1. Bring sections to water.
2. Rinse briefly in cold solution (1).
3. Transfer to solution (1), pre-heated to 60°C, for the optimum period of hydrolysis.
4. Rinse briefly in cold solution (1).
5. Rinse in distilled water.
6. Transfer to solution (2) (Schiff reagent) for 30-90 minutes.
7. Drain and transfer to 3 baths of solution (3) for 1, 2 and 2 minutes in each, respectively.
8. Rinse well in distilled water.
9. Counterstain as desired.
10. Dehydrate, clear and mount.

Results:

Deoxyribonucleic acid **(DNA)—Reddish-Purple;** Other tissues—**according to counterstain.**

VERHOEFF'S ELASTIC FIBRE STAIN

(Verhoeff, F. H. (1908). J.A.M.A. 50, 876)

For demonstration of elastic fibres

Alcoholic hematoxylin (5% w/v)

Hematoxylin	5 g
Ethyl alcohol, absolute	100 ml

Ferric chloride solution (10% w/v)

Ferric chloride	10 g
Distilled water	100 ml

Lugol's Iodine solution (1% w/v)

Iodine	1 g
Potassium iodide	2 g
Distilled water	100 ml

Iodine crystal alone is insoluble in water; pot. iodide makes it soluble. That is why pot. iodide is added to make iodine solution. Mix pot. iodide with distilled water; then mix iodine.

Solution (1)

Alcoholic hematoxylin (as above)	20 ml
Ferric chloride solution (as above)	8 ml
Lugol's iodine solution (as above)	8 ml

Solution (2)

Ferric chloride solution (as above)	20 ml
Distilled water	80 ml

Mode of preparation

ALCOHOLIC hematoxylin

Dissolve the hematoxylin in alcohol with the aid of gentle heat (**not on open flame**). Filter, record date and label.

Ferric chloride solution

Dissolve the ferric chloride (10% w/v) in distilled water and label.

Solution (1)

Add the ferric chloride and Lugol's iodine to alcoholic hematoxylin. This keeps well for 1–2 days.

Solution (2)

Add the ferric chloride to the distilled water and mix well.

Procedure

1. Bring sections to water.
2. Stain in solution (1) for 15–60 minutes.
3. Rinse in water.
4. Differentiate in solution (2), controlling the degree of differentiation microscopically. In case of over-differentiation, before transferring to 95% alcohol, return to Sol. 1, and restain.
5. Transfer to 95% alcohol to remove the trace of iodine.
6. Wash in water.
7. Counterstain with eosin, phloxine, or van Gieson.
8. Dehydrate, clear and mount.

Results:

Elastic fibres — **Black**

Other tissues — **Red.**

MALLORY'S PHOSPHOTUNGSTIC ACID HEMATOXYLIN (PTAH)

Peers, J. H. (1941). *Arch . Path.* 32,446

***A differential stain for* striations of skeletal muscles and myofibrils, collagen, neuroglia cells and fibres.**

Solution (1)

Mercuric chloride saturated aqueous solution (Approx. 7%)

Solution (2) LUGOL'S IODINE: Mordant

Iodine	....	1	g
Potassium iodide	....	2	g
Distilled water	....	100	ml

Iodine crystal is insoluble in water when it is alone. Iodine crystal is made soluble with addition of potassium iodide. Mix pot. iodide with distilled water; mix iodine.

Solution (3)

Sodium thiosulphate, 5% aqueous solution.

Solution (4): Oxidizing agent

Potassium permanganate	.....	0.25	g
Distilled water	.....	100	ml

Solution (5): Bleaching agent

Oxalic acid	.....	5	g
Distilled water	.....	100	ml

Mix and label

Solution (6): Staining agent

Hematoxylin	.....	1	g
Phosphotungstic acid	.....	20	g
Distilled water	.....	1000	ml
Potassium permanganate	.....	0.177	g

Mode of Preparation

Solution (4)

Dissolve potassium permanganate in distilled water and label.

Solution (6)

Dissolve hematoxylin in 500 ml distilled water with gentle heat. Dissolve phosphotungstic acid in remaining 500 ml of distilled water. Combine the two solutions when cool, and add potassium permanganate. Record date and label.

Procedure

1. Bring sections to water.
2. Mordant in **solution (1)** at 37°C for 3 hours.
3. Rinse in water.
4. Transfer to **solution (2)** for 10 minutes.
5. Rinse in water.
6. Bleach in **solution (3)** for 5 minutes.
7. Rinse in distilled water.
8. Oxidize in **solution (4)** for 5 minutes.
9. Rinse in distilled water.
10. Bleach in **solution (5)** for 5 minutes.
11. Wash well in tap water.
12. Stain in **solution (6)** overnight at room temperature.
13. Rinse in tap water.
14. Dehydrate, clear and mount.

Results:

Cell nuclei—**Deep Blue;**

Neuroglia—**Deep Blue;**

Fibroglia and myoglia fibrils—**Deep Blue;**

Red blood corpuscles—**Deep Blue;**

Fibrin—**Deep Blue;**

Collagen—Brownish Red.

GORDON AND SWEETS' RETICULIN STAIN

Gordon, H, and Sweets, H. M. Jr. (1938). ***Amer J. Path.* 12, 545**

A good routine method for **PERICELLULAR RETICULIN** only; does not stain cells.

***Solution (1): Oxidizing agent**

Potassium permanganate, 0.5% aqueous solution	.....	95	ml
Sulphuric acid, 3% aqueous soln.	.....	5	ml

***Solution (2): Bleaching agent**

Oxalic acid	.....	1	g
Distilled water	.....	100	ml

***Solution (3): Mordant**

Iron alum	.....	2.5	g
Distilled water	.....	100	ml

***Solution (4): Impregnation (staining) agent**

Silver nitrate, 10.2% aqueous solution	.....	5	ml
Sodium hydroxide, 3.1% aqueous solution	.....	5	ml
Ammonia (sp. gr. 0.880)	.....	as required	
Glass distilled water	.....	as required	

Solution (5): Reducing agent

Concentrated formaldehyde solution (40%)	.....	100 ml
Distilled water	.....	900 ml

Solution (6): Toner

Gold chloride, 0.2% aqueous solution

Solution (7): For Fixation

Sodium thiosulphate, 5% aqueous solution

Mode of Preparation

***Solution (1): Oxidizing agent**

Add the sulphuric acid to permanganate solution, mix and label.

***Solution (2): Bleaching agent**

Dissolve the oxalic acid in distilled water, and label.

***Solution (3): Mordant**

Dissolve iron-alum in distilled water and label.

***Solution (4): Stain (Impregnation) agent**

Measure the silver nitrate solution into a chemically clean 100-ml graduated cylinder and add ammonia water, drop by drop with constant shaking until the precipitate formed is redissolved. Add the sodium hydroxide solution and again dissolve the precipitate by adding ammonia water drop by drop. The precipitate should be (only) just dissolved and the final solution should be slightly turbid. Make up the volume to 50 ml with (double) glass distilled water. The solution is best prepared at the time of use.

Procedure

1. Bring sections to water.
2. Oxidize in **solution (1)** for 1-5 minutes.
3. Wash in water.
4. Bleach in **solution (2)** for 3-5 minutes.
5. Wash thoroughly in tap water and several changes of distilled water.
6. Mordant in **solution (3)** for a period between 10 minutes and 2 hours (10 minutes should usually suffice).
7. Wash in several changes of distilled water.
8. Impregnate with **solution (4)** for 30 seconds.
9. Wash in several changes of distilled water.
10. Reduce in **solution (5)** for 1 minute.
11. Wash in tap water and then distilled water.
12. Tone in **solution (6)** for 10–15 minutes.
13. Rinse in distilled water.
14. Fix in **solution (7)** for 5 minutes.
15. Wash in water for 1-2 minutes.
16. Counterstain nuclei with safranine (1% aqueous).
17. Dehydrate, clear and mount.

Results:

Reticulin fibres — **Black**

Cell nuclei — **Red.**

PIGMENT STAINING: (PEARL'S) PRUSSIAN BLUE REACTION

(Specific for HEMOSIDERIN only)

Hemosiderin appears chiefly in liver as granules or crystals, when there is excessive destruction of red cells. Also it occurs in lungs in **CVC**.

Make paraffin or frozen section with a **rust-free** knife.

Procedure

1. Take the section down to water; rinse in distilled water (distilled water should be essentially **iron-free**).
2. Put the sections in the following freshly made up solution: for **staining**.

2% Pot. ferrocyanide	.....	2 parts
2% Hydrochloric acid	.....	2 parts

   Leave the section in this solution for 20 to 30 minutes; staining at a temperature above 60°C may cause artefacts.
3. Transfer to distilled water.
4. **Counterstain** with 1% eosin or safranine.
5. Dehydrate, clear and mount; or **after water, mount in glycerine jelly** to which a few drops of H_2O_2 has been added. This **makes the stain more permanent.**

Result:

Hemosiderin is stained **Blue**;

Cells and nuclei appear **Red.**

N.B. The reaction is due to the presence of ferric salts which results in the formation of FERRIC FERROCYANIDE.

Pot. ferrocyanide + Iron (Fe in hemoglobin) = Ferric ferrocyanide + Potassium (K).

Hemozoin (pigment of malaria) is **hematoidin (iron-free pigment** identical with bile), and **HEMOFUSCIN** occurring in **hemochromatosis does not show Prussian Blue reaction.**

GMELIN REACTION

For demonstration of **Bilirubin** and **Hematoidin.**

Nitric acid (sp. gr. 1.42)	....	1 volume
Ethyl alcohol, absolute	....	1 volume

Mode of preparation

Add nitric acid to alcohol slowly in small quantities. Label and put date.

Procedure

1. Bring sections to water.
2. Add a few drops of the **alcoholic nitric acid.**
3. Apply a coverslip and remove excess of fluid carefully.
4. Examine quickly under a microscope.

Results:

Bilirubin and hematoidin crystals turn **Red** to **Purple** and then **Green.**

STEIN'S IODINE METHOD FOR BILIRUBIN

Solution 1: Mordant

(a) ***Lugol's iodine (Liquor iodinitis):***

Iodine	.....	1 g
Potassium iodide	.....	2 g
Distilled water	.....	100 ml

Thus the **formula is 1 : 2 : 1** for Lugol's iodine. Gram's iodine contains 300 ml D/W; the formula is thus **1 : 2 : 3.**

Mix pot. iodide with distilled water. Then mix iodine.

(See for Gram's stain in Practical Microbiology)

(b) *Tincture of iodine* (B.P.) ..... 1 volume

Solution 2: Bleaching agent

Sodium thiosulphate, 5% aqueous solution

Solution 3: Kirkpatrick's carmalum (Stain and a mordanting agent)

Carmine	.....	25 g
Potassium alum	.....	25 g
Acetic acid (glacial)	.....	25 ml
Distilled water	.....	1000 ml
Salicylic acid, as **preservative**	.....	1 g

Mode of preparation

Solution 1

Combine the two solutions (a) and (b), and label.

Solution 3

(a) Preparation of **Acetic-carmine solution:**

Grind carmine in a mortar. Add glacial acetic acid, and 100 ml distilled water. Mix. Transfer to a 2-litre empty flask already kept in a boiling water bath. Add 400 ml of distilled water and gently boil the solution in the flask in the water bath for 60 minutes. Remove the flask, and allow the solution to cool.

(b) Preparation of **Potassium alum solution:**

Dissolve potassium alum separately in 500 ml of distilled water by gently heating.

Combine **(a)** acetic carmine solution with **(b)** potas-alum solution and boil for 60 minutes in a boiling water bath. Cool, filter and dissolve 1 g salicylic acid. Put the label and date. This stain is stable for 1 year at room temperature in an amber bottle.

Procedure

1. Bring sections to water.
2. Immerse in **solution (1)** for 6-12 hours.
3. Bleach in **solution (2)** for 15-30 seconds.
4. Wash in water.
5. Stain with **solution (3)** for 1-3 hours.
6. Dehydrate, clear and mount.

Results:

Cell nuclei — **Red**

Bilirubin — **Green.**

VON KOSSA'S STAIN FOR CALCIUM

Solution 1: Impregnating agent

Silver nitrate	.....	5 g
Double glass distilled water	.....	100 ml

Solution 2: Bleaching agent

Sodium thiosulphate, 5% aqueous solution

Solution 3: Kirkpatrick's carmalum (See above).

A staining and mordanting agent

Carmine	.....	25 g
Potassium alum	.....	25 g
Acetic acid, glacial	.....	25 ml
Distilled water	.....	1000 ml
Salicylic acid, as preservative	.....	1 g

Mix and label as in **Stein's iodine method for bilirubin**, solution (3).

Mode of preparation

Solution 1

Dissolve silver nitrate in (double) glass distilled water. Store in a brown bottle; label and put date.

Procedure

1. Bring sections to distilled water.
2. Immerse in **solution (1)** for 5 minutes or longer, exposing to bright daylight for silver impregnation.
3. Wash in distilled water.
4. Fix in **solution (2)** for 5 minutes.
5. Wash in distilled water.
6. Stain with **solution (3)** for 3-5 minutes.
7. Dehydrate, clear and mount.

Results:

Cell nuclei — **Red**;

Calcium, phosphate and carbonate — **Black**.

AMMONIACAL SILVER NITRATE METHOD FOR ARGENTAFFIN CELLS

(After Fontana)

1. For the demonstration of the **argentaffin cell granules** and **melanin** in formalin fixed tissue.

2. For demonstration of **Tr. pallidum in Cytology smear**.

Solution 1: GRAM'S IODINE (Mordant)

Iodine	1	.....	1 g
Potassium iodide	2	.....	2 g
Distilled water	3	.....	300 ml

The formula is 1 : 2 : 3; formula for Lugol's iodine it is 1 : 2 : 1 (See page 19). Mix potassium iodide with distilled water at first; then mix iodine.

Solution 2: Bleacher

Sodium thiosulphate, 3% aqueous solution.

***Solution 3: Impregnator (See below)**

Silver nitrate, 10% aqueous soln.	.....	25 ml
Distilled water	.....	25 ml
Ammonia (liq. sp. gr. 0.880)	.....	as required

Solution 4: Toner

Gold chloride, 0.2% aqueous solution

Solution 5: Counter-stain

Safranine, 1% aqueous solution

Mode of preparation

***Solution (3)**

Measure the silver nitrate in an absolutely chemically clean 100 ml graduated cylinder. Add ammonia, drop by drop with constant shaking, until the precipitate first formed is almost re-dissolved. Add distilled water. Keep the solution in the dark for 24 hours. Store in a brown bottle, record date and label. The solution is **stable for 14 days**.

Procedure

1. Bring sections to water.
2. Place in **solution (1)** for 5 minutes.
3. Transfer to **solution (2)** for 3 minutes for mordanting.
4. Wash in distilled water.
5. Impregnate with **solution (3)**, in dark for 18-48 hours.
6. Rinse in several changes of distilled water.
7. Tone in **solution (4)** for 10 minutes.
8. Rinse in distilled water.
9. Mordant in **solution (2)** for 2 minutes.
10. Wash in running tap water.
11. Stain with **solution (5)** for 1 minute.
12. Wash in tap water for 30 seconds.
13. Dehydrate, clear and mount.

Results:

Argentaffin cell granules and melanin granules and Treponema pallidum — **Black**;

Other tissue constituents — varying shades of **Red** and **Pink**.

METHENAMINE-SILVER METHOD

For demonstration of **argentaffin cell granules and fungi by Methenamine-silver (nitrate) solution**.

Stock solution:

Methenamine (**hexamethylene tetramine**)	....	3 g
Distilled water	....	100 ml
Silver nitrate, 5% aqueous soln.	....	5 ml

Weigert's (or Lugol's) iodine

Solution 1: Mordant

Iodine	.....	1 g
Potassium iodide	.....	2 g
Distilled water	.....	100 ml

Mix pot. iodide with distilled water; then mix iodine, otherwise iodine crystals won't dissove without pot. iodide (see Page 19 and 20).

Solution 2: Bleacher

Sodium thiosulphate, 5% aqueous solution.

Solution 3: Working Methenamine silver nitrate solution

Stock solution (See above)	.....	30 ml
Holmes borate buffer, pH 7.8	.....	8 ml

Solution 4: Toner

Gold chloride (yellow) 0.1% aqueous solution.

Solution 5: Counter-stain

Safranine	.....	0.1 g
Distilled water	.....	100 ml
Acetic acid, glacial	.....	0.1 ml

Mode of preparation

Stock solution:

Measure distilled water into a chemically clean graduated cylinder and dissolve methenamine in it. Add silver nitrate solution. Store in a brown bottle. Label and put date.

Solution 1

Dissolve the potassium iodide in distilled water; add iodine, and label.

Solution 3: Working Methenamine silver nitrate solution

Measure methenamine-silver solution into a chemically clean graduated cylinder. Add borate buffer solution and mix well.

Solution 5

Dissolve safranine in distilled water (1 g%). Add acetic acid, and label.

Procedure

1. Bring sections to water.
2. Treat with **solution (1)** for 10 minutes.
3. Bleach with **solution (2)** for 2 minutes.
4. Wash in running water for 10 minutes.
5. Rinse in two changes of distilled water.
6. Impregnate with **solution (3)** for 3½ hours at 60 °C.
7. Rinse in distilled water.
8. Tone in **solution (4)** for 10 minutes.
9. Rinse in distilled water.
10. Wash in running water.
11. Stain with **solution (5)** for 5 minutes.
12. Dehydrate with acetone, clear and mount.

Results:

Argentaffin cell granules — **Black;**

Other tissue constituents — **Red.**

N.B. The Fite-Faraco technique demonstrates certain strains of Nocardia as long, thin, red structures on a pale blue background. This technique, in the experience of the members of the staff of this installation, stands out as the most useful of the acid-fast procedures for the demonstration of these particular bacteria for the following reasons:

1. The protection afforded by the combination of peanut oil and xylene, which coats the filament capsule.
2. The elimination of alcohol from both the hydratioin and dehydration process, so that the oil coating applied around the filament through the above procedure is not dissolved.
3. The decolorization of the background with a weak solution of aqueous sulphuric acid (1%) instead of the usual 1% acid alcohol is done.

GOMORI'S METHIENAMINE–SILVER NITRATE (GMS) STAIN

(Grocott's application to fungi)

Fixation: Formalin 10 per cent

Technic: Paraffin, celloidin, or frozen section.

Reagents:

1. *5 per cent Chromic acid solution*

Chromic acid	.....	5 g
Distilled water	.....	100 ml

2. *5 per cent Silver nitrate solution*

Silver nitrate	.....	5 g
Distilled water	.....	100 ml

3. *3 per cent Methenamine solution*

Methenamine*	.....	3 gm
Distilled water	.....	100 ml

4. *5 per cent Borax solution*

Borax (photographic grade)†	.....	5 gm
Distilled water	.....	100 ml

5. *Stock Methenamine Silver nitrate solution*

Silver nitrate (5 per cent sol.)	.....	5 ml
Methenamine (3 per cent sol.)	.....	100 ml

A white precipitate forms but dissolves immediately on shaking. Clear solution keeps well for months at refrigerator temperature.

6. *Working Methenamine—Silver nitrate solution*

Borax (5 per cent solution)	.....	2 ml
Distilled water	.....	25 ml
Mix and add Methenamine-Silver nitrate solution	.....	25 ml

7. *1 per cent Sodium bisulphite solution*

Sodium bisulphite	.....	1 gm
Distilled water	.....	100 ml

8. *0.1 per cent Gold chloride solution*

Gold chloride (1 per cent sol.)	.....	10 gm
Distilled water	.....	90 ml

This solution may be used repeatedly.

9. *2 per cent Sodium thiosulphate (Hypo) solution*

Sodium thiosulphate	.....	2 gm
Distilled water	.....	100 ml

Stock light green solution

Light green, S.F. (yellow)‡	.....	0.2 gm
Distilled water	.....	100.0 ml
Glacial acetic acid	.....	0.2 ml

Working light green solution

Light green, stock solution	.....	10.0 ml
Distilled water	.....	50.0 ml

* To be obtained from Fischer Scientific Co. or Eastman Kodak Co.

† To be obtained from Eastman Kodak Co.

‡ Obtained from National Aniline Company.

Staining Procedure

Run a control slide as well

1. Deparaffinize sections through 2 changes each of xylene, absolute, and 95% alcohols to distilled water as usual. Slides previously stained with most other stains may be used by removing cover glasses in xylol and running through alcohols to water. Subsequently chromic acid treatment will remove any remaining stain.
2. Oxidize in 5% chromic acid solution for 1 hour.
3. Wash in running tap water for a few seconds.
4. Rinse in 1% sodium bisulphite for 1 minute to remove any residual chromic acid.
5. Wash in tap water for 5 to 10 minutes.
6. Wash with 3 or 4 changes of distilled water.
7. Place in **working methenamine-silver nitrate** solution in oven **at 58° to 60°C** for 30–60 minutes until section turns yellowish brown. Use paraffin coated forceps. to remove slide from this solution. Dip slide in distilled water and **check for adequate silver impregnation** with microscope. Fungi should be of **dark brown** color at this stage.
8. Rinse in 6 changes of distilled water.
9. **Tone in 0.1% gold chloride solution** for 2 to 5 minutes.
10. Rinse in distilled water.
11. Remove unreduced silver with 2% sodium thiosulphate **(hypo) solution** for 2 to 5 minutes.
12. Wash thoroughly in tap water.
13. Counterstain with working light green for 30 to 45 seconds.
14. Dehydrate with 2 changes each of 95% alcohol, absolute alcohol, clear with 2 to 3 changes in xylene, and mount.

Results:

Fungi—sharply delineated in **black color.**

Mucin—**mauve** (muddy) to **dark gray**.

Inner parts of mycelia and hyphae—**old rose**.

Background—**pale green.**

N.B. There are several important points to be considered in doing a GMS stain as follows: The technique calls for incubation of slides in a 60°C oven for 30 to 60 minutes (the full time being preferable for all fungi, but not for Nocardia), or until sections turn yellowish-brown. In staining for filaments of Nocardia, it has been found that the incubation time for complete development may vary according to **type** and/or **strain** suspected to be present in the particular section. Therefore, if Nocardia is suspected, two slides should be processed, one for 60 minutes and one for 90 minutes, thereby assuring a positive demonstration of any filaments of Nocardia that may exist.

GRIDLEY'S STAIN FOR FUNGI

Fixation: Any well fixed tissue.

Technique: Cut paraffin sections at 6 microns.

Solutions:

1. ***Chromic acid solution***

Chromic acid	.....	4 g
Distilled water	.....	100 ml

2. ***Coleman's Feulgen Reagent***

Bring 200 ml of distilled water to boil, remove from flame and add 1 g basic fuchsin. When fuchsin is dissolved, cool and filter. Add 2 g sodium metabisulphite and 10 ml of normal hydrochloric acid. Let this bleach for 24 hours, and then add 0.5 g activated carbon (Norit); shake for about 1 minute, and filter through coarse paper. The filtrate should be colorless. Store in refrigerator.

3. ***Normal Hydrochloric acid***

Hydrochloric acid, sp. gr. 1.19	.....	83.5 ml
Distilled water	.....	916.6 ml

4. ***Sodium Metabisulphite solution***

Sodium metabisulphite	.....	10 g
Distilled water	.....	100 ml

5. ***Sulphurous Rinse***

Sodium metabisulphite, 10% solution	.....	6 ml
Normal hydrochloric acid	.....	5 ml
Distilled water	.....	100 ml

6. ***Aldehyde-Fuchsin solution***

Basic fuchsin	.....	1 g
Alcohol, 70%	.....	200 ml
Paraldehyde	.....	2 ml
Hydrochloric acid, conc.(11N)	.....	2 ml

Let it stand at room temperature for 3 days until solution turns deep blue. Keep in refrigerator. Filter and warm to room temperature before using.

7. ***Metanil Yellow solution***

Metanil yellow	.....	0.25 g
Distilled water	.....	100.00 ml
Glacial acetic acid	.....	2 drops

Staining Procedure

1. Xylene, absolute and 95% alcohols to distilled water.
2. Place in 4% chromic acid (oxidizer) for 1 hour.
3. Wash in running tap water for 5 minutes.
4. Place in Coleman's Feulgen reagent for 15 minutes.
5. Rinse in 3 changes of sulphurous acid rinse.
6. Wash for 15 minutes in running tap water.
7. Place slides in aldehyde-fuchsin solution for 15 to 30 minutes.
8. Rinse off excess stain with 95% alcohol.
9. Rinse in tap water.
10. Counterstain lightly with metanil yellow solution for 1 minute.
11. Rinse in tap water.
12. Dehydrate through 95% and absolute alcohols.
13. Clear in xylene and mount.

Results:

Fungi, elastic tissue and mucin—**deep rose to purple.**

Background—**yellow.**

N.B.1. Absolutely fresh Coleman's leuco-fuchsin solution is a **must** for optimum results, especially for the demonstration of *Histoplasma capsulatum*.

2. Special attention must be given to the metanil yellow counterstain, since many of the small fungal bodies can be overshadowed if the counterstain is too dark. If this does happen, however, the excess stain can be removed by washing in running water.

PER-IODIC ACID-SCHIFF REACTIONS (PAS)

Fixation: 10 per cent formalin or Zenker's solution.

Technic: Cut paraffin sections at 6 microns.

Solutions:

1. ***Coleman's Feulgen reagent***

   Dissolve 1 g basic fuchsin in 200 ml hot distilled water. Bring to boiling point. Cool and add 2 g potassium metabisulphite, and 10 ml normal hydrochloric acid. Let it bleach for 24 hours, then add 0.5 g activated carbon (Norit). Shake for 1 minute and filter through coarse filter paper. Repeat filtration until solution is colorless. Store in refrigerator.

   or

2. ***Schiff's Leuco-fuchsin solution***

   Dissolve 1 g basic fuchsin in 200 ml hot distilled water. Bring to boiling point. Cool to 50°C. Filter and add 20 ml normal hydrochloric acid. Cool further and add 1 g anhydrous sodium bisulphite, or sodium metabisulphite. Keep in the dark for 48 hours until solution becomes straw colored. Store in refrigerator.

3. ***Test for Schiff's Leuco-fuchsin solution***

   Pour a few drops of Schiff's solution into 10 ml of (37 to 40)% formaldehyde in a watch glass. If the solution turns **reddish purple rapidly, it is good**. If the reaction is delayed and the resultant color deep blue-purple, then the solution is **breaking down**.

4. ***0.5% Per-iodic acid solution***

Per-iodic acid crystals	.....	0.5 g
Distilled water	.....	100.0 ml

5. ***Normal Hydrochloric acid solution***

Hydrochloric acid, conc. sp. gr. 1.19	.....	83.5 ml
Distilled water	.....	916.5 ml

6. ***0.2% Light Green counterstain***

Light green crystals	.....	0.2 g
Distilled water	.....	100.0 ml
Glacial acetic acid	.....	0.2 ml

   or

   Harris' Haematoxylin

7. ***Diastase solution***

Diastase	.....	0.5 g
Distilled water, sterile	.....	100.0 ml

   Store in refrigerator; stays for 1 week.

Staining Procedure

1. Xylene.
2. Absolute alcohol.
3. Alcohol 95%.
4. If Zenker-fixed, remove mercury precipitate in iodine, wash in water and decolorize in hypo solution.
5. Rinse in distilled water.
6. Periodic acid solution for 5 minutes (oxidizer).
7. Rinse in distilled water.
8. Place in **Coleman's Feulgen** or **Schiff's leucofuchsin** for 15 minutes.
9. Place in running tap water for 10 minutes for pink color to develop.
10. Stain in **Harris' haematoxylin** for 6 minutes, or light green counterstain for a few seconds. Light green is recommended for counterstaining sections in which fungi are to be demonstrated. **Omit steps 11 through 15 if light green is used.**
11. Rinse in tap water.
12. Differentiate in acid alcohol—3 to 10 quick dips.
13. Wash in tap water.
14. Dip in ammonia water for blueing sections.
15. Wash in running tap water—10 minutes.
16. Alcohol, 95%.
17. Absolute alcohol, 2 changes.
18. Xylene, 2 changes.
19. Mount.

> N.B. A solution of 5% aqueous Clorox bleach will reduce overstaining by leuco-fuchsin. Running tap water or ammonia water will decolorise the light green.

Results:

Glycogen, mucin, hyaluronic acid, reticulin, fibrin of thrombi, colloid droplets, hyaline of arteriosclerosis, hyaline deposits in glomeruli, granular cells in the renal arterioles, most basement membranes, colloid of pituitary stalks and thyroid, amyloid infiltration and other elements may **show a positive reaction: (rose to purplish red)**.

Nuclei—**Blue.**

Fungi—**Red.**

Background—**Pale Green** (with light green counterstaining).

GRAM-WEIGERT'S STAIN

Weigert, C. (1887). ***Fortscher. Med.*** **5, 228**

For demonstration of **Gram-positive organisms** and **fibrin**.

Stock solution (A)

Ethyl alcohol, absolute	....	33 ml
Aniline	....	9 ml
Crystal violet		to saturation

Stock solution (B)

Crystal violet, saturated aqueous solution **(approx. 1.7%)**

Mix and filter.

***Solution (1)** ***Lithium carmine solution*:**

Carmine	.....	2.5–5 g
Lithium carbonate, saturated aqueous solution **(approx. 1.25 g per 100 ml)**	....	100 ml
Thymol, as preservative	....	1 g

***Solution (2) Aniline + crystal violet:**

Stock solution (A)	....	3 ml
Stock solution (B)	....	27 ml

Solution (3) Gram's iodine soln. (Mordant): (Gram, 1884)

Iodine	....	3 g
Potassium iodide	....	6 g
Distilled water	....	900 ml

Mix potassium iodide with distilled water. Then mix iodine, otherwise iodine won't dissolve.

***Solution (4)**

Xylene	....	1 volume
Aniline	....	1 volume

Mode of Preparation

Stock solution (A)

Combine aniline with alcohol, and saturate with crystal violet.

Stock solution (B)

As stated above.

***Solution (1)**

Mix carmine to lithium carbonate solution. To this dissolve thymol exystals.

***Solution (2)**

Add solution (A) to solution (B); record date and label. The combined stain remains stable for approximately 7 days.

***Solution (4)**

Add aniline to xylene, mix well and label.

Procedure

1. Bring sections to water.
2. Stain with **solution (1)** for 2-5 minutes.
3. Stain with **solution (2)** for 5-10 minutes.
4. Drain and blot with filter paper.
5. Mordant with **solution (3)** for 5-10 minutes.
6. Drain and blot with filter paper.
7. Differentiate in **solution (4)**.
8. Blot and rinse in xylol.
9. Mount.

Results:

Cell nuclei—**Red;**

Fibrin and Gram-positive organisms—**Blue-Black.**

ZIEHL-NEELSEN'S METHOD

(FOR M. TUBERCULOSIS IN TISSUE SECTION)

ACID FAST or Z-N STAIN (AFS)

Fixative: Fix the tissue in Zenker's fluid; when fixed in 10% formal-saline, treat the section with 0.5% ammonia for a few minutes before staining to make the reaction neutral.

Procedure

1. Take the section in water in the usual manner.
2. Stain with **steaming carbol fuchsin** for 5 minutes.
3. Rinse in water.
4. Decolorize with 1% HCl in 70% alcohol or **5% H_2SO_4 for 1 minute** and continue decolorization with neutral 70% alcohol for 2 to 3 minutes, until the section is pinkish on washing. For *Myco, leprae,* strictly decolorize in acid only.

5. Counterstain in 2% aqueous methylene blue for 2 minutes.
6. Rinse in water, dehydrate in absolute alcohol, clear in xylol and mount.

Result:

Acid Fast Bacilli **(AFB) are stained red,** and other organisms and tissues—**Blue.**

LEVADITI'S METHOD FOR TREPONEMA PALLIDUM, OTHER SPIROCHETA AND FUNGI IN HISTOPATHOLOGICAL SECTIONS

Solution 1 (Fixative)

Ethyl alcohol (95%).

Solution 2

Silver nitrate, 1.5% aqueous solution.

***Solution 3**

Pyrogallic acid (reducing agent)....	2-4	g
Distilled water	100	ml
Concentrated formaldehyde solution (40%)	5	ml

Mode of Preparation

***Solution 3 (Reducing Solution)**

Pour pyrogallic acid in distilled water and add concentrated (40%) formaldehyde solution. Record date and label. The solution is best prepared just before use.

Procedure

1. Dissect small pieces of tissue of 1 mm in thickness; and fix in 10% formalin for 24 hours.
2. Rinse in distilled water.
3. Place in **solution (1)** for 24 hours.
4. Return to distilled water, until the tissue sinks to the bottom of the vessel.
5. Impregnate with **solution (2)** for **3-5 days** at 37°C in the dark (in incubator).
6. Wash in distilled water.
7. Reduce in **solution (3)** for 24-72 hours in dark.
8. Wash thoroughly in distilled water.
9. Dehydrate, clear in cedar wood oil and embed in paraffin wax.
10. Cut sections at 5 μ thickness.
11. De-wax in xylene and mount in Canada balsam.

Results:

Spirochaeta — **Black.**

Background — **Yellow to Brown.**

N.B.(a) For living tissue a stronger solution of silver nitrate (3 per cent) is recommended for solution (2).

(b) The silver nitrate is deposited on the surface of Treponema with the result that they appear larger than their true size.

(c) This method is not only for *Treponema*, but also for all other spirochaetes.

METHOD OF GIEMSA'S STAIN

Dilute 10 drops of stain in 10 ml of distilled water (neutral pH), or in phosphate buffer pH 6.8 to 7.0.

The film is fixed with pure acetone-free (absolute) methyl alcohol for 2.5 minutes. Wash with neutral distilled water. Put the slide with the film side down on a special staining dish containing two ridges to support the slide. Put 10 ml of dilute Giemsa's stain in the dish so that the film side is in contact with the stain; keep for 30 to 45 minutes, wash and differentiate in distilled water by two changes in one minute time, when the film has a pinkish grey tinge.

PANOPTIC STAIN (PAPPENHEIM'S) OR MAY-GRUENWALD AND GIEMSA STAIN FOR *H. PYLORI* BACTERIA

This is a **combined May-Gruenwald and Giemsa's stain**. For this, film is at first stained with May-Gruenwald's stain for 5 minutes; washed thoroughly with distilled water and then stained with dilute Giemsa for 30 minutes. **Wright's or Leishman's stain may be used instead of May-Gruenwald's,** before staining with dilute Giemsa. But a simplified method which gives satisfactory result is as follows:

Place the slide with film-side up on a staining rack and cover the smear with Leishman's stain and allow the stain to act for 30 seconds. Dilute it with double the quantity of dilute Giemsa's stain (**one drop of Giemsa to 2 ml of distilled water**) and mix. Stain for 10 minutes and the staining is completed as in Leishman's stain.

This stain gives an admirable result and is better than any one of these stains individually.

MAY GRUENWALD—GIEMSA STAIN FOR *H. PYLORI* IN TISSUE (STOMACH)

Procedure

1. Take the section in water in the usual manner.
2. Stain with hot carbol fuchsin for 5 minutes.
3. Rinse in water.
4. **Decolorize** with Acid-alcohol (1% HCl in 70% alcohol) or 5% H_2SO_4 (36 N) for 1 minute or a few dips and continue decolorization with neutral 70% alcohol for 2 to 3 minutes, until **the section is pinkish on washing**. For **M. leprae, strictly decolorize in acid only.**
5. **Counterstain** in 2% aqueous methylene blue or 2% light green for 2–4 minutes.
6. **Rinse in water**, dehydrate by ascending alcoholic (grading) procedure; clear in xylol and mount.

Result:

Acid Fast Bacilli (AFB) are stained **Red** and other organisms and tissues — **Blue**.

The alternative stain is **Warthin-Starry stain.**

WARTHIN-STARRY METHOD FOR HELICOBACTER PYLORI AND SPIROCHAETES

(After Kerr)[1]

The demonstration of spirochaetes in individual paraffin sections of formalin-fixed tissue.

Acidulated water pH 3.8-4.4

Stock solution:

Triple distilled water	....	1 litre
Citric acid, 1% aqueous solution	....	as required

Solution (1)

Silver nitrate	....	1 g
Acidulated water (*see* above)	....	100 ml

Solution (2)

Gelatin, 5% solution in acidulated water	....	37.5 ml
Hydroquinone, 0.15% solution in acidulated water	....	20 ml
Silver nitrate, 1% solution in acidulated water	....	11.5 ml

1 Kerr, D. A. (1938), *Amer. J. clin. Path.*, 8, 63.

Mode of Preparation:

Stock Solution

Adjust the **reaction of the distilled water to** ***p*****H 3.8-4.4** by the addition of the **citric acid solution.**

Solution (1)

Weigh the silver nitrate into the acidulated water. Store in a brown reagent bottle, record date and label.

Solution (2)

Heat all of the ingredients to 56°C. Add the silver nitrate solution to the gelatin and then incorporate the hydroquinone. **Prepare only as required** and use immediately.

Procedure

1. Bring sections and a known positive control **slide to triple distilled water.**
2. Impregnate with **solution (1)** for 30 minutes at 43°C.
3. Develop in **solution (2)** until sections are light brown or yellow. Check the control slide microscopically.
4. Rinse quickly in warm tap water at approximately 56°C.
5. Rinse in distilled water.
6. Dehydrate, clear and mount.

Results:

Spirochaetes and H. pylori—**Black;** background—**Pale yellow** to **Light brown.**

N.B. (a) **Overdevelopment in solution (3)** produces thickened spirochaetes and a black precipitate.

(b) Sections may be **toned in 1 per cent gold chloride** after step 5 if desired.

(c) **Faulkner** used an acetate buffer of *p*H 3.6 in place of the acidulated distilled water throughout. His developer was prepared by mixing 15 ml of 5 per cent gelatin in *p*H 3.6 acetate buffer with 3 ml of 2 per cent silver nitrate and 1 ml of 3 per cent hydroquinone, both of which are dissolved in *p*H 3.6 acetate buffer. The procedure is similar but the sections are first rinsed in a 1 in 25 dilution of *p*H 3.6 acetate buffer and the staining period in solution (2) is prolonged to 45 minutes at 60°C.

(d) For a report on the merits of various Warthin-Starry modifications the reader is referred to an article by Bridges and Luna[2].

FITE-FARACO METHOD FOR ACID FAST BACILLI

The demonstration of acid-fast bacilli, particularly *Mycobacterium leprae.*

Solution 1: Paraffin remover

Peanut oil	...	1 vol
Xylene	....	2 vol

Solution 2

Basic fuchsin	....	0.5 g
Phenol crystals, melted	...	2.5 ml
Ethyl alcohol, absolute	...	5.0 ml
Distilled water	...	42.5 ml

Solution 3

Acid alcohol (**HCl**; Sp. gr. 1.19—**1 ml** plus **70% Ethyl alcohol 99 ml.**

Solution 4: Counter-stain

Methylene blue	....	0.5 g
Acetic acid, glacial	...	0.5 ml
Tap water	...	100 ml

MACHIAVELLO'S RICKETTSIAL STAIN FOR MITOCHONDRIAL FIXATION AND STAIN

The demonstration of rickettsiae in sections.

Solution 1

Methylene blue, 1% aqueous solution, or

Solution 2

Basic fuchsin, 0.25% aqueous solution

Solution 3: Sörensen's Phosphate buffer

Citric acid, 0.5% aqueous solution

Procedure

1. Bring fixed sections and a control slide to water after fixing in **Regaud's solution**. For Regaud solution fixation technic is upto 3" only (see below).
2. Stain with **solution 1** overnight.
3. Differentiate in 95 per cent alcohol.
4. Wash quickly in distilled water.
5. Stain with **solution 2** for 30 minutes.
6. Differentiate very rapidly in **solution 3** for 1–2 seconds.
7. Dehydrate rapidly in absolute alcohol, clear and mount.

Results

Cell nuclei, **blue**; rickettsiae, **bright red**.

> N.B. Differentiation in solution 3 is critical and the time period is upto or within 2 seconds.

REGAUD'S SOLUTION

A cytoplasmic fixative widely used for the fixation of mitochondria and rickettsiae.

Fixative:

Potassium dichromate, 3% aqueous solution 80 ml

Concentrated formaldehyde solution (40%) 20 ml

Mode of Preparation

Add the concentrated formaldehyde (40%) solution to 3% solution of potassium dichromate immediately before use. Mix well and label.

Mode of Preparation

Fix tissues for **4 days**.

> N.B. (a) Fixation is followed by 4–8 days post-chroming in 3% aqueous potassium dichromate. The dichromate solution is changed every other day during this period. Following post-chroming, blocks of tissue are washed in running tap water for 24 hours. Dehydration should commence in 50% alcohol. (b) The composition of this solution, is widely used for the **fixation of mitochondria and rickettsiae**. (c) Regaud's fluid is recommended by Pearse for the **fixation of chromaffin granules**.

SILVER METHOD FOR SPIROCHAETES AND DONOVAN BODIES[3]

(STEINER AND STEINER, 1957)

The demonstration of spirochaetes and Donovan bodies in individual paraffin sections.

Stock solution (A)

Silver nitrate	....	2 gm
Distilled water	....	1 litre
Sodium potassium tartrate powder		1.65 g

Stock solution (B)

Hydroquinone	....	1.0 g
Double distilled water	....	60 ml

Solution (1)

Uranium nitrate, 1% aqueous solution

Solution (2)

Silver nitrate, 1% aqueous solution

Solution (3)

Gum mastic powder	....	2.5 g
Ethyl alcohol, absolute	....	100 ml

Solution (4)

Stock solution (A)	....	20 ml
Solution (3)	....	20 ml
Stock solution (B)	....	60 ml

Mode of Preparation

Stock solution (A)

Boil the distilled water and dissolve the silver nitrate. Add the sodium potassium tartrate while the solution is still boiling. Filter into a brown reagent bottle, record date and label. The solution remains milky.

Stock solution (B)

Dissolve the hydroquinone in the distilled water just before use.

Solution (3)

Measure the ethyl alcohol into a 250 ml. flask and dissolve the gum mastic. Filter, store in a suitable bottle, record date and label. The gum mastic takes at least 24 hours to dissolve.

Solution (4)

Add stock solution (A) to solution (3) and then incorporate stock solution (B). This solution, which is milky, can be used once only and should be prepared at the time of use.

Procedure

1. Bring sections and a known positive control slide to distilled water.
2. Sensitize with solution **(1)** for 3 minutes.
3. Wash in two changes of distilled water.
4. Impregnate with solution **(2)** for 2 hours at 56°C.
5. Wash thoroughly in distilled water.
6. Dehydrate with 95 per cent and absolute ethyl alcohol—two baths of each.
7. Transfer to solution **(3)** for 5 minutes.
8. Reduce in solution **(4)** for 5-15, minutes examining the control slide under the microscope periodically.
9. Wash in several changes of distilled water.
10. Dehydrate, clear and mount.

Results

Spirochaetes, Donovan bodies, fungi and bacteria—**Black**; background—**Yellow** to **Brown**.

METHENAMINE-SILVER NITRATE METHOD (ORIGINAL GMS STAIN) FOR FUNGI[1]

The demonstration of fungi in sections. **Grocott's application to fungi.**

Stock methenamine-silver nitrate solution

Stock solution

Silver nitrate, 5% aqueous soln.	....	5 ml
Hexamethylene-tetramine, 3% aqueous solution	....	100 ml

Solution (1)

Chromic acid, CrO_3, 5% aqueous solution

Solution (2)

Sodium bisulphite, 1% aqueous solution

Solution (3)

Borax, 5% aqueous solution	....	2 ml
Distilled water	....	15 ml
Stock solution (*see* above)	....	25 ml

Solution (4)

Gold chloride, yellow, 0.1% aqueous solution

Solution (5)

Sodium thiosulphate, 2% aqueous solution

Solution (6)

Light green, 0.2% aqueous soln.	....	10 ml
Distilled water	....	50 ml
Acetic acid, glacial	....	0.1 ml

Mode of Preparation

Stock Solution

Add the silver nitrate to the methenamine solution. A white precipitate forms which dissolves on

1 Faulkner, R. R., and Lillie, R. D. (1945). *Stain Tech.*, **20**, 81.
2 Bridges, C. H., and Luna, L. (1957), *Lab. Invest.*, **6**, 357.
3 Steiner, G., and Steiner, G. (1944). *J. Lab. clin. Med.*, **29**, 868.

1 Grocott, R. G. (1955). *Aner. J. clin. Path.*, **25** 975.

shaking. Record date and label. The solution remains stable for several months if stored at 4°C.

Solution (3)

Dissolve the borax in distilled water and add the **methenamine-silver nitrate stock solution.** The solution should be prepared as required.

Solution (6)

Add the light green to distilled water, incorporate the acetic acid and label.

Procedure

1. Bring sections and a control slide to water.
2. Oxidize in **solution (1)** for 60 minutes.
3. Wash in running tap water.
4. Transfer to **solution (2)** for 1 minute to remove residual chromic acid.
5. Wash in tap water for 5-10 minutes.
6. Rinse in several changes of distilled water.
7. Impregnate with **solution (3)** for 30-60 minutes at 58°C. Examine the control slide under the microscope to check for adequate impregnation.
8. Rinse in several changes of distilled water.
9. Tone in **solution (4)** for 2-5 minutes.
10. Rinse in distilled water.
11. Fix in **solution (5)** for 2-5 minutes.
12. Wash thoroughly in tap water.
13. Stain with **solution (6)** for 30-45 seconds.
14. Dehydrate, clear and mount.

Results

Fungi, sharply outlined in **Black**; inner parts of hyphae and mycelia—**Reddish**; background—**Pale Green.**

SCHLEIFSTEIN'S STAIN[1]

The demonstration of Negri bodies.

Stock solution (A)

Basic fuchsin	....	1.8 g
Methylene blue	....	1 g
Glycerol	....	100 ml
Methyl alcohol, absolute	....	100 ml

Stock solution (B)

Potassium hydroxide 1 : 40,000 aqueous solution

Solution (1)

Stock solution (A)	....	10 drops
Stock solution (B)	.	20 ml

Solution (2)

Ethyl alcohol, 90%

Mode of Preparation

Stock solution (A)

Dissolve the basic fuchsin and methylene blue in the methyl alcohol and add the glycerol. Record date and label. The solution keeps indefinitely.

Stock solution (B)

Prepare a stock 0.25 per cent solution of potassium hydroxide and dilute this solution 1 : 100 for use.

Solution (1)

Add stock solution (A) to stock solution (B). Prepare upto requirement only.

Procedure

1. Bring Zenker (soln.) fixed tissue sections to water.
2. Remove mercuric chloride precipitate by the following procedure
   Immerse in Lygol's iodine (soln.) for 10 minutes.
3. Then rinse in water.
4. Bleach in 5% sodium thiosulphate soln. for 3 to 5 minutes.
5. Wash thoroughly.
6. Warm the section in staining soln. 1 upto steaming; keep there for 5 minutes.
7. Wash quickly in tap water to cool the section.
8. Differentiate in solution 2 till appearance of a pale violet color.
9. Dehydrate in ascending grades of alcohol, clear in xylol (2 changes) and mount in bex mountant.

Results

Negribodies—**Deep magenta**; Cytoplasm of cell—**Bluish**; Red cells—**Copper color.**

1 Schleifstein. J. (1937). *Aner. J. Publ. Hlth*, 27, 1283.

ADDITIONAL LEARNING:

THE COLLAGENS

There are many major types of collagen and several minor types as well.

Usually collagen is the secretory fibrillar product of fibroblasts and some other cells.

The variation of types occurs by **Genetic control** resulting in slight variation in the **composition of alpha-chain**. Each of the collagen type has their own characteristic amino acid content.

Type I Collagen

(a) the thick collagen fibres constitute, the **bulk of collagen** material of the body.

(b) Type I collagen **forms the organic matrix of bases**.

(c) Type I collagen is a major **structural protein in the lung.**

Electron microscopic study

Type I collagen is composed of tightly packed bundles, with **thick fibrils of 75 nm diameter** along with interfibrillar material (**ground substances**). Longitudinally the fibrils show 64 nm axial periodicity.

There are prominent cross bandings in Type I collagen that indicate the **lack of interference of the zones** from (interfibrillar) ground substance.

The **thickness** on the diameter **of Type I collagen fibrils is regulated by the presence of a partially processed form of Type III precollagens.**

Type II Collagen

Type II collagen forms some basis of:

(a) **Hyaline cartilage** and

(b) **Elastic cartilage**

The (a & b) are produced by certain **chondroblastic activity**. Type II collagen fibres are made up of fibrils which are arranged in a **meshwork form** along **with** large amounts of **proteoglycans** (N-acetyl muramic acid and N-acetyl glycosamine in many layers in Gram positive cell wall). The type II fibres are **hardly seen under a light microscope** due to masking effect of abundant interfibrillar material. Electron microscopy shows hardly any difference between Type II and Type I fibres. Prior hyaluronidase (hyalase) treatment may unmask Type II fibres and make it readily accessible for **immunohistochemical evaluation**.

Type III Collagen

Presence of Type III collagen is exclusively found in those tissues and organs, **where Type I collagen tissue occurs**: (a) the **Kidneys, liver, lung** and **spleen,** and (b) the classical **reticular fibres contain Type III collagen.** Electron microscopic (E/M) study of reticular fibres shows loosely packed (Type III) fibrils which are surrounded by plentiful of carbohydrate-rich interfibrillar material. The **reticulin fibres are argyrophilic** which is due to the abundant **proteoglycan content of (Type III collagen) fibres;** this is not dependent upon the proteins of the (Type III collagen) fibrils.

The functions of Type III collagen fibres are to:

(a) provide limited supports and

(b) (i) allow some motility; (ii) for easy diffusion and (iii) for exchange of metabolites.

Type III collagen is also called **fetal collagen,** as **60% of collagen** in the **fetal skin is Type III collagen** as opposed to only **20% of Type III collagen is present in the adult skin.**

Type IV Collagen

Type IV collagen is a part and parcel of the (defined) structures **of all basement membranes** of the body tissues with special reference to basement membrane of kidney substances (basement membrane of Bowman's capsule).

Under the **light microscopy, no fibre** and fibril of Type IV collagen **is visible.**

E/M study shows very **fine fibrils of Type IV collagen** forming a felt-work-like structure in all the basement membranes at various sites. Type IV collagen is closely associated with significant amount of carbohydrate complex. This explains the strong reaction of basement membranes to PAS (Per-iodic acid Schiff) stain.

Type V Collagen

This Type V collagen is **produced by** a wide variety of cells, notably (i) **endothelial cell,** (ii) **connective tissue cells,** and (iii) **some epithelial cells.**

Functions:

1. It remains in close contact with the cell surface so that it is involved in the attachment of cells to the adjacent structures.
2. It is involved in maintenance of tissue.

Type VI Collagen

Type VI collagen is disulfide-rich variant identified in the boundary zone where **interstitial collagenous fibres (Type I and Type II)** are linked to non-collagenous elements.

Mode of Preparation

Solution 1

Add the peanut oil to xylene, mix well and label.

Solution 2

HCl (HCl; Sp. gr. 1.19)—1 ml plus 70% (v/v) Ethyl alcohol 99 ml.

Solution 3

Combine the alcohol and phenol, and the basic fuchsin and when solution is effected make up the volume to 50 ml with distilled water. Filter, store in a suitable bottle, record date and label.

Solution 4

Measure the tap water into a 250 ml flask, dissolve the methylene blue and add the acetic acid. Record date and label.

Procedure

1. Deparaffinize sections with two baths of solution (1) for 12 minutes in each
2. Drain and blot.
3. Stain with solution (2) for 20–30 minutes at room temperature.
4. Wash in tap water.
5. Differentiate in solution (3) for approximately 60 seconds.
6. Wash in tap water.
7. Counterstain in solution (4) for 30–60 seconds.
8. Remove excess of solution 4 with tap water.
9. Blot and dry in air.
10. Mount.

Results

Acid-fast bacilli—**Red**; background—**Light blue.**

N.B. Wade[1] advocated the use of **rectified turpentine** in place of xylene in **solution 1** and differentiated in 20 per cent aqueous sulphuric acid.

Diagrams/Notes

B. GENERAL AND SPECIAL PATHOLOGY

CHAPTER 2

INFLAMMATION

Inflammation is a series of pathological changes associated with local vascular reaction and cellular response of the living tissue to an injury insufficient to kill the tissue. Features of acute inflammation in any organ or tissues of the body is:

(a) **Congestion and dilation of vessels** with *infiltration* of (i) red cells, (diapedesis), and (ii) neutrophilic leukocytes (due to emigration and transmigration).

(b) Due to the accumulation of fluid exudate, there is formation of ***edema*** at the site.

(c) After 3 to 4 days, macrophages infiltrate.

(d) At about the end of a week, granulation tissue forms, which comprises young capillary buds (endothelial proliferation followed later by canalization), and young fibroblasts. It indicates the start of apparent repair.

In repair, fibrosis is the last event. During examining a section, note changes under these headings.

ACUTE INFLAMMATION IS CHARACTERIZED BY:

1. **Congestion of blood vessels** marked by their dilation packed with red cells; leukocytes fall out of the axial stream i.e., rolling and tend to adhere to the vessel wall (emigration or migration of leucocytes).

2. **Dead necrosed cells** forming a homogeneous mass.

3. **Exudate** consists of **fibrin, neutrophils** and **red cells** that pass out into the edematous tissues.

4. Later, accumulation of leukocytes, plasma cells, lymphocytes and histiocytes (macrophages) occur in the **circular muscular layer of appendix.**

Neutrophils are characteristic cells of acute inflammation, that is found in the muscular layer of tubular organs, e.g. appendix in acute appendicitis.

Subacute and chronic stages are characterized by the following:

1. **Exudative changes** of acute inflammation may still be present. In addition, there is **eosinophilic infiltration** in **subacute inflammation.**

2. **Repairing process** is characterized by the appearance of:

(a) **Histiocytes** (macrophages) to clear the debris.

(b) **Lymphocytes, plasma cells** and may be a few neutrophils, may be some eosinophils.

(c) **Fibroblasts.**

(d) Formation of new capillaries (**neoangiogenesis**).

(e) Finally, formation of **scar tissue** (fibrous tissue)—pale and avascular.

Chronic stage of the inflammation is characterized by the presence of **lymphocytic** and / or **plasma cell** infiltration, and **fibrosis**. There may be presence of some eosinophils.

PYEMIC ABSCESS—LIVER

Two types of Pyemia:

1. **Portal**: from **infective emboli; via mesenteric veins** (infected piles); liver is the victimized organ.

2. **Systemic Pyemia**: from **infected emboli of systemic** vascular **origin** affecting any organ.

Microscopic appearance:

1. Note the structure of the liver.

2. The **central zone** of abscess shows:

(a) **Densely packed leukocytes** [mainly poly**morphonuclear leukocytes (PMN** or neutro**phils)].**

(b) **Mixed with them are masses of dark-blue stained organisms** (Staph., Strepto, etc.).

3. **Peripheral area**: The abscess is surrounded by a zone of hyperemia.

INFLAMMATION OF THE SEROUS MEMBRANE

Acute Pleurisy, Pericarditis, Peritonitis, Synovitis, Tenosynovitis, Meningitis, etc.

Naked-eye appearance:

Pleura looks **rough, lustureless**, opaque and **shaggy** due to fibrinous exudate.

Microscopic appearance:

1. Active congestion of pleura with dilation of vessels; and alveoli are packed with blood and exudate.

2. Pleural surface is covered with exudate consisting of:

(a) pale pink strands of fibrin in the deeper parts;

(b) fibrin mixed with neutrophilic leukocytes in superficial parts;

(c) when organization commences serosal (Mesothelial) cells are absent.

3. Newly formed young, sprouting (budding) capillaries (vascular hair pin bend loops) are marked (neovascularization).

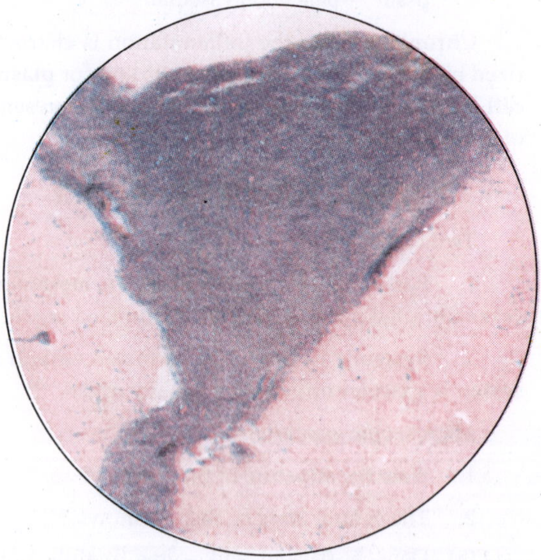

Fig. 2.1: Acute suppurative meningitis—two cerebral convolutions (pink) occur right and left and between these the subarachnoid space is filled with an exudate of many leukocytes (purple). H & E × 40

4. The adjacent lung tissue shows congestion of capillaries, and consolidation with fibrinous exudation in the alveoli (neovascularization).

ACUTE (NONSPECIFIC) PYOGENIC LEPTOMENINGITIS

'**Lepto**' means 'Thin'; the meningitis of the **Pia** and **Arachnoid**; as opposed to **Pacchymeningitis** ('**Pacchy**' means 'Thick' = dura) that occurs by Traumatic or Syphilitic cause.

History: A 13 years old boy was presented in a toxic condition with high fever, neck rigidity (positive Kernig sign), leukocytosis and adrenal hemorrhage (**Waterhouse-Friderichsen syndrome**).

Naked-eye or Gross appearance:

1 Rosy-red coloration of the meninges, due to distention of the surface vessels.

2. There may be a few petechial or larger hemorrhagic areas.

3. A turbid inflammatory exudate covers the surface of the brain.

Microscopic appearance (Fig. 2.1):

1. Limitation of the exudate by the arachnoid meninx and its extension into sulci. Vessels are greatly distended.

2. A fine network of fibrin is present.

3. Entangled in the fibrinous network, are neutrophils, a few lymphocytes and large mononuclear phagocytes (histiocytes i.e. macrophages); these (exudate) fill the subarachnoid space.

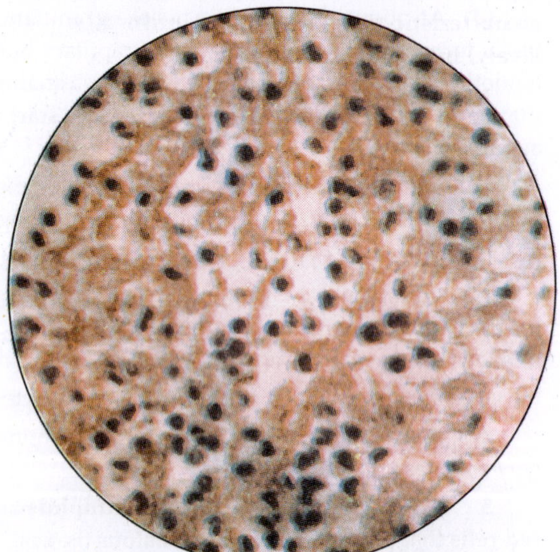

Fig. 2.2: Acute fibrinous pericarditis—The exudate consists of numerous neutrophils (polymorphonuclear leukocytes) and a network of fibrin. H & E × 400

ACUTE FIBRINOUS PERICARDITIS

History: A 12 years old girl had an old history of follicular tonsillitis; now she presented with left-sided chest pain, rise of temperature. On investigation ESR, and ASO titer are elevated (ESR = 110 mm).

Naked-eye or gross appearance:

A thick sero-fibrinous exudate presenting a typical appearance of RHEUMATIC PERICARDITIS.

Microscopic appearence (Fig. 2.2):

1. Exudate mainly consists of fibrin with a varying number of neutrophilic leukocytes and red cells in its **fibrin** meshes.

2. The surface endothelium is absent at places. The capillaries (vessels) are dilated.

3. Tendency to organization by formation of new young sprouting (budding) capillaries and fibroblasts and collagen laid down along the successive layers of fibrin.

ACUTE APPENDICITIS

History: Sixteen years old girl complaining of excruciating pain on right iliac fossa. On examination McBurney's point was tender. There was fever, vomiting and leukocytosis.

Determination of (acute, sub-acute and chronic) type of inflammation in appendix is judged by the characteristic type of cellular infiltration (exclusively) in the circular muscle layer.

Naked-eye or gross appearance:

1. The organ is swollen, enlarged, congested (red in color) and inflamed.

2. Surface is covered with a fibrinous or purulent exudate.

3. On cutting open, longitudinally the mucous membrane looks swollen (edematous), very congested and may be ulcerated; lumen may be narrowed due to edema. Fecal concretions may be present.

Microscopic appearance (Fig. 2.3):

1. The mucous layer is ulcerated but a few intact portions are seen.

2. It is covered with inflammatory exudate (**neutrophils and fibrin**), and necrotic cells.

3. All the coats with special reference to the **muscle coat show heavy infiltration with only neutrophilic leukocytes (in tubular organs)**.

4. Acute congestion of blood vessels with red cell and neutrophilic exudate is seen specially in the peritoneal coat which is thickened.

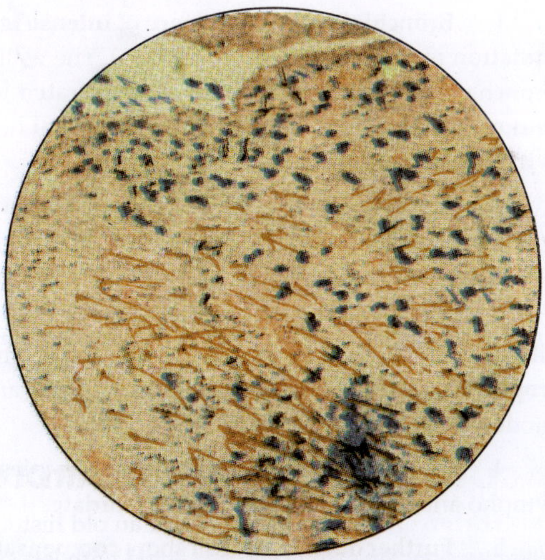

Fig. 2.3: **Acute Appendicitis.** Muscular coat is infiltrated with neutrophils: H & E × 400

ACUTE LOBAR PNEUMONIA

History: A 2 years old child showed high fever, dyspnea, toxicity with absence of lung sound along a wide area at back on the right side; pulse: respiration rate ratio is altered 3 : 2 (normal is 3 : 1).

Three important pathological stages are:

I. THE STAGE OF CONGESTION

Gross appearance:

[Erythrocytic preponderance (98%) and acute congestion leading to consolidation of lung]

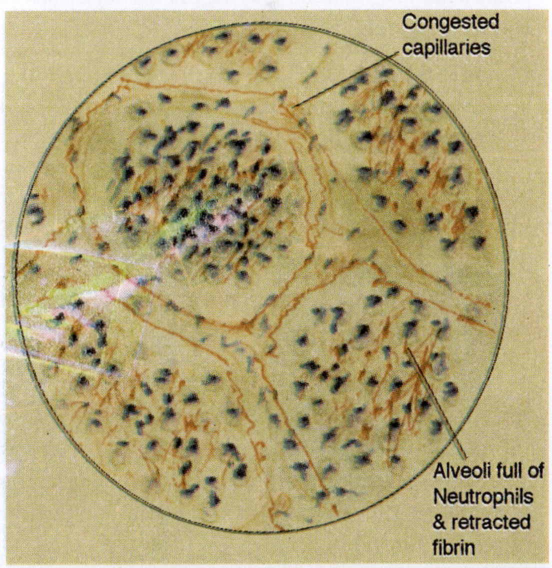

Fig. 2.4: **Acute Lobar Pneumonia**—Stage of Grey hepatization: H & E × 400

[The consolidation in lobar pneumonia produces an appearance resembling that of liver; hence the term **'HEPATIZATION'**, meaning liver-like look and solidification (consolidation) of lung that sinks in water].

Microscopic appearance:

1. Capillaries in the alveolar walls are intensely congested and distended with red cells.

2. The alveoli show early acute inflammatory exudate, consisting mostly of **fibrin, red cells** and a few **neutrophilic leukocytes** (actually whole blood is the exudate).

II. THE STAGE OF RED HEPATIZATION (Erythrocytic preponderance)

Naked-eye or Gross appearance:

1. The affected part is consolidated, voluminous, reddish-brown in colour, very friable and cut bits of lung sink in water.
2. Surface is covered by sticky, fibrinous exudate.
3. Cut surface is dry, granular, reddish-brown and granite-like in appearance.

Microscopic appearance:

1. Alveoli are full of fibrinous network containing red cells and only a few leukocytes in their meshes.

2. Walls of alveoli are congested with dilated capillaries and infiltrated with fair number of neutrophilic leukocytes. Swelling of the pneumocytes (alveolar epithelium) is seen.

III. THE STAGE OF GREY HEPATIZATION [Neutrophilic preponderance and retraction of fibrin (Fig. 2.4)]

Naked-eye or Gross appearance:

1. Hepatization of lung is grey in color; more friable.

2. Cut surface is grey, dry and finely granular.

Microscopic appearance (Fig. 2.4):

1. Fibrin contents of alveoli are seen to be retracted from the walls. Red cells are negligible (so no reddish appearance): neutrophilic leukocytes are present in large number; most of them have undergone degeneration (pus cell formation). Note excess of cells on fibrin network.

2. The congestion of the vessels in the interalveolar walls is diminished.

3. Partial organization of the exudate is recognized on the pleural surface.

IV. THE STAGE OF RESOLUTION (Healthy Stage)

No sign of any inflammation. Microscopically normal alveoli show absorption of exudate. Clinically, there is **complete restoration of function**.

BRONCHOPNEUMONIA

(A condition of Bronchiolitis)

History: A mildly toxic child had fever, dyspnea and patchy areas of consolidation (solidification; dullness = absence of respiratory sound).

Naked-eye or Gross appearance:

1. **Both lungs** are found to be involved; **lower lobes** [in their posterior parts (basal) are usually **affected]. Patchy consolidated areas scattered throughout** the lung tissue **with** alternate **areas of compensatory emphysema** (c.f. massive lesions of lobar pneumonia). Little or **no exudate** is present on the pleural surface.

2. On section, there are dark areas, corresponding to the (i) **zone of congestion round** the **bronchioles**, beyond which is the (ii) **zone of emphysema** and then (iii) **normal lung tissue**.

3. Tiny beads of **pus** can be squeezed out from the bronchioles which form in the **centre of the consolidated areas**.

4. Bronchial **lymph nodes** are **enlarged** and **soft**.

Microscopic appearance:

1. **Bronchioles show** evidence of **intense inflammation** of bronchioles (**bronchiolitis**). The walls of bronchioles are **swollen, thickened, infiltrated** with **leukocytes** and show erosion of the epithelial lining **with desquamation**.

2. The **lumina** of the bronchioles is **filled with purulent exudate** with shed **epithelium, neutrophils** and **organisms** (Staph., Strep., Klebs.) with little **fibrin**.

3. **Surrounding** the bronchiole, **alveoli** are **filled with inflammatory exudate** comprising **neutrophils, 'catarrhal' cells** (large epithelial cells) and a moderate amount of **fibrin**.

4. **Alveoli** contain **mononuclear cells** (plasma, lympho and macro) and **edematous exudate**.

5. **Further outside**, alveoli show **compensatory emphysema**, and then reach the normal lung tissue (respiratory and terminal bronchii).

6. **Blood vessels** in the inter-alveolar septa (alveolar walls) are **intensely congested.**

Tuberculous bronchopneumonia or **bronchopneumonic type of Tb**, shows marked **fibrosis** and mononuclear infiltration making the bronchus non-elastic and rigid. The sputum contains shed elastic fibres.

BRONCHIECTASIS (Fig. 2.5)

History: A 40 years old man who had past history of pulmonary Tb now presents with posterior chest pain with massive foul smelling expectoration (sputum) with discomfort in the chest.

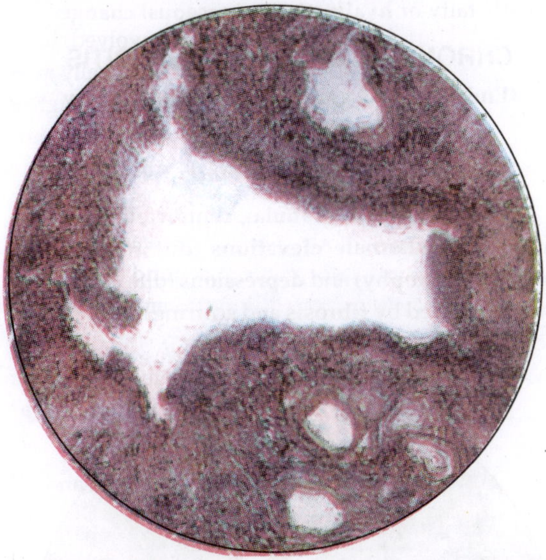

Fig. 2.5: Bronchiectatic cavity—The cavity is lined by a darkly stained layer of chronically inflamed granulation tissue, while the surrounding lung is irregularly fibrosed. Hematoxylin and eosin. × 5

Naked-eye or Gross appearance:

Usually the lower lobes of the lungs are bilaterally affected. Bronchi and bronchioles are dilated 3 to 4 times more than their normal calibers, which contain mucopurulent exudates with very much offensive, foul smell.

Microscopic Appearance (Fig. 2.5 and 2.6):

In a full blown active case following features are noted:

1. **Marked acute and chronic inflammatory cellular exudates** (neutrophils, lymphocytes and occasional plasma cells).

2. **Pseudostratification** of ciliated and non-ciliated columnar epithelial cells mostly.

3. **Squamous metaplasia** of remaining columnar cells.

4. **Fibrosis of bronchial and bronchiolar walls.**

5. **Peribronchial fibrosis.**

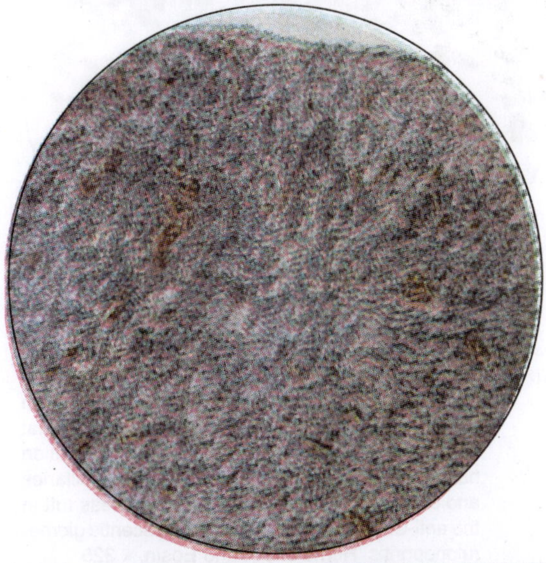

Fig. 2.6: Wall of Bronchiectatic cavity—Adjacent to the cavity (top) the wall consists of granulation tissue which is congested and infiltrated with many inflammatory cells. Further out (bottom) the tissue is more fibrous and less infiltrated with cells. The cavity is lined by a thin layer of squamous epithelium. H & E × 80

THE GLOMERULO-NEPHRITIS (GN)

DIFFUSE GLOMERULO-NEPHRITIS

It is an inflammatory condition of the kidney without pus formation but ultimately after years inflammatory process results in scarring of the kidney due to fibrosis.

ACUTE OR POSTSTREPTOCOCCAL (PS) GLOMERULO-NEPHRITIS (GN)

It is a condition of generalized capillaritis (glomerulitis) of the kidney. It is an immunological injury that occurs at the surface and periphery, i.e., at the capillary level (at the peripheral distribution of the arterial system), where mostly immunological interaction occurs.

***Naked-eye or Gross appearance*:**

Kidney is **enlarged, capsule strips off easily** leaving a smooth surface which shows petechial **hemorrhagic spots.**

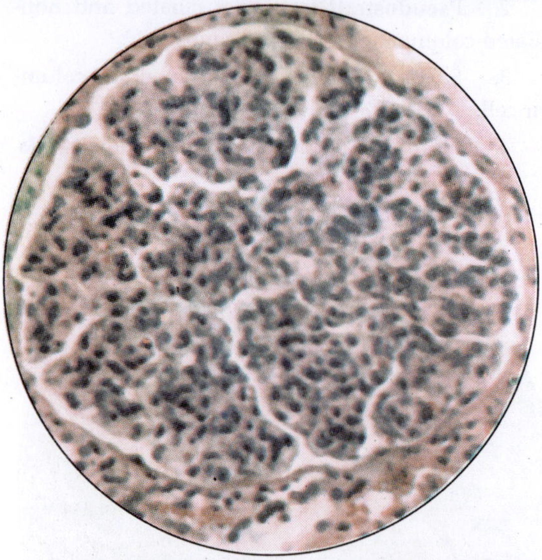

Fig. 2.7: Acute glomerulonephritis—the tuft of the glomerulus is swollen so as to fill the space within which it lies. Its increased number of nuclei indicates that the tuft is also unduly cellular. Such proliferation has resulted in occlusion of many of the capillaries and consequently in a (relatively) bloodless tuft in the anti-GBM antibody-mediated crescentic glomerulonephritis. Hematoxylin and Eosin. × 325

Cut Section:

Cortex—Pale with minute hemorrhage; **Medulla**—Deeply congested and differentiated from the cortex.

Microscopic appearance (Fig. 2.7):

1. **Glomerular tufts**—greatly swollen and enlarged by **cellular proliferation** (of the endothelial cells) lining the capillaries; number of nuclei is increased due to proliferation.

2. **Capsular space**—Fibrinous **exudate** contains **red cells** and **neutrophils**.

3. **Tubules**—Show **cloudy swelling** or fatty change. The lumen contains cellular debris and blood **(red cell) casts (Cellular cast or RBC cast)**.

RAPIDLY PROGRESSIVE GLOMERULO-NEPHRITIS GN: (an early concept) (SUBACUTE)

(Large white kidney; alike nephrosis)

Naked-eye or gross appearance:

Kidney is greatly **enlarged** and **pale**, firm or **soft** in consistency; the **capsule strips off easily**.

Cut Section:

Cortex—Swollen, pale with yellow streaks of fatty or lipoid deposition; **pyramids**—Often **congested**.

Microscopic appearance:

1. Uniform involvement of all **glomeruli** which are **swollen**.

2. **Endothelial proliferation** more marked.

3. **Proliferation of capsular epithelium** forming **'crescents' (Epithelial crescents)**.

4. **Basement membrane swollen** with early hyalinization giving rise to **lobulation**.

5. **Tubules** show **cloudy swelling** and occasionally fatty or **hyaline (proteinaceous) change**.

CHRONIC GLOMERULO-NEPHRITIS

(End stage and granular contracted kidney or end stage kidney)

Naked-eye or Gross appearance:

Kidney is **small, granular, contracted, firm and pitted with** alternate **elevations** (due to **compensatory hypertrophy**) and **depressions** (due to degeneration followed by **fibrosis** and scarring). Pelvic fat is increased.

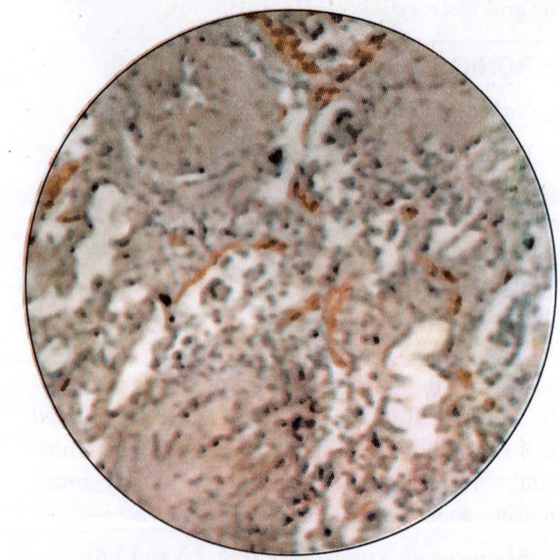

Fig. 2.8: Chronic glomerulonephritis—Glomeruli (two top and one bottom) show advanced fibrosis. The tubules in neighbourhood of glomeruli are atrophied and replaced by fibrous tissue, while some tubules are also dilated. The fibrous tissue is infiltrated with lymphocytes. Hematoxylin and Eosin. × 240

Capsule—adherent to the cortex.

Cut Surface:

Cortex is scarred, thinned out and pale. **Demarcation** between cortex and medulla is **lost**. There may be scattered **cystic spaces** in the **cortex** (or 1 or 2).

An attempt to peel off the capsule causes **decortication** (capsule is adherent to the cortex due to fibrosis, which breaks down).

Microscopic appearance (Fig. 2.8):

1. **Glomeruli**—A large proportion of them are partially or completely hyalinized giving ONION SCALE appearance. Connective tissue between the glomeruli is greatly increased.

2. **Tubules—Atrophied and replaced by fibrous tissues**, but there are areas where tubules have **hypertrophied** (compensatory).

3. **Blood vessels**—Medium and small sized interlobular arteries show intimal proliferation and hypertrophy of the media. Afferent arterioles to the glomeruli show hyaline thickening. Renal **ischemia is due to glomerular and vascular changes.**

4. **Kidney interstitium**—Marked **interstitial fibrosis** with **mononuclear (lymphocytic, plasmacytic and histiocytic) cellular infiltration.**

CHRONIC PYELO-NEPHRITIS (Chronic PN)

Naked-eye or Gross appearance:

Usually the change is seen more in one kidney (unlike chronic nephritis where there is diffuse scarring in both kidneys). In chronic PN, scarring occurs only in one or 2 regions mostly in the upper and lower poles with the frequency of reflux in these sites.

Microscopic appearance:

1. Periglomerular fibrosis.
2. Hyalinization of Glomeruli.
3. Thyroidization of tubules; tubular lumina are full of colloid (alike follicles of the thyroid gland).
4. Increased fibrosis in interstitial tissue.
5. Dense lymphocytic infiltration in interstitial tissue.
6. Onion skin appearance of the blood vessels.

REPAIR

GRANULATION TISSUE

Granulation tissue occurs in all types of acute inflammation. It means (i) proliferation and hyperplasia of supporting fibroblasts and side by side (ii) capillary endothelial proliferation and **capillary budding**, their organization, and bending loops, i.e., **neoangiogenesis** (canalization and vascularization).

The vascular thin-walled **capillary hair-pin (bends) on the surface looks like red granules on a velvety bed**. As it looks **(red and) granular**, it is called **granulation tissue**.

Microscopic appearance:

1. **Surface** necrotic **layer of fibrin** showing degenerating **leukocytes and red cells**.

2. Intermediate layers—Under the surface layer, **hair-pin-bend-like vascular** loops (newly formed blood vessels) which grow as protoplasmic buds from the pre-existing vascular endothelium are canalized later on. **Vascular loops** are **perpendicular to the surface** and **fibroblasts are parallel to the surface.**

3. **Deeper layers**—Numerous newly formed blood vessels which are thin-walled capillary loops;

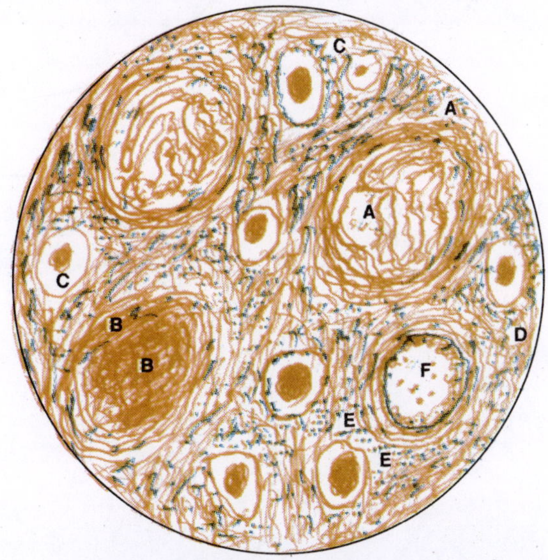

Fig. 2.9: **CHRONIC PYELONEPHRITIS**—A. Periglomerular Fibrosis, B. Hyalinizatiion of Glomeruli, C. Thyroidization of the Tubules (due to deposition of colloid), D. Increased Interstitial Fibrosis, E. Lymphocytic Infiltration of the Interstitial Tissue, F. Onion skin appearance of Blood vessels

proliferating **fibroblasts are parallel to the vessels** (in the deeper layers).

4. **Still deeper layers** are infiltrated with **plasma cells** and young, and developing **fibroblasts** are **at right angles** (perpendicular) **to the vessels (alike intermediate layers).**

5. **Infiltration with neutrophils, macrophages and lymphocytes occur.**

6. Normal tissue is at the deepest of all the layers [1. Surface layers; 2. Intermediate layers; 3. Deeper layers; 4. Still deeper layers; 5. Normal tissue (deepest) layers].

Diagrams/Notes

Diagrams/Notes

Diagrams/Notes

Diagrams/Notes

Diagrams/Notes

CHAPTER 3

DISTURBANCES OF NUTRITION (Retrograde changes)

DEGENERATION (CELL INJURY & DAMAGE)

Degeneration indicates pathological changes which occur in the cell or tissues in the process of sickness of cells. The term degeneration today is confusing and even may also denote localized cytoplasmic lesion. For fatty degeneration or infiltration it should be better expressed as fatty change. However, degeneration is characterized by the conversion of cell protoplasm or tissue structures which is visible in those degenerated cells. **Degeneration** is usually **defined according to the nature of the abnormally accumulated material in the cells**, e.g. fatty change and is one of the important criteria of **reversible cell injury**.

Phases of degeneration:

1. Hydropic change
2. Fatty change
3. Lipid accumulation, e.g., Gaucher's and Niemann-Pick (or Pick) disease.
4. Cloudy swelling
5. Hyaline change
6. Mucinous change
7. Amyloid change (always extracellular)
8. Glycogen accumulation, e.g., von Gierkie's disease

Causes of degeneration

Poison (toxins)

1. **Bacterial: Acute**—diphtheria; **Chronic**—tuberculosis.
2. **Metabolic products**—Acetone, acetoacetic acid, etc., in diabetes.
3. **Chemical**—Phosphorus, chloroform, alcohol, arsenic, etc.

Deficient oxygenation—Anemia; impaired circulation—**Chronic (passive) venous congestion** (CVC).

Physical agents—Trauma, excess of heat or cold, electricity, X-ray, radium, etc.

Immunological (Hypersensitivity) agents—various allergic and hypersensitive factors. Other immunological injurious agents.

However, strictly speaking, when the term degeneration should be used, it should signify irreversible cellular changes. But we do not restrict ourselves to that strict definition always.

PROTEINOUS DEGENERATION

Cloudy swelling

Synonyms: Parenchymatous, granular or albuminous degeneration. It is the commonest and **mildest form of detectable cell changes as a result of injury to the cell**. Principal organs affected are **heart, kidney, liver, muscle,** etc.

CLOUDY SWELLING OF THE KIDNEY

Gross appearance:

1. The organ is slightly **enlarged and swollen**.
2. It is **pale due to compression of blood vessels** by swollen cells.
3. The surface is slightly opaque, cloudy, turbid, and gives a **parboiled appearance.**
4. *Cut surfaces* bulge out through the capsule.

Microscopic appearance:

1. **Cells** are unusually **granular** (crowded with albuminous granules). These **granules obscure the nucleus** of the cell.
2. Affected **cells** are swollen, ill-defined, larger than normal and **project into the lumen of the convoluted tubules making it** narrow and **star-shaped.**
3. Proteinaceous substance accumulation: (i) outside the cells—in amyloidosis, (ii) Reabsorption droplets in proximal tubules in kidney appear as pink hyaline droplets, (iii) **Hugely distended ER produces** large, homogeneous, **eosinophilic inclusions—Russel bodies.**
4. **Nuclei** are either normal or stain faintly.
5. **Globules of fat** may begin to appear.

HYALINE DEGENERATION

This is not a distinct pathological entity; the term is used to describe a **reversible** physical appearance of tissues, e.g., **the tissues are clear, translucent, glossy** in appearance and stain brightly with acid dyes: eosin, fuchsin, etc. It is a type of proteinous change. Hyaline degeneration may be cellular (epithelial), myxomatous (connective tissue), or intramuscular tissues [**Zenker's degeneration** (Fig. 3.1)]. This includes a number of conditions with common features, e.g., hyaline degeneration in fibromyoma; **Zenker's degeneration** of the rectus abdominis muscle after typhoid fever due to Salmonella endotoxin action including Leiomyoma [Fibromyoma (Fibroid-uterus) i.e., Leiomyoma].

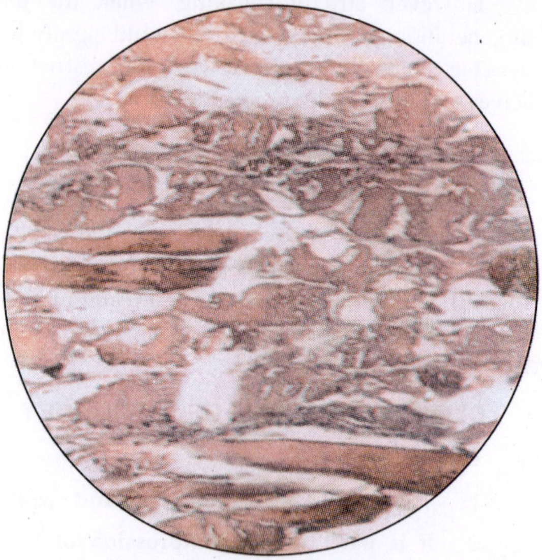

Fig. 3.1: Zenker's degeneration (necrosis) of muscle—Section of abdominis rectus from a case of typhoid fever. The fibres middle left and bottom right are hyaline and acidophilic and show pyknotic nuclei, while the others are poorly stained, vacuolated and broken up as a result of autolysis. Hematoxylin and Eosin. × 100

Amyloid (Amylum = starch; oid = like) is the combination of glycoprotein with acid mucopolysaccharides. A state of hypergammaglobulinemia (**macroglobulinemia, 19s**) precedes amyloid (secondary deposition) change. Amyloid is stained by (a) **PAS,** (b) **Lugol's iodine** (starch-like reaction, so it is called **amyloid**), (c) **Methyl violet** and (d) **Congo red**.

FATTY CHANGE—LIVER

Synonyms: Fatty infiltration, fatty degeneration.

The fatty change of the cells shows the appearance of fat droplets in the cytoplasm. It indicates an interference with the normal function of the cells or tissues as a result of which **fat becomes visible histologically as droplets** or globules **in the cell.** Organs usually affected are **liver, kidney** and **heart**. Later on the cells may be filled with fat, giving the **appearance of signet-rings.**

Gross appearance:

1. Liver is **paler** and more **yellowish** than normal; soft and friable—**floats on water (fat is lighter than water).**

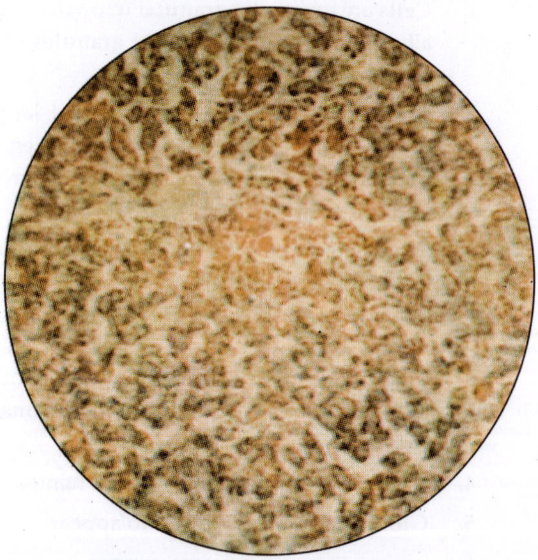

Fig. 3.2: Fatty change of Liver—All the liver cells contain globules of fat. In most, the fat globules are minute and situated at the cell margin, but in some the globules are of large size. The cells around the portal tract (near top left) are more affected than those in the central zone of the lobule. Scharlach R and Hematoxylin × 100

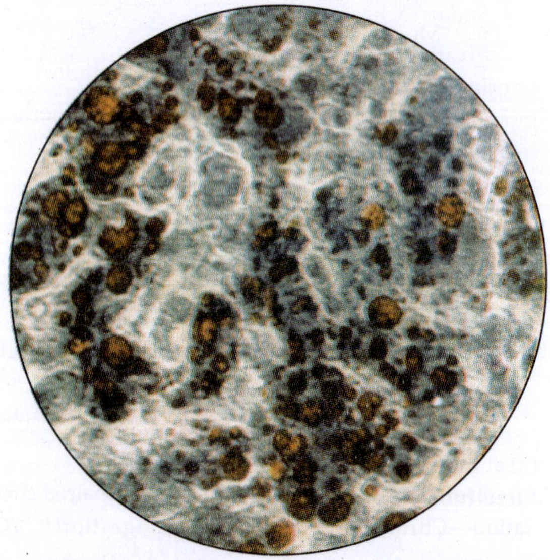

Fig. 3.3: Fatty change of Liver—Many of the cells contain a mixture of small and large globules of fat. Scharlach R and Hematoxylin × 400

2. The **edges are rounded** and the **cut surface** is **greasy** with yellowish specks due to bulging out of tissue.

Microscopic appearance **(Fig. 2.2 and 2.3):**

1. **Polygonal cells** of the liver lobules are **distended with fat**. Such accumulation may be either in the cells **near the central vein** (centrizonal), or in cells of the **peripheral zone**, and **midzone**.

Central zone is affected—in chloroform poisoning, **thyrotoxicosis**.

Midzone—in infective conditions, like **viral infections (hepatitis)**.

Peripheral zone—in eclampsia, phosphorus and **carbon tetrachloride poisoning**.

2. Fat droplets may push the nucleus to one corner, offering a '**signet-ring**' appearance of cells.

3. The nucleus is normal or pyknotic.

With **Sudan III** and **IV stain**, fat droplets are stained orange colour (Draw diagram). **Scharlach R** stains fat droplets **Scarlet red; Osmium Tetroxide**, a fixative and a stain offers **black colour**.

FATTY CHANGE—HEART

(Sudan IV stain and H & E; for procedure, see Ch. 1)

Gross: Tabby cat or Thrush breast appearance.

Microscopic appearance:

Transverse striations of muscle fibres are lost.

Sudan **IV** *Stain*

Fixative is boiling formalin (for) 5 minutes. Groups of muscle fibres containing numerous fat globules are stained **orange**. They vary in size, appear to be in rows along the length of muscle cells and also around the nuclei.

Osmic Acid Fixative and Stain

It is both a fixative and a stain.

With this fat globules are stained **black**.

FATTY CHANGE—KIDNEY

Microscopic appearance:

Observe—collection of lipid and fat globules (a) at the base of the **epithelial cells** lining the **convoluted tubules**, and (b) in the **nucleus**.

AMYLOIDOSIS—LIVER

Naked-eye or Gross appearance:

1. The **organ** is **enlarged** to a varying degree.

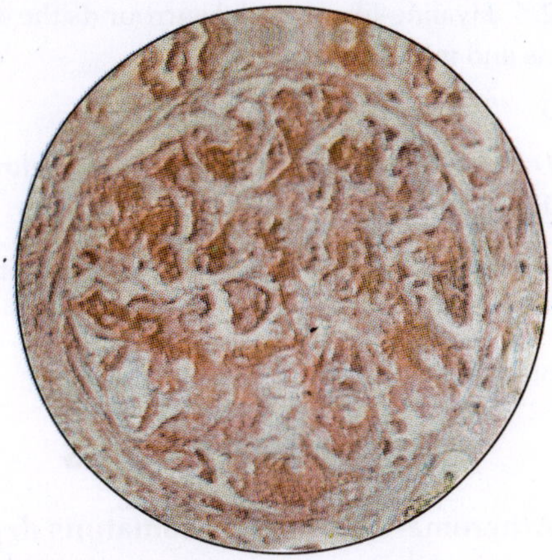

Fig. 3.4: **Amyloid Kidney**

2. **Firm** (rather elastic), resembling India rubber; **edges**—hard and smooth.

Microscopic appearance:

1. **Amyloid deposition** or change is **always extracellular**, and never within a cell.

2. Mid-zone in the liver lobule is homogeneous and pink (H & E).

3. **Capillaries of the intermediate zone** have undergone **amyloid changes**. They offer amyloid reaction. Smaller vessels in the portal areas may also be affected.

4. **Amyloid is deposited between Kupffer (macrophage) cells and liver cells.**

5. The involved tissue becomes enormously swollen, where **liver cells are compressed, atrophied** or they may disappear altogether.

6. In the peripheral and central zones, unaffected capillaries are seen along with the liver cells.

AMYLOIDOSIS—SPLEEN

Naked-eye or Gross appearance (Sago spleen):

Organ is enlarged; on section it shows translucent structures resembling half-boiled sago grains (sago spleen) due to accumulation of extracellular amyloid material. Hyaline (amyloid changed) areas stain purple (**metachromatic reaction) with methyl violet**.

Microscopic appearance:

In focal types:

1. **Malpighian bodies show** prominent **amyloid** (hyaline-like) **changes round the central arteries.**

2. Hyaline-like material surrounds the smaller vessels and infiltrates their walls.

3. The deposit is **extracellular.**

***Draw a diagram from a section of amyloid kidney* (Fig. 3.4).**

> **N.B.** Amyloid (pink, homogeneous material) deposit is seen in the glomeruli and peritubular regions. Amyloid deposit (change) is always extracellular.

ARTERIOSCLEROSIS

I. Atheroma—Aorta (Atheromatous deposit)

Atherosclerosis is primarily a degenerative lesion affecting especially the large vessels—like aorta, but coronary and cerebral arteries are also usually affected. **Atheroma may be localized or generalized.**

Naked-eye or gross appearance (Fig. 3.5):

1. Aorta has lost its elasticity and tunica interna (intima) is tortuous and dilated (elastosis or reduplication of internal elastic lamina by elastosis, i.e., elastic degeneration).

2. Intima shows a number of distinct elevated plaques with well defined edges, pale-yellowish in colour with **cholesterol or calcareous deposit (calcification).**

3. **Intima is thickened, necrotic and ulcerated at places.**

Microscopic appearance (Fig. 3.6):

1. **Atheromatous plaques** or *bullae* in the intima are seen which is thickened due to laminated fibrils. In the plaques, cells are vacuolated (foamy cells). Some calcification may be evident in the atheromatous areas. Calcium can be stained as **black areas** with **von Kossa's Calcium stain.**

2. The *internal elastic lamina* has undergone degeneration and shows large spaces containing granular materials and lipid substances.

3. The **media** is either normal or shows slight **atrophic change** towards its inner part, specially **where the thickening of the intima is highest.**

4. The adventitia does not show any significant change.

With *Sudan* IV *staining*: The intima contains a large amount of Sudan positive material. **Cholesterol** is present **in the atheromatous plaques.**

II. Monckeberg's Sclerosis (Medial Sclerosis)

1. Middle sized arteries, 2. Medial coat of arteries in 3. middle aged persons—3 Ms.

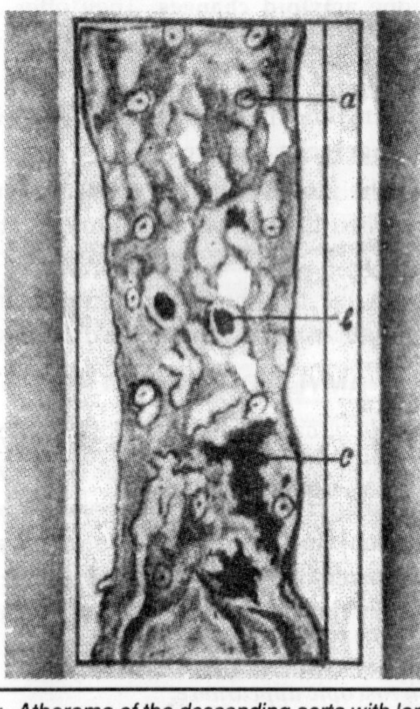

Fig. 3.5: *Atheroma of the descending aorta with longitudinal streaking,* and (a) atheromatous plaque at the branching of the artery; (b) ulcer; (c) ulcer with calcification, with deformity of the intima and a mural thrombus

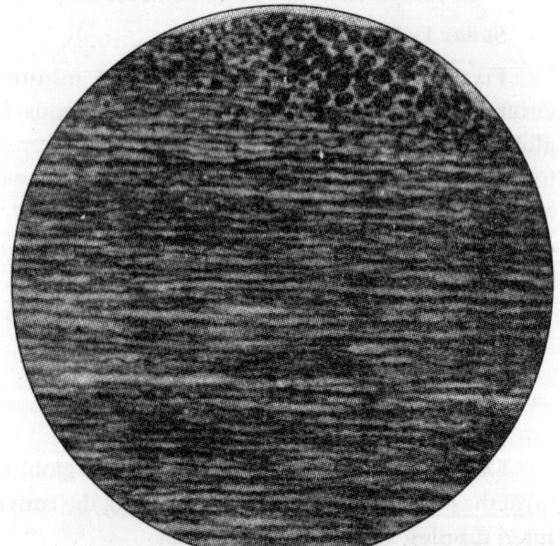

Fig. 3.6: Section of atheromatous plaque of the aorta. The endothelium is raised, thickened and contains lipoid matter with subendothelial proliferation of fibrous tissue (stained with Sudan III)

Found in medium sized arteries. Degenerative changes occur in the media i.e., where muscle coat is present. Deposit of calcium salts forms irregular rings. *Internal elastic lamina* is stretched over them. Arteries turn into rigid, non-elastic tubes.

III. Medial Calcification of Arteries

This usually corresponds to Monkeberg's medial sclerosis type of arteriosclerosis. It occurs near about or after the middle age. Some authors coated this to occur after 50 years of age. The cause is not known but ageing process is a related factor. The lesion is attributed by 3 Ms, e.g., it is seen in

1. **Middle aged** persons, affecting **medial coat** of **middle-sized arteries.**
2. The medium sized (or muscular) arteries, whose
3. Medial coat is affected

Clinically it has least significance.

Naked-eye or Gross appearance:

1. Arteries turn into **rigid, non-elastic tubes.**
2. **Calcium** is deposited in the media (either **intracellular** or **extracellular**) and hardening of the artery occurs.

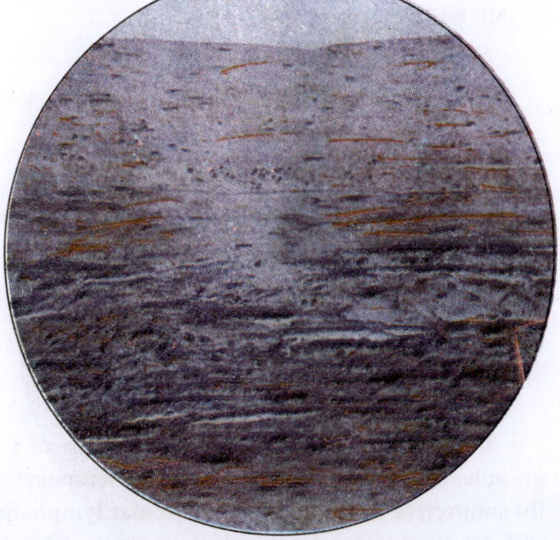

Fig. 3.7: Calcification of Media of Femoral Artery—The media is degenerated and extensively infiltrated with lime salts in granular form (Purple), while the intima shows definite fibrous thickening.
* Hematoxylin and Eosin. × 100

Calcium salts appear as fine, white granules (or clumps and aggregates).

The feel is hard and while cutting open the artery, there is a gritty sensation. This is an example of **dystrophic calcification.**

Microscopic appearance (Fig. 3.7):

Under **H & E stain**:

1. Calcium salt has a **bluish to blackish** amorphous or granular, and aggregated or **clumped appearance**.

von Kossa special stain offers a **black** appearance to calcium salts.

2. Deposits of calcium salts form irregular rings.
3. Internal elastic lamina is stretched over the rings.
4. The lesion does not extend upto the lumen in the intima.

NECROSIS

Necrosis means **molecular or microscopic death** of local cells or tissues from any cause. It may be a primary phenomenon or a sequela of degenerative process. **Necrosis is the molecular or microscopic death of cells.**

Varieties

Coagulative, liquefactive (colliquative), caseous, gummatous (in syphilis), fat, fibrinoid (oid = like; fibrin-like) and gangrenous and focal. Structural changes occur both in the cell-body and in the nucleus. **Grossly**, the appearance varies in different types of necrosis (See Authors' Textbook).

Microscopic appearance:

Cytoplasmic changes

1. **Swelling of cells** associated with *homogeneous and acidophilic* cytoplasm.
2. The cellular outline is lost or indistinct.

Nuclear changes (3 changes)

1. The nuclear chromatin undergoes gradual dissolution and loses affinity for nuclear stains—**Karyolysis.**
2. The nuclear chromatin is **broken up** into a number of irregular fragments—**Karyorrhexis** (Karyo = nucleus; rrhexis = fragmentation).

3. Nucleus is condensed into a small, deeply stained chromatin mass—**Pyknosis** (inkspot-like nucleus).

FOCAL NECROSIS—LIVER

Causes: Typhoid fever, pneumonia, diphtheria, mushroom poisoning, etc.

Microscopic appearance:

1. **Loss of cellular structure** in the affected areas (acidophilic or eosinophilic).

2. Cells often show **nuclear changes**—karyolysis, pyknosis, karyorrhexis, depending on the degree of affection.

3. Granular and fatty change of many cells.

4. Regeneration or fibrosis (scarring) in certain areas.

PATHOLOGICAL PIGMENTATION

I. ENDOGENOUS PIGMENT

Melanin pigment: See later, "malignant melanoma—liver, see under **Epithelial Tumors**".

A. HEMOSIDERIN PIGMENT AND CVC

1. **Liver in Pernicious anemia** (**HEMOSIDERIN**) (stained by pot. ferrocyanide in HCl—**Prussian blue** or **Pearl's reaction**)

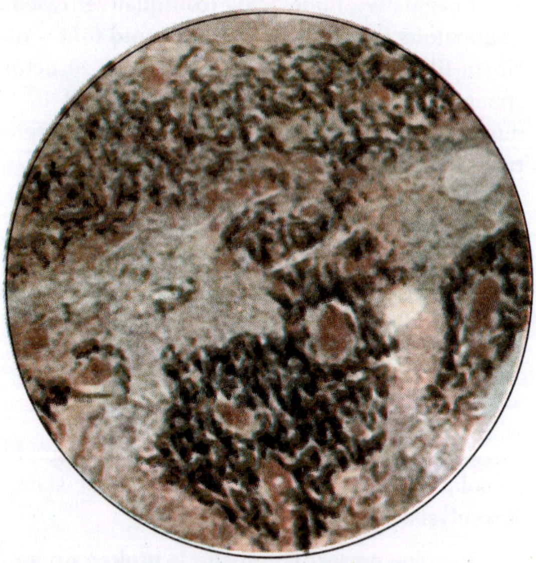

Fig. 3.8: Anthracosis—Large amount of carbon particles are present around the vessels and in the deep layer of the pleura. Hematoxylin and Eosin. × 80

(a) The cells of the **peripheral zone** of the liver lobule **show fine blue pigment** (containing **iron**).

(b) It (blue pigment) is present within the **liver cells** and phagocytic **Kupffer's cells** lying on the sinusoids.

B. HEMOCHROME PIGMENT

2. **Liver showing hemochrome pigment (hemochromatosis) causing bronzed diabetes**

C. HEMOZOIN PIGMENT

3. **Malarial liver (hemozoin pigment)**

The pigment is limited to the cells of the **reticuloendothelial system** and is not found in the liver cells. The cells **containing hemozoin** are: (a) **Kupffer's cells**, (b) Cells lining the dilated hepatic sinusoids (**endothelial cells**).

> **N.B.** In case of excessive hemolysis and in chronic venous congestion (CVC), hemosiderin pigment is present in the liver cells.

The pigment may also be present in the large **mononuclear cells, and in the endothelial cells** of the capillaries of **brain, spleen, heart,** etc.

II. EXOGENOUS PIGMENT

Inhalation of the materials causes PNEUMOKONIOSES.

A. ANTHRACOSIS—LUNG

The condition is due to inhalation of particles of coal dust working in a coal mine.

Naked-eye or Gross appearance:

1. **Lungs are voluminous** and **emphysematous**, and become intensely **black** (in patches).

2. Bronchial lymph nodes are black and show masses of carbon pigment.

3. *Cut surface* is finely gritty.

Microscopic appearance **(Fig. 3.8):**

1. **Deposition of carbon** in the form of fine granules in the **(a) alveolar cells (pneumocytes)**, **(b) connective tissue**, in the **perivascular lymphatics**, and **(c) histiocytes** (macrophages) in the alveolar spaces (**heart failure cells**).

2. Fibrosis encloses the irritant pigment **(Fig. 3.8)**.

> **N.B.** Anthracosis of the lung does not predispose to tuberculosis.

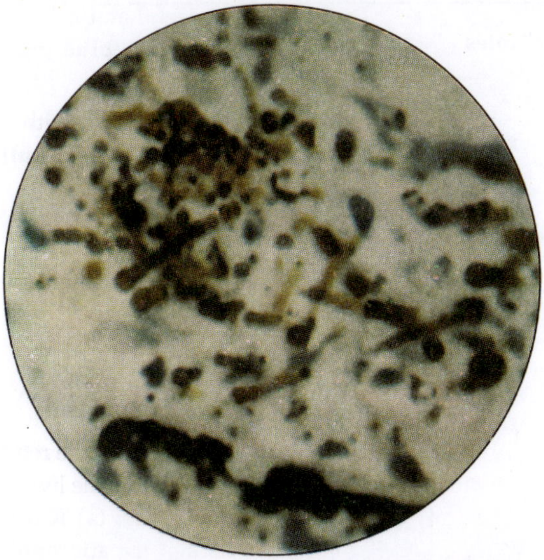

Fig. 3.9: Asbestosis—The field shows an accumulation of golden brown pigment in the form of granules and "**Asbestos bodies**" variable in length; these bodies consist of closely arranged discs and may be swollen at one or both ends. Hematoxylin and Eosin. × 800

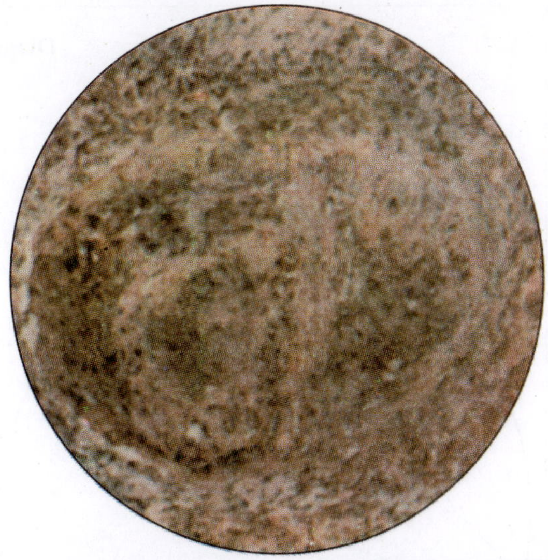

Fig. 3.10: Silicotic nodule—The dense fibrous laminae on which the nodule is composed are concentrically arranged and infiltrated with brown siliceous pigment. Hematoxylin and Eosin. × 80

B. ASBESTOSIS—LUNG

Asbestosis occurs by inhalation of asbestos particles that produce PNEUMOKONIOSIS.

Microscopic appearance (Fig. 3.9):

1. Diffuse interstitial fibrosis with multiple asbestos bodies (Fig. 3.9).

2. Formation of beaded rods with a translucent center that consists of asbestos fibers coated with an iron-containing proteinaceous **golden brown** pigment called **ferruginous bodies** that contain (iron + protein + asbestos).

Complication:

Malignancy, e.g., mesothelioma.

C. SILICOTIC NODULES (SILICOSIS)—LUNGS

They are not related to any pigment but are one of the important pneumokoniotic elements.

This is due to **inhalation of silicon dioxide** and is a world-wide occupational disease.

Naked-eye or Gross appearance:

Greyish pale nodules are present as hard, collagenous scars in the upper zones of the lungs. **Radiographic eggshell calcification** is present.

Microscopic appearance **(Figs. 3.10 and 3.11):**

Presence of silicotic nodule (**Fig. 3.10**) is made of concentric layers of hyalinized collagen surrounded by a dense capsule of more condensed collagen (**Fig. 3.11**).

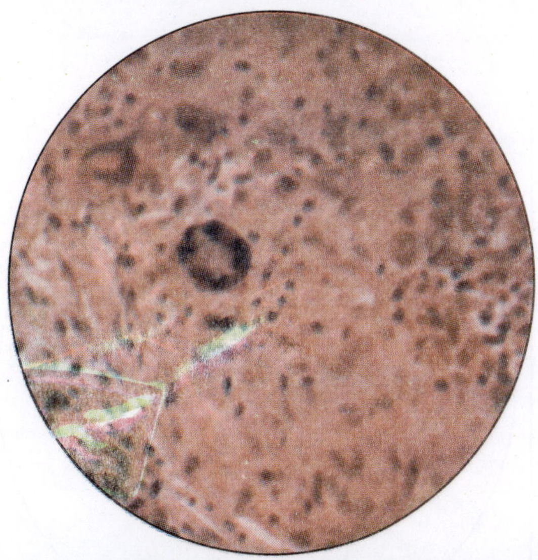

Fig. 3.11: Traumatic silicosis—The dark particles of copying-ink pencil scattered throughout the field are surrounded by specialised granulation tissue consisting of endothelioid cells, lymphocytes, plasma cells and giant cells. The picture closely resembles tuberculous granulation tissue. Hematoxylin and Eosin. × 275

Diagrams/Notes

Diagrams/Notes

Diagrams/Notes

Diagrams/Notes

Diagrams/Notes

CHAPTER 4

CHANGES DUE TO DISTURBANCES OF CIRCULATION

CHRONIC (Passive) VENOUS CONGESTION (Nutmeg Liver)

CVC—LIVER (Fig. 4.1)

It occurs in Right Ventricular, [i.e., Congestive Cardiac Failure (CCF)].

Naked-eye or Gross appearance:

1. **Liver** is often **enlarged, firm** or may become smaller; in later stage, shrunken owing to atrophy of the parenchymal cells (hepatocytes).

2. **Cut surface** shows undue distinctness of lobules and a **mottled** appearance with alternate dark and light areas; the **dark areas represent** the **dilated, engorged central vein**, and the **light (yellowish) areas** are the **fatty change in liver cells in the peripheral zone (parts)**.

Microscopic appearance:

1. **Dilation of central vein** of the lobule and engorgement of the sinusoids.

2. **Atrophy** of the cells of the **central zone** near the central vein showing necrosis from hypoxic effect.

3. **Fatty changes** may be present in the **peripheral parts** of the lobules.

4. **Glisson's capsule** is sometimes **thickened**.

BROWN INDURATION OF THE LUNG

Naked-eye or Gross appearance:

Lungs are voluminous, russet (rusty) brown in colour, tough and indurated (thickened and hard).

Microscopic appearance:

1. **Pulmonary capillaries** in internal veolar septum are congested, dilated and tortuous to form projections into the pulmonary alveoli. Alveoli are filled with red cells.

2. **Alveolar walls** are thickened and characteristically beaded.

3. **Large mononuclear cells** (macrophages) are abundant with weakly stained cytoplasm and a central reticulated nucleus.

4. **"Heart-failure cells"** (wandering histiocytes) derived from walls of the alveoli (interalveolar septa) are laden with brown iron pigment. The pigment is **haemosiderin** giving positive prussian blue reaction.

5. Marked increase in fibrous (interstitial) tissue of the lungs occur.

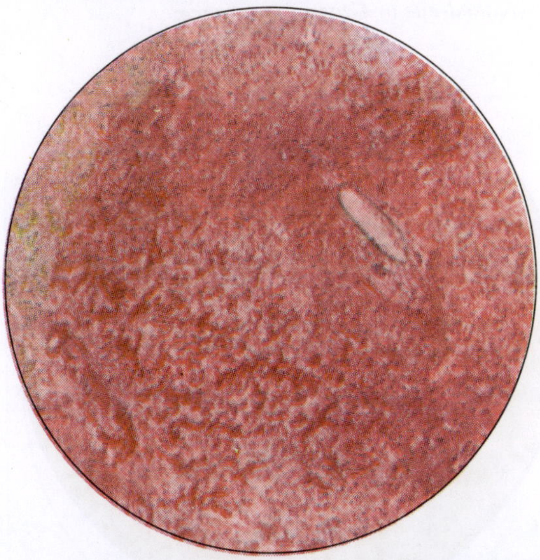

Fig. 4.1: Chronic venous congestion of Liver (Nutmeg Liver)—The Liver cells still survive in the peripheral zone of the lobules, but the intermediate and central zones have been replaced by engorged sinusoids. A dilated intralobular vein in longitudinal section is present (towards bottom left). Hematoxylin and Eosin. × 75

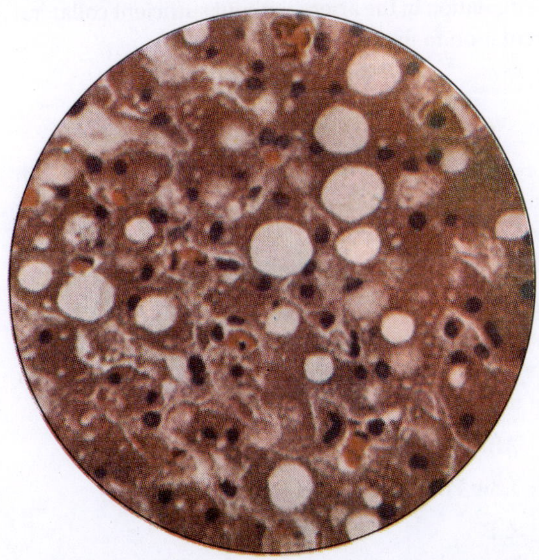

Fig. 4.2: Chronic venous congestion of Liver—Peripheral zone of lobule shows the presence of fat spaces of various sizes in liver cells. The fat has been washed out by fat solvents during the tissue processing. Hematoxylin and Eosin. × 350

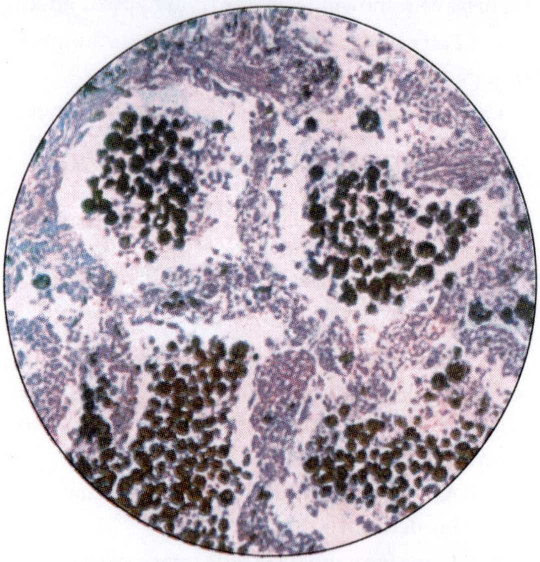

Fig. 4.3: Chronic Venous Congestion (CVC) of Lung—while their walls are congested and swollen, the alveoli contain large number of histiocytes ladened with brown iron pigment. Hematoxylin and Eosin/and prussian blue reaction(+) × 100

INFARCTION

An infarct is an ischemic area of (**coagulation or liquefactive**) **necrosis** resulting from a sudden arrest of circulation in the artery without sufficient collateral circulation to that particular part.

INFARCT—SPLEEN

Naked-eye or Gross appearance:

1. An irregular slightly depressed, pale area on the surface; **capsule—adherent** and surrounded by a **pink zone of hyperemia**.

2. **Cut surface** shows a dry opaque (fan- or) wedge-shaped or **irregular area, pale** in color with **base directed to the surface of the organ**. The area is demarcated by a **hemorrhagic zone**. (Scar formation is a useful finding in postmortem examination).

Microscopic appearance:

Low Power (**L.P.**) and High Power (**H.P.**).

L.P.

Affected area shows 3 zones:

1. **Coagulation necrosis (acidophilic)** where general architecture is preserved but nuclei are obscure. Interstitial tissue may be unaffected being more resistant and less specialized.

2. **Zone of hyperemia** proximal to the area of infarction. This zone shows frank hemorrhage.

3. **Normal tissue.**

H.P.

1. **Cells** may be **swollen** eosinophilic where nuclei are obscure.

2. Minute granules are uniformly distributed.

3. Arteries, veins and capillaries contain homogeneous, eosinophilic substance.

4. **Marked congestion of capillaries** proximal to the infarct area, which shows an attempt for collateral circulation. Proximal tissue to infarct area shows hemorrhage for blockage ahead.

5. Beyond the congested area, inflammatory cells (neutrophils) and macrophages are present. Neutrophils appear after 6–12 hours; macrophages appear later after 24 hours.

6. Signs of repair occurs from the hyperemic zone and are characterized by:

Proliferation of fibroblasts and formation of **new capillaries** (neoangiogenesis).

INFARCT—KIDNEY

Naked-eye or Gross appearance:

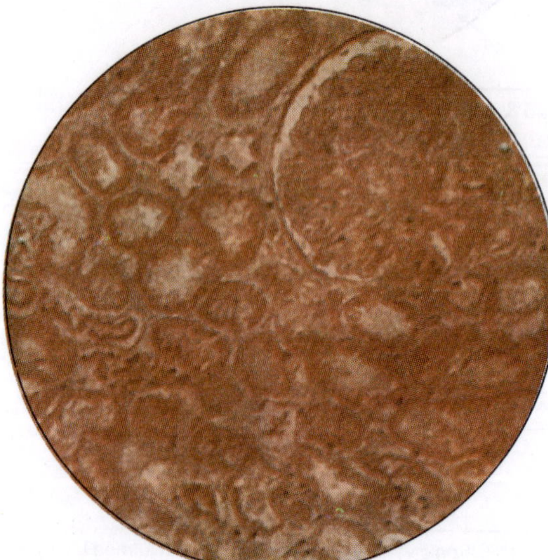

Fig. 4.4: Infarct of Kidney—All the elements in the field—Glomeruli, tubules and interstitial tissues being devoid of nuclear staining (obscure nuclei) and unusually acidophilic cytoplasm indicating necrosis. Hematoxylin and Eosin. × 200

Cut-surface shows a **wedge-shaped** area, involving the whole width of the cortex and the corresponding part of the medulla.

Microscopic appearance **(Fig. 4.4):**

L.P.

1. **Glomeruli:** Exhibit normal architecture with loss of nuclei (**karyolysis**). Cytoplasm is abnormally eosinophilic. **Fibrin** may be present in **glomerular spaces** (**ghost tissue appearance**).

2. **Tubules:** Convoluted and collecting tubules are similarly affected; some undergo **necrosis near the edge** of the infarct.

3. **Blood-vessels:** Homogeneous, eosinophilic.

H.P.

1. Many of the nuclei in cells at the periphery of the infarct area show **pyknosis** and **karyorrhexis** (necrotic change).

2. **Signs of hyperemia and repair** are present at the periphery (as in the spleen).

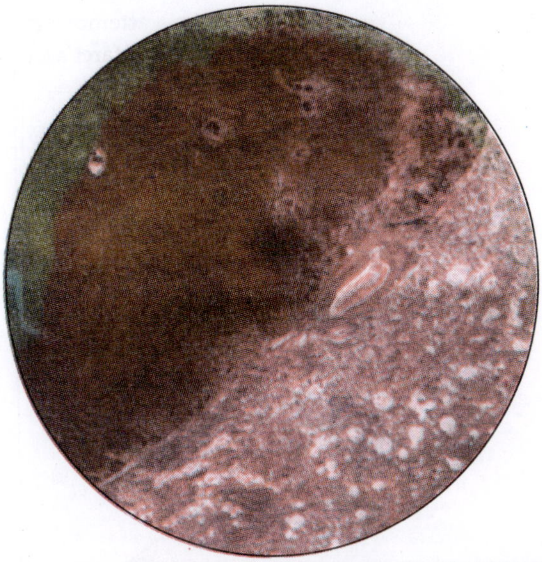

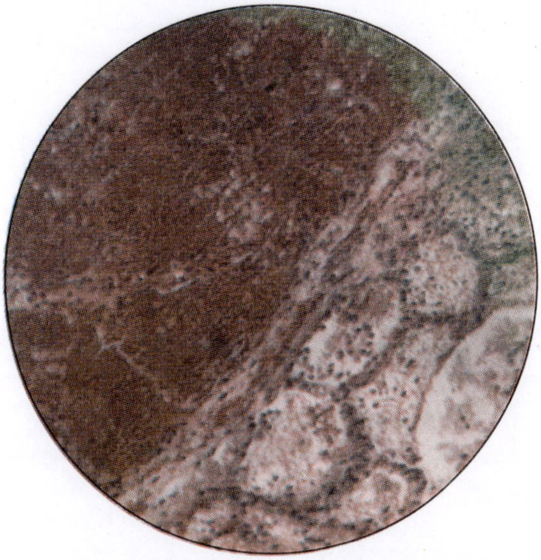

Fig. 4.5 & 4.6: Hemorrhagic and red infarct of Lung—Field is taken from edge of infarct in Fig. 4.5. In Figure 4.6 the Alveolar walls in the damaged region are necrotic and lysed, while the air spaces are filled with fresh blood. The lesion is sharply demarcated from the neighbouring edematous lung. Hematoxylin and Eosin. × 100

Diagrams/Notes

Diagrams/Notes

Diagrams/Notes

Diagrams/Notes

CHAPTER 5

GRANULOMATOUS AND INFECTIVE DISEASES

(SPECIFIC INFECTIVE GRANULOMAS)

Infective granulomas are characterized by chronic inflammatory conditions produced as a result of a subacute and chronic infections caused by some specific agent. In such cases, lesions are healed by formation of granulation tissue (vascular and cellular) associated with various protective and reparative process. Common granulomas are—**tuberculosis, syphilis, leprosy (bacterial); actinomycosis, histoplasmosis (mycotic), dermal leishmanoid and ameboma (protozoal), lymphogranuloma inguinale (chlamydial),** etc.

A. TUBERCULOSIS

TUBERCULOSIS OF THE SKIN

Tuberculosis verrucosus cutis and **lupus vulgaris**:

1. **Acanthosis** of the skin (thckening of the rete malpighii layer).

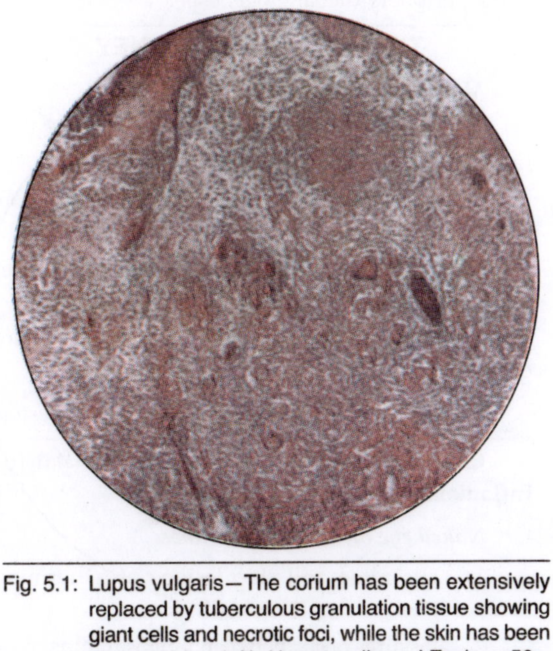

Fig. 5.1: Lupus vulgaris—The corium has been extensively replaced by tuberculous granulation tissue showing giant cells and necrotic foci, while the skin has been ulcerated (top left). Hematoxylin and Eosin. × 50

2. **Papillomatosis** (downward growth of the rete pegs; downward epidermal papillomatosis).

3. **Dermis** shows:

   (a) Central (caseous) **necrotic mass;**

   (b) Zone of **epithelioid cells** and **giant cells** of **Langhans** type (nuclei arranged at the **periphery, or in one or both poles, or semicircular in a horseshoe manner**);

   (c) Peripherally **Lymphocytic** and occasional plasma cellular infiltration forming defensive barrier of 25 to 30 layers or more.

   (d) **Fibroblastic** and **capillary endothelial proliferation** (neoangiogenesis-sprouting capillaries).

   (e) Laying down of collagen (collagenization).

Draw a diagram of a microscopic tubercle.

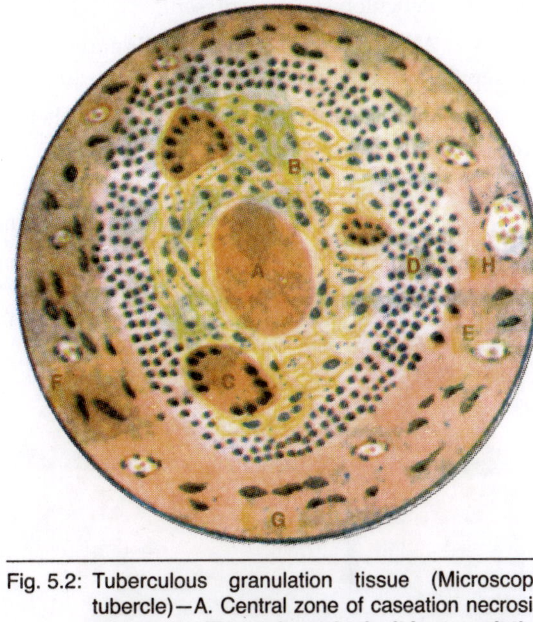

Fig. 5.2: Tuberculous granulation tissue (Microscopic tubercle)—A. Central zone of caseation necrosis; in case of **miliary tuberculosis, it is coagulation necrosis**). It is characterized by homogeneous eosinophilic (acidophilic) area near about the centre of the granulation tissue; B. Epithelioid reticulum (network) formation in the area surrounding the zone of necrosis. This is characterized by the presence of pale stained (indefinite) lipid laden epithelioid cells (macrophages) with pale stained vesicular hematoxylin stained nucleus within them; C. Presence of Langhans' type of giant cells (foreign body giant cells with polar or peripheral distribution of the nuclei); D. Barrier (zone) of lymphocytes and may be occasional plasma cells; E. Young capillaries and blood vessels (neoangiogenesis); F. Zone of fibrosis and young fibroblastic proliferation (collagenization); G. Fibrocytes (mature fibroblast) and collagen tissue; H. Young capillaries.

TUBERCULOSIS OF LYMPH NODE

Lymph nodes are **matted** together due to **tuberculous peri-adenitis**:

1. A **central** area of **caseation** with destruction of much of the structure of the node is present staining homogeneous eosinophilic.

2. Surrounding this area, there are multinucleated **giant-cells of Langhans'** type.

3. A zone of **epithelioid cells** or **epithelioid reticulum** present. They are relatively pale looking cells with somewhat vesicular nuclei. [**Epithelioid cells are characteristic cells of Tb. granuloma**; they are **RE cells or modified macrophages** produced after their engulfment of mycolic (fatty) acid in the cell wall of AFB--Reticulohistiocytes present].

4. At places **Langhans giant cells** are studed in the epithelioid reticulum.

5. **Zone of lymphocytes** around the epithelioid cells are seen with occasional plasma cells (30–40 layers).

6. **Proliferation of fibroblasts** and laying down of secreted collagen.

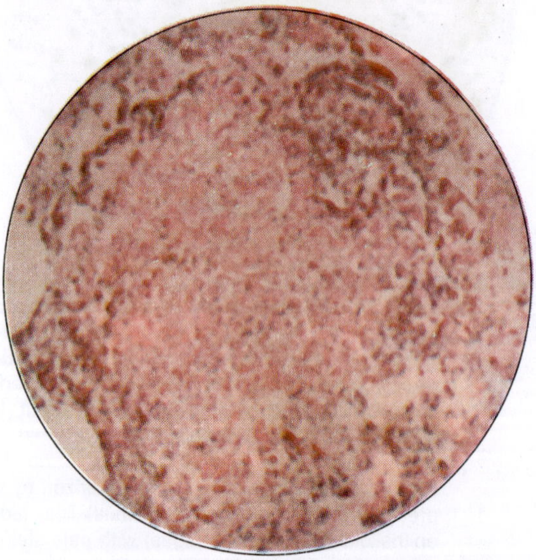

Fig. 5.3: Acute miliary tuberculosis of Lung—The field contains a young folicle (microscopic tubercle) of which many similar tubercles were present throughout the tissue. The follicle consists of numerous feebly stained endothelioid cells surrounded by a zone of lymphocytes, but shows **no caseation**, Giant cell or fibrosis. The necrosis type in **miliary Tb. is coagulative** and not caseous. Hematoxylin and Eosin. × 75

7. **Capillary endothelial cells** budding at the periphery are present (**neoangiogenesis**).

8. Presence of **fibroblasts** (secreting collagen is present).

9. **Fibrocytes** (hyper-mature fibroblast) are present.

10. **Collagen bundles** present.

ACUTE MILIARY TUBERCULOSIS—LUNG

Naked-eye or Gross appearance:

Scattered pearl-like areas of coagulation necrosis are distributed on the surface; cut surface of the lung offers a miliary (submiliary size like a pinhead millet seed) appearance.

Microscopic appearance:

A tubercle consists of

1. Non-vascular mass of **coagulative necrosis** in the centre (no caseation), surounded by

2. Epithelioid cells with round or oval vesicular nuclei and pale cytoplasm.

3. Occasional multinucleated Langhans giant-cells.

4. Lymphocytic infiltration beyond the zone of epithelioid cells and occasional plasma cells.

5. Fibrobastic and capillary proliferation occurs at the periphery (neoangiogenesis).

TUBERCULOSIS—KIDNEY

Microscopic appearance:

1. A central area of caseation destroying the kidney **parenchyma (functional part)**.

2. Epithelioid cells and giant-cell formations occur.

3. Lymphocytic and occasional plasma cell infiltration.

4. In the periphery, areas of fibrosis and young capillary proliferation occur.

Draw diagram of tuberculous ulcer of small intestine.

CROHN'S DISEASE, Synonym: Regional ileitis, Inflammatory Bowel Disease

Naked eye or Gross appearance:

1. Ulcerated and skip lesions of (i) terminal ileum, (ii) ileocecal valve and (iii) cecum.

2. Fissures occur between mucosal folds.

3. Fistulous track is a common finding.

4. Intestinal wall is thickened, rubbery in consistency due to transmural edema.

5. Submucosal fibrosis, and

6. Hypertrophy of muscularis proprio.

Microscopic appearance:

The process is diffuse and hyperplastic.

1. Lymphoid tissue is involved in the process.
2. Caseation is absent.
3. Giant-cells of Langhans type are present in the granulation tissue.
4. Metaplasia of (i) Epithelium, and (ii) Paneth cells.
5. Mucosal ulceration occurs.
6. Crypt abscess form.
7. Destruction of crypts occur.

EPITHELIOID CELLS ARE CHARACTERISTICS OF TUBERCULOSIS (TUBERCULOUS GRANULATION TISSUE), AND MICROSCOPIC TUBERCLE.

B. SYPHILIS

PLASMA CELLS ARE CHARACTERISTIC INFLAMMATORY CELLS OF SYPHILIS.

GUMMA—LIVER

It occurs in **acquired syphilis.**

Naked-eye or Gross appearance:

Necrotic material in the cut section of the liver; *hepar lobatum*. Gummatous lesions cause parenchymal necrosis into irregular masses dividing the liver artificially into many lobes; the lobes (lobatum) of liver (hepar).

Microscopic appearance:

1. **Central mass** of gummatous necrotic material forming major portion of the gumma (**coagulation necrosis with gummy substance**).

2. **Peripheral zone** of granulation tissue containing *Plasma cells* lymphocytes and macrophages.

3. Beyond this area, layers of dense fibrous tissue is present.

4. Giant cells may be present.

5. Thickened arteries (**endarteritis obliterans**) are seen.

Pericellular cirrhosis occurs in congenital syphilis (Fig. 5.4).

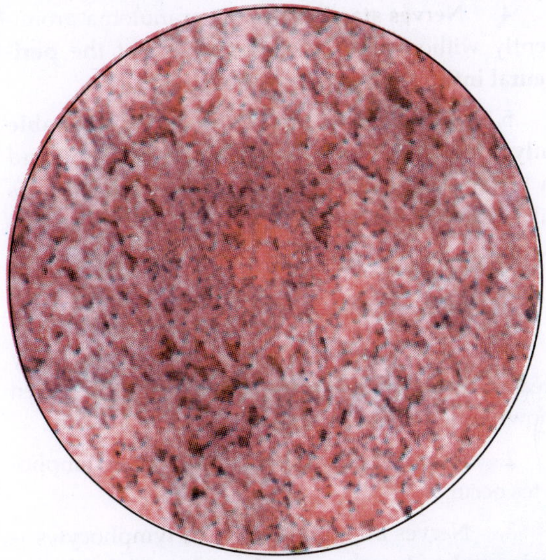

Fig. 5.4: Congenital syphilitic pericellular cirrhosis of Liver—The field shows a central focus of necrosis and mononuclear cell inflitration—A miliary gumma. The tissue elsewhere consists of isolated or small groups of liver cells separated by loose fibre distribution of connective tissue around each cell—"Pericellular cirrhosis," due to the presence of **reticulin fibre shown by silver impregnation method.** Hematoxylin and Eosin. × 80

GUMMA—TESTIS
(In Syphilis)

Microscopic appearance:

1. There are areas of **central necrosis** and a **peripheral zone of granulation tissue** with scattered *Plasma cells.*

2. Beyond it, there is connective tissue proliferation, fibrosis as well **as perivascular cuffing** with infiltration of lymphocytes and *Plasma cells.*

3. Giant cells are usually absent.

C. LEPROSY

LEPROMATOUS (POLAR) TYPE

Microscopic appearance:

1. Epidermis is thinned and flattened out.

2. Clear papillary **Green zone** without inflammatory cells seen between epidermis and dermis.

3. Characteristic cells are HISTIOCYTES (**macrophages**), in which the protoplasm frequently undergoes **fatty change with vacuoles formation** (foamy or **Lepra cells** of **Virchow in lepromatous type**).

4. **Nerves stand** out in the granuloma prominently without any involvement except the **perineural infiltration** with lymphocytes.

5. Ziehl-Neelsen stain shows **innumerable only acid-fast bacilli in smears** (not alcohol fast) and in histopathological sections bacilli are in bundles (like a pack of cigars).

TUBERCULOID (POLAR) TYPE OF LEPROSY

Microscopic appearance:

1. **Small foci** of epithelioid cells surrounded by areas of **lymphocytic infiltration** present, which often shows **Langhans' type of giant cells** in the centre.

2. Focal and compact infiltration with lymphocytes occur.

3. Nerves are infiltrated with lymphocytes—**perineural and ENDONEURAL Lymphocytic infiltrate.**

4. **Bacilli** are few, and difficult to detect in smears or histopathological sections.

D. MYCOTIC GRANULOMA

It is caused by fungi. A group of fungi especially form **multiple discharging sinuses**, through which granules of **sulphur yellow, black,** and **red colour** come out. The causative organisms under **Actinomycetoma** (Mycelia < 1 μm): **Actinomyces israeli** (ANAEROBIC), or **Nocardia (aerobic)**, e.g., *A. israeli, A bovis, N. asteroides;* under EUMYCETOMA (Mycelia > 1 μm): They are: Madurella mycetomatis, M. griseus, Pseudoallescheria boydii, Acremonium falciforme, Cephalosporium falciforme, etc. most of which are **Acid Fast**.

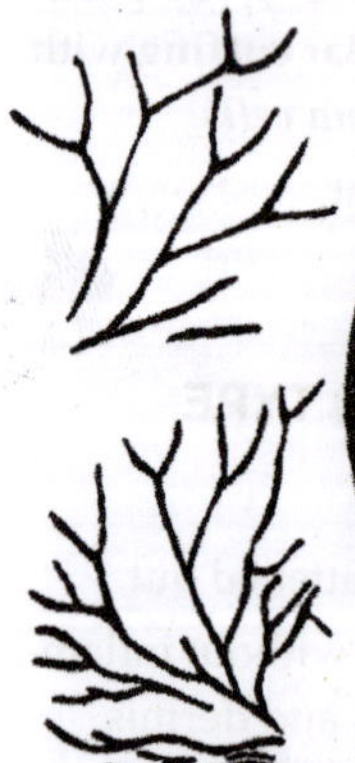

Fig. 5.5

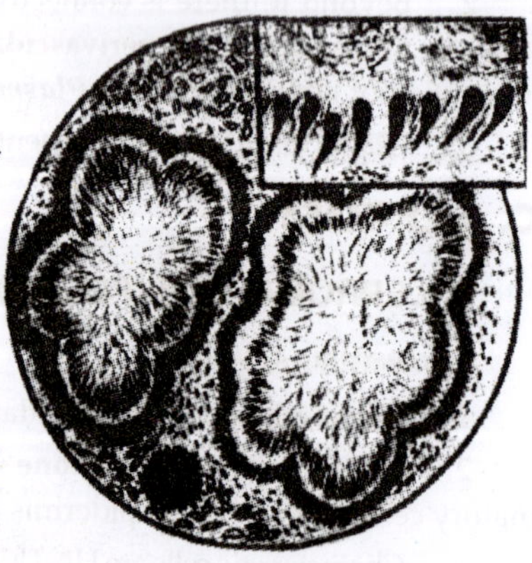

Fig. 5.6

Fig. 5.5: Branching of mycelia of *A. israeli*

Fig. 5.6: Ray fungus (inset—showing clubs)

ACTINOMYCOSIS

(Non-Acid Fast)

Microscopic appearance:

1. The granuloma contains the **ray fungus** which consists of — (a) **Central mycelial threads;** (b) **Characteristic radiating clubs at the periphery**.

2. Zone of suppuration containing Actinomyces colony, **neutrophils**, surrounded by a layer of granulation tissue rich in **large fat-laden phagocytic (macrophage) cells** and occasional giant cells (**microabscess**).

3. A framework of dense fibrous tissue encircles the whole granuloma.

E. PROTOZOAL GRANULOMA

SKIN—DERMAL LEISHMANOID

(Post K-A Dermal Leishmaniasis)

This is caused by **L. donovani** (amastigote). Oriental sore is caused by **L. tropica**.

Naked eye or gross appearance of Dermal leishmanoid is NODULAR.

Microscopic appearance:

1. **Epidermis** is thin, and papillae of the skin are **flattened**.

2. The sub-papillary layer is edematous; vessels are dilated and proliferating.

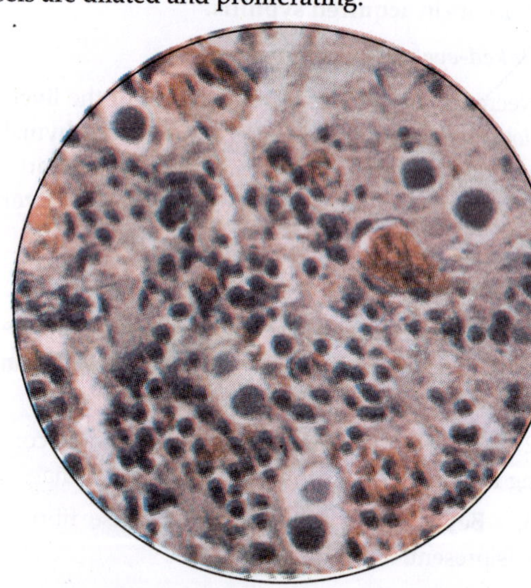

Fig. 5.7: Floor of Amoebic ulcer of colon—Several entamoebae histolytica (large, round, purple structures) are present in the field. The tissue in the neighbourhood is congested and infiltrated with lymphocytes, while an area of necrosis is seen (top right). Hematoxylin and Eosin. × 400

3. There is a dense infiltration of epithelioid cells in the dermis. These contain **L-D bodies** when seen under high power immersion.

Draw a diagram of amoebic granuloma (colon).

LARGE INTESTINE—AMOEBIC GRANULOMA

Naked-eye or Gross appearance:

It shows undermined (flask-shaped ulcer of colonic mucosa.

Microscopic appearance:

1. Scattered ulcers with **sloughs**.
2. **Trophozoite and cystic forms** of *E. histolytica* in the ulcer.
3. The **floor** is infiltrated with **mononuclear cells** (histiocytes, lymphocytes and few plasma cells).
4. **Thickened blood vessels** are seen.

Diagrams/Notes

Diagrams/Notes

Diagrams/Notes

Diagrams/Notes

CHAPTER 6

MISCELLANEOUS LESIONS

HEPATOBILLIARY SYSTEM

FATTY LIVER

History:

History of regular and heavy drinking, high intake of fat in food, e.g., all types of fried food, chips, red meat daily or in short intervals. History of Lipoid nephrosis or minimal change disease; on examination it conforms with the history.

Pathologic Features

Naked-eye **or** *gross appearance*:

Liver is **enlarged** with rounded margins. On cutting through, the **cut margins bulge out**. It is **yellowish** and **greasy** to touch.

Microscopic view:

1. **There are different sizes of fat vacuoles in liver cell cytoplasm called**

(a) **Microvesicles** around the nucleus, and

(b) **Large macro-vesicles** which push the nucleus to the periphery offering the **cells signet ring appearance**.

2. The **vacuoles** in the cells on coalescing **form** very **larger vacuoles** which assume like a cyst called **fat cysts**.

3. Formation of **lipogranulomas** occur when granulomatous cellular elements, the lymphocytes and macrophages infiltrate the neighbouring area of the fat cyst, with formation and **appearance of multinucleate giant cells**.

4. Demonstration of fat is done in frozen sections which when are stained by the following stains:

(a) Sudan IV—*Orange colour*

(b) Scharlach R—*Scarlet red*

(c) Oil Red 'O'—*Red*

(d) Sudan Black 'B'—*Black*

(e) Osmic acid [fixative and stain (both)]—*Black*.

CIRRHOSIS-LIVER

A. PORTAL CIRRHOSIS

(*Gr. Kirros = tawny*, a portwine colour like that of dilute cocacola)

Synonyms

(Hobnail liver; Laennec's or **multilobular** or **nutritional** or **alcoholic** or **micronodular cirrhosis**).

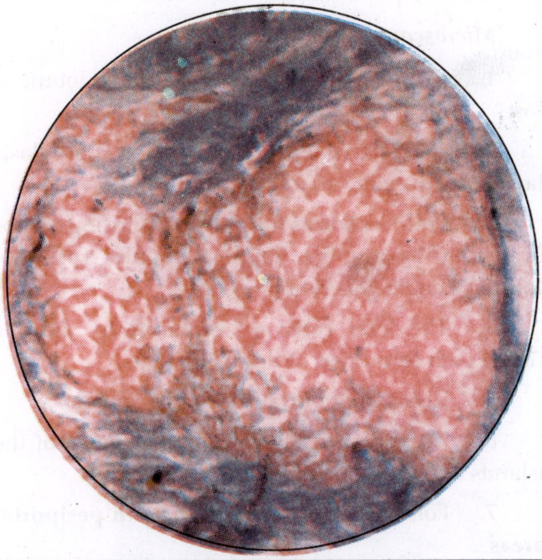

Fig. 6.1: Common (portal) Cirrhosis of Liver—An islet of Liver (pink) is surrounded by dense fibrous tissue (bluish). The islet has no central vein and the trabeculae are irregularly arranged—Features characteristic of regenerated tissue. Heidenhain's Azan method. × 65

History:

A 40 years old male known to be heavy drunkard presented himself with malnutrition and impaired digestive function related to chronic gastric acidosis, and mucosal damage, and pancreatitis. There is history of blood vomiting.

Fundamentally, cirrhosis is a degenerative disease causing massive, irregular, progressive, diffuse fibrosis with structural alterations of lobules. Relation of central vein to portal tracts are deranged and also vascular perfusion is markedly deranged.

Naked-eye or Gross appearance:

The liver is atrophic in later stage. It gives a **hobnail appearance**, particularly on its inferior surface (which are regenerated nodules). Weight—usually 1,200 to 1,300 g. The colour is brownish (tawny). *Cut* *surface.* The cut surface is correspondingly nodular. The nodules are variable in size, usually 2-4 mm to < 1 cm in diameter. **The nodules are due to regenerative hyperplasia** of the liver cells, and the **depressions** are due to **fibrosis.**

It should be differentiated from **Post-necrotic cirrhosis** in which **nodules** are much **larger** (1-2 cm) than those of portal cirrhosis (2-4 mm).

Microscopic view:

1. Normal architecture of the liver lobule is lost.

2. **Connective tissue** proliferation (fibroblasts laying down collagen) in the **portal spaces.**

3. **Proliferation of fibroblasts** encircling groups of liver cells forming fictitious lobules (**pseudo-lobules**), and regenerating nodules.

4. The liver **cells are replaced by fibrous tissue** with **formation of new bile ducts.**

5. **Relation of portal triads** may be **lost.**

6. **Central veins are not in the centre** of the islands of proliferating liver cells.

7. Formation of new **bile ducts in periportal areas.**

8. Portal vein does not drain into new nodules.

9. **Mallory's hyaline bodies** are seen in some liver cells and it is characteristic of alcoholic cirrhosis (**Mallory bodies**).

B. POST NECROTIC CIRRHOSIS

History:

A 35 years old lady had history of deep jaundice 2 years back. Before that she had received blood transfusion.

The liver is atrophic and small with coarse nodules. The weight is 1 kg or less (normal 1.7 kg). Nodules are 1 to 2 cms in diameter. Size of nodules is variable. Color of nodules his paler than normal because **regenerated liver lacks in lipochrome pigment.**

Microscopically

1. Lobular architecture is lost.

2. **Fibrous bands** are mostly thick and **wide** and not uniform.

3. They (fibrous septa) are densely **infiltrated with lymphocytes and plasma cells.**

4. The lobules contain many proliferating bile ducts, histiocytes (macrophages), lymphocytes and plasma cells (**mononuclear cellular infiltration**).

5. **Regenerating nodules** are variable in size.

6. Their junction with fibrous bands are sharp.

7. Veins are compressed at the edge of the nodules.

8. Within the nodules, persisting liver lobules may be seen to have normal relation with portal tracts and central veins (cf. portal cirrhosis No. 5). **Relation of portal triad is intact.**

9. **Liver cells** within the regenerated nodules vary in size and show large, bizarre nuclei.

INFECTIVE HEPATITIS

History:

A jaundiced patient complaining of severe anorexia and vomitting. Bilirubin estimation showed 8 mg/dl.

Usually the HBV, HCV as well as HDV infections show significant features and produce characteristic changes clinically for various (named), hepatitis.

Piecemeal necrosis:

1. The **viruses** cause piecemeal necrosis. To start with, a few cells in peripheral areas show necrosis with infiltration of the area.

2. **Lesion in the portal tract itself.** Clinically the lesion progresses to chronic (active and persistent) hepatitis stage.

Then the portal tract lesions are seen. In the portal areas there is *hepatic artery, portal vein* and *bile duct* which also are inflamed, it is called **Triad-itis** (inflammation of the portal triad with infiltration by mononuclear cells).

Histopathological changes in Portal tract lesions:

(a) **Triad-itis** (hepatic artery portal rein and bile duct).

(b) **Bile capillaries** in the **portal tracts** are expanded and portal tracts are infiltrated by mononuclear cells. These are the changes caused in **HBV, HCV, HDV infections.**

(c) HCV infection causes lymphocytic aggregate and lymphoid follicle formation with **germinal centre**, and moderate **fatty change**.

3. **Intralobular lesions:**

(a) In moderate infections, **focal** areas of **inflammation** and **necrosis** occur.

(b) Scattered acidophilic bodies present in the lobules.

(c) Kupffer's cell hyperplasia and hypertrophy.

(d) In long standing advanced HBV bridging hepatitis cases, there is widespread **bridging necrosis** meaning bands of necrosed liver cells that bridge the

i) **Portal tract to portal tract**

ii) **Central vein to central vein** and

iii) **Portal tract to central vein.**

(e) Regeneration of liver cells at the site of persistent liver cell necrosis.

(f) In case of chronic HBV (hepatitis B) infection, scattered ground glass appearances of liver cells are seen all over, which indicate the presence of abundant hepatitis B surface antigen **(HBsAg) in the cytoplasm of liver cells.**

(g) Moderate fatty change occurs within liver cells in case of **HCV** infection only.

4. The terminal event is the **Bridging Fibrosis** that occurs in an existing chronic (active and progressive) hepatitis in the case where, there occurs the irreversible type of damage. **Bridging fibrosis** consists of:

(a) **Periportal fibrosis** offering the portal tract a characteristic **stellate-like look** studded with mononuclear cells (lymphocytes, histiocytes and occasional plasma cells).

(b) The terminal stage of chronic (active and persistent) hepatitis shows dense fibrous septa destroying the lobular architecture and forms large sized nodules (**macro-nodular**); post-necrotic regenerating irregular nodules of proliferating liver cells are termed as post-necrotic nodules of **post-necrotic cirrhosis** (**PNC**).

CHRONIC CHOLECYSTITIS

History:

A 40 years **fair** looking, **fatty, fertile female** (the **5 Fs**) was brought to the emergency department at 6 AM with severe colicky pain at the right hypochondrial region. She had a high fatty diet last night.

Gross:

1. Gall bladder is frequently **small, fibrosed** and **contracted**, or may be enlarged, or normal in size. The external bluish transluscence is lost, and looks dull and opaque due to **subserosal fibrosis**, or **yellow** color occurs due to the presence of **sub-serous fat** that grows sometimes. On cutting open, the wall is found thickened due to fibrous tissue proliferation and contraction. Excessive scarring can give rise to **hourglass deformity**. Sometimes there is impregnation of the inner wall with calcium, which is termed as **porcelain gall bladder**.

2. The gall bladder content may be healthy bile, or the bile may be pale and turbid. There may be mucopus, stone, or cholesterol-rich brownish debris called **biliary mud**.

Microscopically:

1. The gall bladder is always found **infiltrated** in its muscle layer **by lymphocytes** and occasional **plasma cells**. The surface epithelial cells show harmonizing lining with the mucosal folds which look wavy on the surface. The **mucosal glands** in many cases **penetrate deep down**, up to **the muscle layer**, (which lies isolated, or in groups). This condition is called *cholecystitis glandularis proliferans*. Along with this **Aschoff-Rokitansky sinus** is formed. Dense fibrosis occurs.

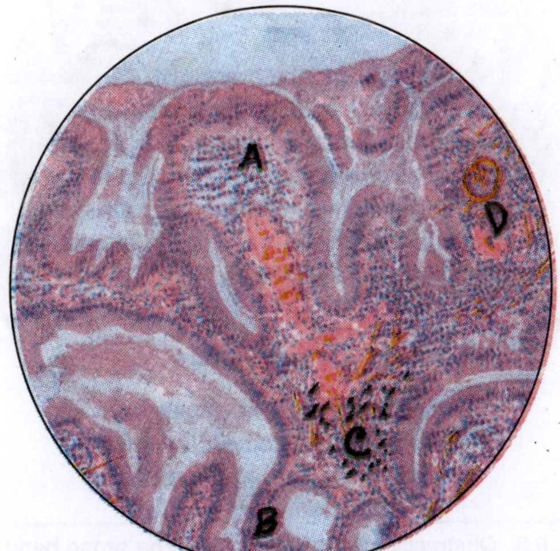

Fig. 6.2: The chronically inflamed proliferated mucosal glands of gall bladder shows: A. Mucosal (papillary) folds; B. Aschoff-Rokitansky sinus; C. Fibromuscular coat showing lymphocytic infiltration; D. Dense fibrosis

2. Sometimes the mucosal **glandular epithelia contain imbibed cholesterol** in the gall bladder. This imbibition and absorption of cholesterol into the gall bladder may be due to:

(i) Local disturbance of cholesterol metabolism, or

(ii) Obstruction to the lymphatic and venous channels predisposing to the accumulation of cholesterol absorbed from bile. The mucosal epithelial cell fail to **secrete cholesterol from the cell**, which when gets retained and trapped in the cell and that causes cholesterolosis of the gall bladder along with *(cholecystitis) glandularis proliferans*.

BILIARY CIRRHOSIS

(Unilobular cirrhosis)

Synonyms

Monolobular cirrhosis, Hanot's cirrhosis. This is secondary to:

1. **Biliary obstruction by**
   - (a) **Tumours** of the head of the pancreas.
   - (b) **Stone** in the common bile duct.
   - (c) Benign **stricture** of the hepatic ductules.

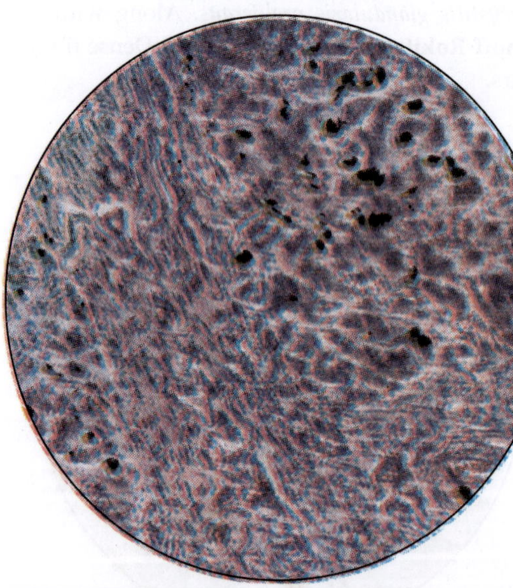

Fig. 6.3: Obstructive Biliary Cirrhosis—The broad band of fibrous tissue to left and bottom represents a thickened portal tract. It contains several bile ducts seen both in cross and longitudinal section. Darkly stained masses of bile pigment are evident among the liver cells (top right and bottom left). Hematoxylin and Eosin. × 100

2. **Infection**, or
3. **Pericholangiolitic conditions** causing inflammation of the small bile ducts in portal areas that may give rise to ***primary biliary cirrhosis.***

Naked-eye or Gross appearance:

The liver is often enlarged. The **surface** is very **finely granular** and the color is **intense green.**

Microscopic appearance:

1. Intrahepatic **bile ducts are dilated,** often infiltrated with **neutrophils.**
2. **Connective tissue** (collagen) is increased in the portal tract and **encircles each lobule.**
3. **Newly formed ducts** are present in the portal tract.
4. Bile **canaliculi are distended** with **inspissated bile.**
5. Chronic inflammatory cells **(lymphocytes** and **plasma cells)** infiltrate the **fibrous tissue.**

THYROID–GOITER

Definition

Goiter is the **non-inflammatory, non-neoplastic enlargement** of the thyroid gland due to deficiency of iodine with the binding protein **[Protein bound iodine (PBI)].**

PARENCHYMATOUS GOITER

Microscopically:

1. The **follicles** are **increased** in number.
2. They are **lined by cuboidal** or **low columnar cells.**

SIMPLE COLLOID GOITER (Fig. 6.4)

Naked-eye or gross appearance:

The thyroid is uniformly and **diffusely enlarged** and **soft** in consistency. *Cut surface* presents a finely **honeycombed** appearance. The **space contains** glistening, clear, amber colored **colloid matter.**

Microscopic appearance:

1. The **acini** are **widely dilated** and **irregular** in appearance.
2. Deeply stained, **acidophilic colloid** is present in the acini.

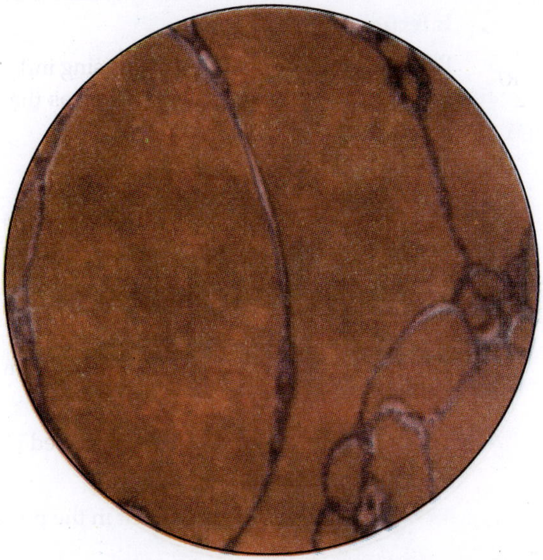

Fig. 6.4: Simple goiter—Some of the acini are greatly distended, and all the acini are lined by cubical or flattened epithelium and filled with strikingly acidophilic colloid devoid of peripheral vacuolation. Hematoxylin and Eosin. × 70

3. The **epithelium** is **flattened** out.
4. Areas of **active hyperplasia** are usually **scanty**.

MULTINODULAR GOITER

Multinodular goiter involves both hyperplasia and involution that causes irregular **enlargement of the thyroid gland** giving rise to **nodularity**.

Naked-eye or Gross appearance:

1. The size is enlarged and the gland may weigh 200 g.
2. Enlargement may exert lateral pressure and midline structures like the esophagus and trachea may be pushed laterally. When the enlargement occurs posterior to the sternum and the clavicle, it causes **intrathoracic plugging goiter.**
3. **Hyalinized stroma** runs amongst the territory of the follicles and multiple nodules.
4. **Cut surface** shows presence of **brown** (due to hemorrhage), **gelatinous colloid**. Older lesions have **variegated appearance** with **areas of hemorrhage, fibrosis, calcification** and **cystic degeneration.**

Microscopic appearance:

1. **Follicular hyperplasia** showing **colloid** in the follicles.
2. There is **scalloping** (moth-eaten appearance) **of the colloid.**
3. Follicles are lined by **cuboidal epithelial cell with intact** basement membrane **(B.M.)**.
4. **Degenerative changes** may occur in follicles.
5. The **follicles show clear boundary** created by the stroma around them **with intact B.M.**
6. Each **hyperplastic nodule is bounded by** a capsule, and the compressed parenchymal **(epithelial) cells** lie at the periphery.

NODULAR OR ADENOMATOUS GOITERS

Naked-eye or Gross appearance:

The appearance is extremely varied. The surface is nodular and irregular.

Cut section may show one or more capsulated adenomas. They may be numerous, scattered throughout both lobes. Each **adenoma is larger than a pea, or as large as an orange.** It has a well-formed capsule. A solid adenoma may undergo necrosis. A **colloid adenoma** frequently becomes cystic. The cyst may be chocolate in color due to extravasated blood. **Cholesterol crystals** may be present; **calcification** may occur in the fibrous septa of an adenoma.

Microscopic types and appearance:

Two types are seen, such as:

1. **Colloid adenoma**
2. **Fetal adenoma**

COLLOID ADENOMA

1. Acini are filled with **colloid matter** often with interspersed islets of **hyperplasia** of cubical epithelial cells.
2. There is (moth-eaten **scalloping appearance) of the colloid** matter.
3. The **capsule is well formed** and the surrounding **acini are compressed.**

FETAL ADENOMA

This occurs in middle aged female and likely to **undergo malignant change.**

1. Usually it is a **single adenoma** in which **acinar structure** is seldom seen **(lost)**.
2. The **cells are cuboidal** and spheroidal with **dark staining nuclei.**

3. **Cells are arranged compactly**, or in strands or columns often **interspaced with hyaline stroma**.

The **capsule** is seen, often **well-formed**.

THYROID

PRIMARY HYPERPLASIA OF THE THYROID GLAND or Diffuse Toxic Goiter or Thyrotoxicosis or Grave's Disease or Exophthalmic Goiter (Ophthalmopathy)

The characteristic **Triad features** are:

1. **Diffuse bilateral symmetrical** moderate **enlargement** of the thyroid.
2. **Thyroid causing toxicosis** or hyperthyroidism with toxic features.
3. **Exophthalmia** or **ophthalmopathy**.

Naked eye or gross features:

There is diffuse, moderate and symmetrical bilateral thyroid enlargement weighing up to 80 g weight.

The cut surface is reddish-brown and homogeneous, meat-like, but there is no normal translucency of the surface.

Microscopic features:

1. Marked **epithelial hyperplasia and hypertrophy** causing considerable height of the follicular lining epithelial cells with **papillary infolding** formations as a result of **heaped up epithelium** into the small follicular lumen.

2. Follicular **colloid liquidity is decreased**, becomes **finely vacuolated** with weakly eosinophilic staining property.

3. There is more vascularity in the stroma of the gland with lymphocytic (focal) accumulations.

Iodine administration causes **hypoplastic type of changes**, i.e., (a) diminished vascularity of the part, with (b) increase in the follicular cells and (c) hypoplastic change in follicular cells with lowering of the height of the follicular lining epithelial cells. The opposite situation, i.e., the **hyperplastic type of changes** are caused by **thiouracil group** of (antithyroid drug) is marked.

TOXIC GOITERS (Fig. 6.5)

It may be:

1. **Primary hyperplasia of thyroid** (Exophthalmic or **primary toxic goiter—primary hyperplasia**).

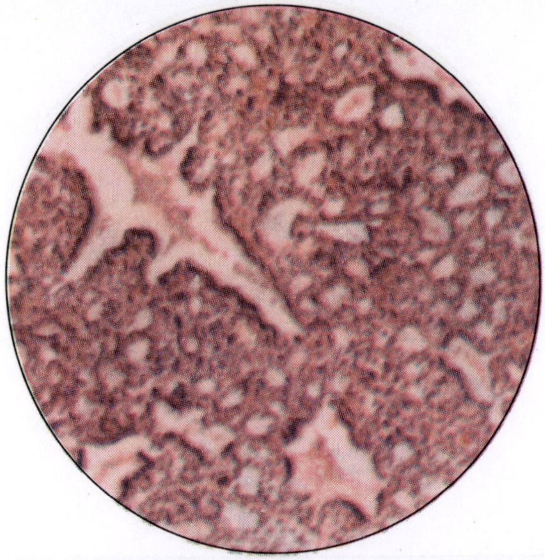

Fig. 6.5: Primary hyperplasia of the thyroid (Exophthalmic goiter)—Tissue consists of many small round, or oval acini and a few larger acint of irregular shape. While the small acini are lined by cubical or low columnar cells. Hematoxylin and Eosin. × 70

2. **Secondary (Toxic adenoma)**.

Naked-eye or Gross appearance:

In primary condition, glands are uniformly enlarged to a moderate degree. The thyroid is **highly vascular, granular and friable**. The colour is like that of flesh. The thymus may show hyperplasia.

Microscopically:

1. **Reduction** in amount of **colloid**, and vacuoles are seen at the periphery of the acini (**scalloping** or **moth-eaten appearance** present).

2. Acinar cells are increased in number and **tall columnar** in appearance.

3. **Infolding** of the wall of the acini is a striking feature and acini lose their normal outlines. There may be extensive **lymphocytic infiltration** in the stroma forming lymphoid follicles at places.

4. In the **involution form**, cellular hyperplasia is less with **restoration of colloid** in the vesicles.

BENIGN PROSTATIC HYPERTROPHY (BENIGN NODULAR HYPERPLASIA OR BENIGN ENLARGEMENT OF THE PROSTATE) BPH/BNH/BEP:

The prostate may be **large and soft**, or relatively smaller, even, and harder. **Nodularity is characteristic**. The **lateral lobes** are usually enlarged.

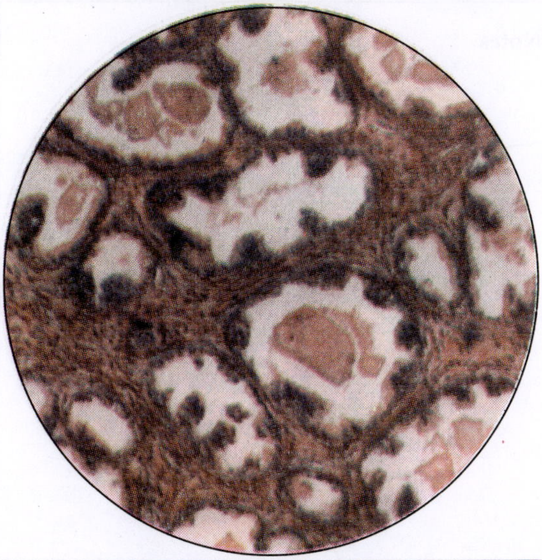

Fig. 6.6: Hypertrophy of Prostate—The acini are increased in number and of variable size and shape. They frequently are papilliform and sometimes contain pink-stained corpora amylacea. Hematoxylin and Eosin. × 80

Microscopic appearance:

1. There is **glandular hyperplasia** with **overgrowth of fibromuscular tissues**.
2. The **acini** are **enlarged**. The **papillary processes** of epithelium may **project** into the lumen; or the epithelium may project into the lumen of the gland (acini).
3. There are two types of epithelial cells forming two layers that line the acini:
   (a) the inner one is tall columnar, mucus-secreting cells with ill-defined cell-outline.
   (b) the outer layer of cubical/squamous epithelium.

Often the glandular hyperplasia dominates the fibromuscular hyperplasia.

4. Formation of **corpora amylacea** is seen in the glandular space.

Diagrams/Notes

Diagrams/Notes

Diagrams/Notes

Diagrams/Notes

PART TWO
Special Pathology

CHAPTER 7
HISTOPATHOLOGY (SYSTEMIC)

GASTROINTESTINAL SYSTEM

1. PLEOMORPHIC ADENOMA (Mixed Parotid Tumor)

History:

Painful swelling in parotid region.

Microscopic appearance:

1. Structure is diverse and pleomorphic.
2. Cord and masses of epithelial cells embedded in a hyalinized connective tissue matrix, enclosed with a well developed fibrous capsule.
3. **Cuboidal epithelial cells** showing glandular arrangement (acinar structure).
4. **Mucoid connective tissue** producing **mucin**.
5. **Myxomatous material** simulating **cartilage** cells (pseudocartilage) is homogeneous.
6. **True cartilage cells** may be present.
7. **Malignant changes** may be seen with **hyperchromatism of nuclei** and **atypical mitosis** in them.

2. CHRONIC GASTRITIS

History:

Patient complaining of belching, erructation and heart burn.

Three types:

I. TYPE A:

Autoimmune gastritis site of affection is the **body- and fundal-mucosa**. It may be associated with Addison's disease and Hashimoto's thyroiditis. Circulating **autoimmune bodies** are formed **against parietal cells** and the **Castle's intrinsic factor**. Parietal cells are depleted. **Castle's intrinsic factor** secretion is **impaired, gastric mucosal atrophy** occurs with development of **pernicious anemia**. There is associated **hypochlorhydria and achlorhydria.**

Hyperplasia of gastrin producing **'G' cells** occur in the **pyloric antrum** that **cause Hypergastrinemia.**

II. TYPE B:

***H. pylori* related Hypersecretory gastritis**:

Antral mucosa is affected. The excessive secretion of acid by H. pylori infection is called **Hypersecretory gastritis.**

Cells look without any change except more number of *Zymogen granules*.

III. TYPE AB:

Chronic atrophic gastritis (Environmental gastritis): Any type of environmental condition may cause this condition at any age. Even there may be **conversion of body and fundal type** gastritis as well as **antral 'B' type** gastritis to this form.

A. Chronic Superficial Gastritis

Pathological changes in Type A Gastritis:

***Grossly,* the mucosa** may be

(a) Normal
(b) Atrophied
(c) Edematous

Microscopic changes:

1. **Acute** and active **inflammatory changes** in the mucosa with vascular prominences. This may be superficial and deep.
2. **Metaplastic cellular change** may be present, which may be as under:

i) **Intestinal type** (taller or **high cuboidal** cells)

ii) **Pseudopyloric type:** Medium or high cuboidal.

SIMPLE CLASSIFICATION OF GASTRITIS:

1. Chronic **superficial gastritis.**
2. Chronic **atrophic gastritis** with gastric mucosal atrophy.
3. Chronic **hypertrophic gastritis.**
4. **Uncommon forms** of gastritis.

Microscopically:

Chronic superficial gastritis: Changes occur in the **superficial (mucosal)** layer showing **lymphocytic** and plasma cellular **infiltration**, without any change in the deeper layer.

H. pylori (spiral bacterial) **invasion** occurs which is seen **on the epithelial cell layer** (and not in area with intestinal type tall columnar epithelial cells metaplasia).

Fate of Chronic Superficial Gastritis:

1. Good Prognosis—(**Cure**).
2. Development of **Atrophic gastritis** by gastric mucosal atrophy.
3. Peptic ulcer disease.
4. **Malignant change.**

B. Gastric Mucosal Atrophy

Microscopic appearance:

Deeper layer of mucosa shows epithelial elements: (i) **atrophy and destruction** of mucosal glands, and (ii) **epithelial metaplasia.**

Metaplasia are of two types in the stomach:

1. ***Intestinal type metaplasia:*** This occurs in **pyloric antral cuboidal epithelial cells** converting them into mucus-secreting Goblet (columnar) cells. In addition, there are **Paneth cells** and **Endocrine cells** present as well. The extensive metaplasia is indicative of **Gastritic precancerous** and **cancerous conditions.** ***H. pylori* is absent in the metaplastic area.**

2. **Pseudopyloric metaplasia:** This **Epithelial metaplasia** simulates the epithelial cells of glands of the pyloric area and the metaplasia that affects the epithelial cells of the glands belonging to the glands of the body of the stomach below the fundus.

The metaplastic cells look like the proliferated mucosal neck cells.

3. GASTRIC ULCER

History:

Acidity and pain in the abdomen (gastric and pyloric region); on taking food the existing pain

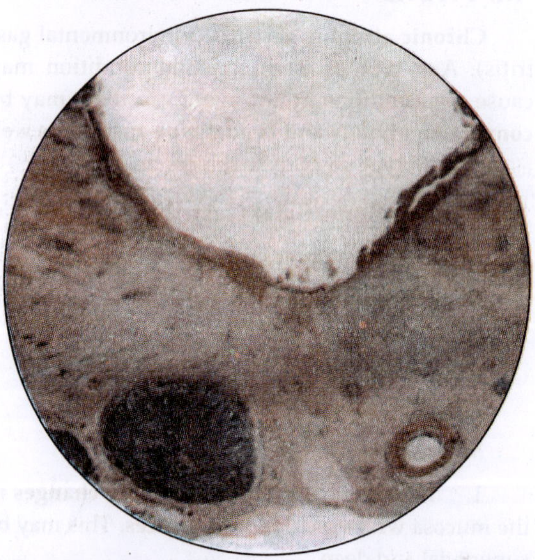

Fig. 7.1: Chronic Gastric Ulcer—The ulcer has penetrated the mucous, submucous and muscular coats and is bounded externally by a thickened subserous layer. It is lined by a thin band of necrotic material. Hematoxylin and Eosin. × 50

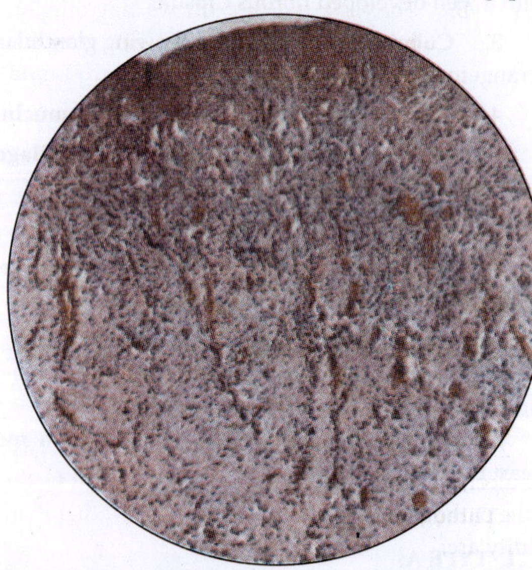

Fig. 7.2: Floor of Chronic Gastric Ulcer—The floor of the ulcer consists of granulation tissue which is congested and infiltrated with inflammatory cells. A narrow zone of necrosis is present at the surface (top). Hematoxylin and Eosin. × 80

increases and replacement of surface epithelia occurs by Goblet cells at the pylorus (cf. duodenal ulcer where pain is relieved with food).

Grossly (Macroscopically):

It is a chronic spherical or oval ulcer, small or large, measuring **1 cm to 7 cm** in its longest dimension and **subserous layer** of the gastric wall reaches the liver and pancreas. The **ulcer walls** are precipitous or overhanging and the **floor** is smooth or nodular. Both the walls and the floor are composed of (i) **superficial necrotic** as well as (ii) **deep fibrotic layers.** The serous aspect may show adhesion to the neighbouring structures.

Complications are like:

1. **Hemorrhage**
2. **Perforation**
3. **Fibrous contraction,** and
4. **Malignant transformation**
5. Pyloric stenosis and obstruction
6. Subphrenic abscess between the liver and the diaphragm.

A. *HEMORRHAGE* occurs from erosion of a larger blood vessel that is incorporated in the ulcer.

B. The *FIBROUS CONTRACTIONS* may offer an **hour** *GLASS* **(deformity of)** *STOMACH* **(contracture causing deformity),** and *PYLORIC OBSTRUCTION.*

The fundamental pathogenesis occurs due to impaired gastric mucosal defense against the **acid-pepsin secretion** of the stomach.

PATHOGENESIS:

Hyperacidity

1. **High serum gastrin level** occurs by the ingested food in an atonic stomach leading to hyperacidity.

2. **Low acidity and normal acidity** causes gastric ulcer; **hyperacidity is not that an important factor** in the pathogenesis of gastric ulcer. Factors other than acidity are:

(i) **Smoking**
(ii) **Gastritis** and
(iii) **Bile reflux** from the duodenum.

3. The protective gastric mucus (mucin) against **gastric acid-pepsin derangement** occurs in the formation of gastric ulcer.

There is quantitative **reduction in the production of gastric mucus**. Side by side there is **quantitative** and qualitative (altered) production of the gastric mucus which has inferior (-ve) grade of protection to the gastric mucosa.

PATHOLOGICAL FEATURES

SITE OF ULCER:

Along the **lesser curvature** and near the **pyloric antrum** on the **posterior wall;** whereas **duodenal** ulcers occur **on the anterior wall of the first part of duodenum (postpyloric region)**. Gastric ulcer may occasionally occur on the **cardia** and in ***Meckel's diverticulum***.

Gross appearance:

Single, small (usually 1-2.5 cm), spherical to oval **punched out ulcers with flat margins** occur in the stomach. Ulcers may be superficial and also deep. In 20% cases, an associated duodenal ulcer may occur as well. Gastric ulcer may underego **malignant change—bowl-shaped** with **central cupping** (depression) with **rolled up elevated margin,** and **indurated** (thickened) **mucosa**. The ulcer is larger and excavating.

Duodenal ulcer does not undergo malignant change.

Microscopic appearance:

There are **four types of changes** showing four different areas of (fibrinous and cellular) exudate.

1. **The Necrotic Zone:** It is on the floor of the ulcer, comprising **little exudate—Leukocytes** and the **necrotic material.**

2. **Superficial Exudative Zone:** It contains **Nuclear remnants** in **necrosed** cytoplasmic eosinophilic **granular and smudgy areas.**

3. **Zone of Granulation Tissue:** It comprises the (i) chronic nonspecific **inflammatory infiltrate** and the (ii) proliferating **budding capillaries** of neoangiogenesis.

4. **The Cicatrix Zone:** This is present at the bottom of the thick layer of granulation tissue and is made up of **dense fibrocollagen scar tissue.**

4. INTESTINAL TUBERCULOSIS

History:

Abdominal discomfort; on clinical examination, there is a **doughy feel** (consistency) on the abdomen.

Two types of infection occurs:

1. **Primary type (Tuberculosis)** occurs by drinking raw infected milk; this type is **disappearing** fast **due to** the reason for consumption of **pasteurized milk**. It occurs in infants and young children in a similar way like the development of Ghon's focus. **Ulceration is not a rule.**

2. **Secondary [Tuberculosis (Tb.)] infection:** This occurs by ingestion of (coughed out) infective sputum secondary to the open type pulmonary Tb. or direct infection by taking unhygienic infected food and drinks.

Mode of infection:

Massive dose of ingested organism passes through the intestinal mucosal tubular glands with production of inflammatory exudates in the depth of the glands. Macrophages carry the tubercle bacillus with the exudates to the deeper tissue in the **submucosa** where they produce **granulomatous lesions** with denudation of the mucosa and **ulceration**. Next the bacilli by lymphatic spread settle at the regional mesenteric lymph nodes to cause caseation. Tremendous granulomatous **Proliferative lesion** in the lymph node produces huge enlargement of mesenteric lymph nodes called **Tabes mesenterica** (Tabes means destruction).

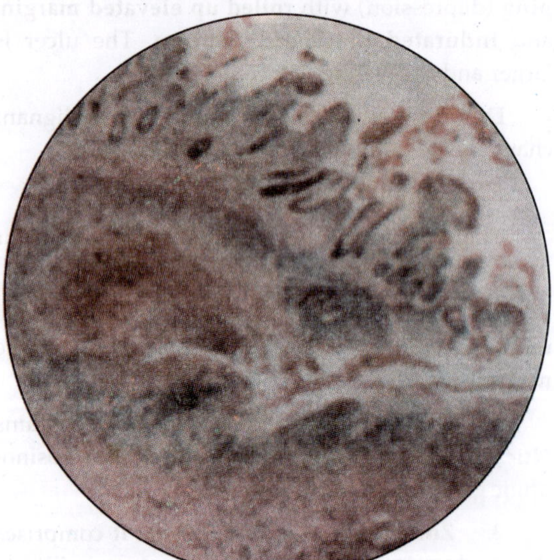

Fig. 7.3: Tuberculous ulcer of small intestine—On right: The mucous membrane is sloughed out to form an ulcer the floor of which consists of submucosa. Towards left: The submucosa shows an area of **caseation** (red) surrounded by the remains of a Peyer's patch. Hematoxylin and Eosin × 35

Gross appearance:

The common site of intestinal Tb (ulcerative lesion) is the terminal part of the ileum. To start with small grayish white tubercles in the lymphoid **follicles** (Peyer's patches) develop, many of which **coalesce** and undergo **caseation and softening**; breakdown of these lesions results in **ulcer formations**.

Characteristics of small intestinal Tb

The FLOOR (formed by serosa seen from outside) contains **tubercles.**

EDGE: Undermined (indurated).

Margin: **Irregular.**

The process spreads from the mucosal surface to the serous surface. Aggregates of tubercles are seen on the peritoneal surface which is covered with plastic **exudate (thick, fibrinous, dried).**

The overlying peritoneum is thickened. The ulcers (inflammatory immune response) spread along the **transverse axis** of the gut in the same line. Excessive collagen tissue forms thickened **"girdle ulcers"**. The lesion spreads to the cecum. In the plastic exudation of the serosa, adhesions of the bowel segments are common that form kinks which lead to **subacute intestinal obstruction.** The healing of a deep and extensive ulcer by collagen tissue may cause marked contraction and stenosis of the bowel leading to subacute intestinal obstruction.

Microscopic appearance:

The characteristic microscopic picture is one of a microscopic tubercle with central caseation, and formation of epithelioid reticulum.

5. JUVENILE RECTAL POLYP

History:

10-year old boy complaining of passage of blood in the stool. Endoscopic rectal biopsy material is put forth for histopathological examination.

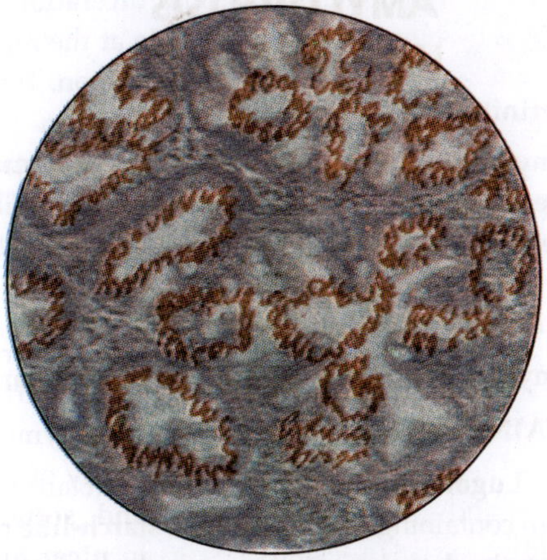

Fig. 7.4A: Juvenile polyp—Non-neoplastic colonic polyp

They are multiple, colorectal hamartomatous retention polyps which occur below 15 years of age in children. Solitary polyp of this type occurs in the rectum. This is a benign condition. They are **sessile non-inflammatory, non-neoplastic polyps. Adenomatous polyps are stalked**.

Pathological Features

Grossly, the polyps are often pedunculated; 2 cm in size, spherical with smooth surface.

Microscopic Features:

They are glands with cystic dilation lined by goblet cells. The dilated cyst contains mucus. The stroma is made of fibroconnective tissue, and infiltrated with chronic inflammatory cellular infiltrate when the surface shows ulceration. These polyps are **not precancerous**.

6. ADENOCARCINOMA OF COLON

History:

Patient complaining of passage of blood in stool, weight loss, tiredness and alternate loose motion and normal stool.

Occasional pain in the colonic region. Operated colon is submitted for histopathological examination.

The **tumor** almost always **arises from pre-existing adenoma** of the colon.

Adenoma → hyperplasia of epithelial cells → dysplasia → carcinoma in situ → invasive carcinoma.

PATHOLOGICAL FEATURES

Grossly, right sided colonic growth is large.

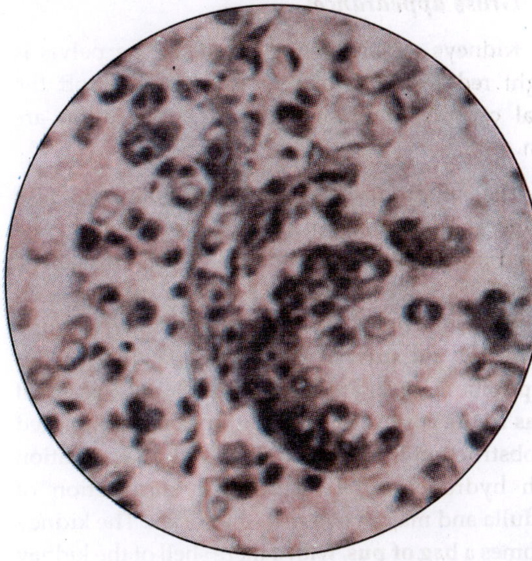

Fig. 7.4B: Carcinoma of Colon showing mucoid degeneration —Numerous cells, isolated and in masses, are separated by abundant, feebly stained mucin. Many cells are distended by a large globule of mucin, while the nucleus is flattened out at one side—**"Signet-ring" forms**. Hematoxylin and Eosin. × 360

cauliflower-like, soft, friable, fungating, polypoid carcinomatous growth projecting into the lumen of the colon.

The **left sided** colonic carcinomas have a **napkin ring configuration** which encircles the luminal (mucosal) bowel wall circumferentially with increased amount of fibrous tissue forming the **annular ring** with **ulceration** of the central portion **at the surface** with **elevated margins**—typical of carcinomatous ulcer.

Microscopic Features:

The malignant **acini show back to back arrangement**. The acini are lined by Goblet cells. Two acini join together by a **breakthrough the basement membrane** and fuse together. Nuclei show atypism. Mitotic figures are encountered.

RENAL SYSTEM

7. CHRONIC PYELONEPHRITIS (Pyelo = pelvis; Nephro = kidney)

History:

65 years old lady gives repeated history of UTI. She is an old case of **Diabetes mellitus**.

Gross appearance:

Kidneys are swollen, congested. The pelvis is bright red with full of pus. On stripping off the renal capsule, multiple areas of suppuration are seen.

The **cut surface** shows **dark irregular**, and also **wedge shaped areas** in the renal substance. The healed areas are represented by **'V', 'U'** or **saddle shaped scars. Perinephric abscesses** may be seen when the infection spreads through the perinephric tissue. The **cut surface** also shows patchy areas of suppuration: **linear areas in pyramids**, and **spherical areas in the cortex**. Calyceal outlines are obliterated by obstruction in pyelonephritis and in association with hydronephrosis resulting in destruction of medulla and major portion of the cortex. The kidney becomes a **bag of pus**, with a mere shell of the kidney tissue (**pyonephrosis**). It is a slow and gradual process producing fibrosis. Scarring and contraction of the kidney resulting in a granular contracted kidney-like condition, alike the **granular contracted kidney** of chronic gomerulonephritis and arteriolar nephrosclerosis, i.e., the **end-stage kidney**.

Renal tubules are destroyed and are replaced by dense scar tissue. The **tubules** in the intervening areas are dilated, lined by flattened epithelium, and **filled with acidophilic, colloid material**; resembling the structures of thyroid acini. There are presence of **microabscesses** with **interstitial infiltration by neutrophils**, which are admixed with the common finding of streaks of **lymphocytic and plasma cellular infiltrations**.

The clinching **Microscopic Diagnostic Points** for chronic pyelonephritis are:

1. **Periglomerular fibrosis**, otherwise the glomeruli look normal.
2. **Hyalinization of glomeruli**.
3. **Thyroidization of renal tubules** due to colloid cast formation in the lumen.
4. **Onion-scale (skin) appearance of the arterioles**.
5. **Interstitial infiltration with lymphocytes**, occasional plasma cells, sometimes admixed with neutrophils.
6. **Dense interstitial fibrosis**.

AMYLOIDOSIS
(Amyloid change)

Definition:

Amyloid (amylum = starch; oid = like; starch-like) degeneration represents a waxy, translucent hyaline change in the walls of the blood vessels of spleen, liver, kidney, etc. It is characterized by the deposition of amyloid substance in *intercellular spaces*.

Amyloid deposition is always extracellular.

STAINING REACTIONS (only)

1. **Lugol's iodine** poured on the cut surface of the organ containing amyloid gives a **starch-like reaction,** namely; **dark-brown areas,** which change into a **blue** or **violet color, when diluted sulphuric acid is applied on them**. Amyloid is a glycoprotein and gives a **polychroming effect** when stained with methyl violet, giving a pale, rosy-purple color.

It is a mucopolysaccharide-protein complex which is nicely demonstrated by

2. **Per-iodic Acid Schiff (PAS)** method. Periodic acid **oxidizes carbohydrate to aldehyde, and amyloid is stained purple with leukofuchsin present in Schiff's reagent.**

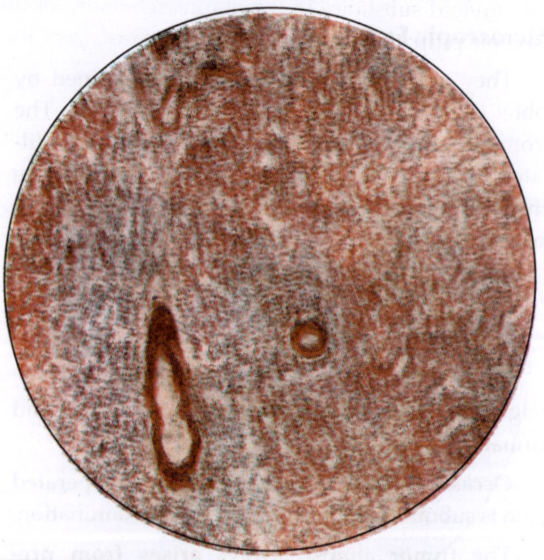

Fig. 7.5: Amyloid degeneration of Spleen—Diffuse type—The connective tissue in the walls of the venous sinuses and the reticulum of the pulp spaces are impregnated with amyloid substance. The lymphoid tissue of the malpighian bodies **toward left** is unaffected, but their central arteries are involved. Congo-red and Hematoxylin × 60

3. **Metachromatic staining reaction with methyl violet** (pink) is **due to the presence of sulphuric acid groups.**

4. Amyloid has an affinity for *Congo-red*, which is selectively retained and stians amyloid, and forms the basis of **Paunz Benhold test**. When 10 ml of 1 per cent sterile congo-red is injected intravenously in amyloidosis patient; 60–80 per cent or more of the dye disappears from blood in an hour after the injection, by its (congo-red) deposition in amyloid tissue.

5. The **Polarizing microscopy** for Congo-red-stained amyloid materials show **green birefringence.**

8. AMYLOID SPLEEN (Fig. 7.5)

Gross appearance:

Spleen (Fig. 7.5, 7.6 & 7.7). The spleen is enlarged, firm, elastic, India rubber-like in consistencey.

There are two types of splenic lesions: (a) *diffuse*, (b) *focal*

In the **DIFFUSE TYPE**, the ***cut surface*** shows a characteristic homogeneous, translucent, glossy and smooth appearance.

Microscopically, there is widespread deposition of amyloid substance in the fibrous reticulum of the splenic pulp; the follicles tend to be spared from this change. The **amyloid deposit starts** from the venous sinuses and **spreads towards the reticulum of the pulp**.

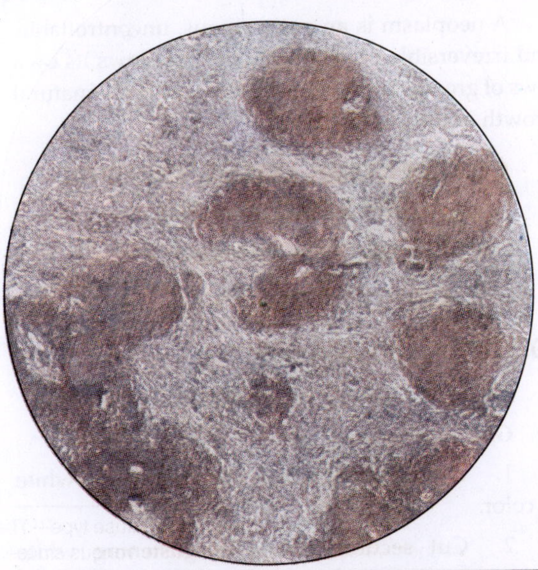

Fig. 7.6: Amyloid degeneration of Spleen—**Localized type**: All the malpighian bodies in the field have been replaced by amyloid substance, but there is little or no affection of the pulp. Methyl violet × 20

In the **FOCAL TYPE**, the ***cut surface*** shows areas resembling **half-boiled sago grains (sago spleen)** due to accumulation of amyloid material in the arteriolar walls, which extends into the surrounding lymph follicles. These extend into the surrounding lymphoid follicles. These areas stian **purple with methyl** violet **(metachromatic reaction)**. The Malpighian bodies show prominent amyloid deposits in the central arteries (**Fig. 7.6**). The deposit is **extracellular**, which gradually replaces the lymphoid tissues of the follicle.

The X-ray diffraction study of amyloid reveals the ***beta-pleated sheet conformation***.

Liver. The organ is enlarged, firm and unusually transluscent. The deposit starts from the **midzone** of the lobule and appears in the space between the **sinus endothelium and the liver cells**. The deposit of amyloid causes narrowing of the sinuses with pressure atrophy of the parenchyma cells.

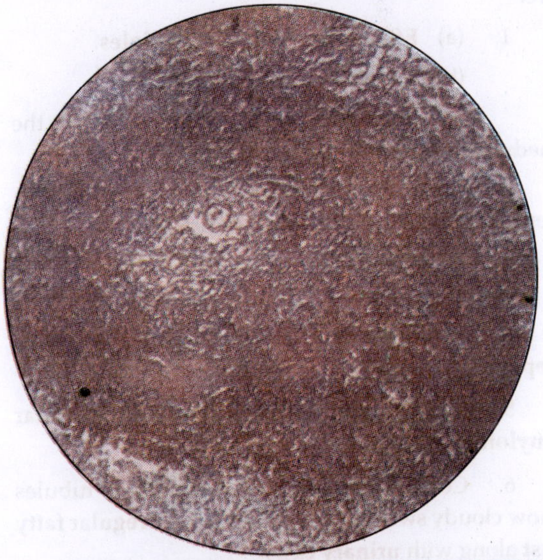

Fig. 7.7: Amyloid degeneration of Spleen—**Localized type**: The lymphoid tissue of the malpighian body illustrated has largely disappeared following impregnation of its **reticulum with amyloid substance**. The central artery and a narrow zone of lymphoid tissue around it have escaped. The pulp is also unaffected. Methyl violet × 80

Pancreas. Hyaline material, found in the **islets** of Langerhans in the pancreas in old diabetics appears to be a kind of amyloid change.

9. AMYLOIDOSIS OF KIDNEY

History:

40 years old male has pain in loins. On examination with **1% Congo Red Dye injection** shows 80% of the dye that has disappeared from circulation within one hour. Kidney biopsy was submitted for histopathology.

Chief Features:

Amyloid deposit is Extracellular.

1. Amyloid deposit occurs in the **media of the afferent glomerular arterioles.**

2. Amyloid deposit is in the glomeruli and back in the interlobular artrioles in advanced stage. Amyloid is deposited in the delicate fibro-connective reticulum supporting the glomerular tufts of capillaries. Ultimately, swollen capillary tufts are replaced by thick, convoluted waxy strands obliterating the capillary lumens.

In advanced stage, the site of amyloid deposits are:

1. (a) **Efferent glomerular arterioles.**
   (b) **Intertubular plexus.**
   (c) **Arcuate arteries; vasa recta** in the medulla are affected.
2. **Medial muscle layer** is replaced by homogeneous, **pink amyloid material.**
3. Bowman's capsular lining epithelial cells and
4. The tubular **basement membranes** (TBM) of lining cuboidal epithelial cells **show amyloid-deposit.**
5. **Peritubular regions show extracellular amyloid deposit.**
6. Cells of the proximal convoluted tubules show cloudy swelling and excretion of **irregular fatty cast** along with **urinary casts:**
   (a) Granular
   (b) Fatty, and
   (c) Hyaline, tubular casts.

Amyloid is stained

(a) **In vitro by:**
   (i) **Methyl (gentian or crystal) violet**
   (ii) **Lugol's iodine solution**

(b) **In vitro and in vivo (both) by Congo-red.**

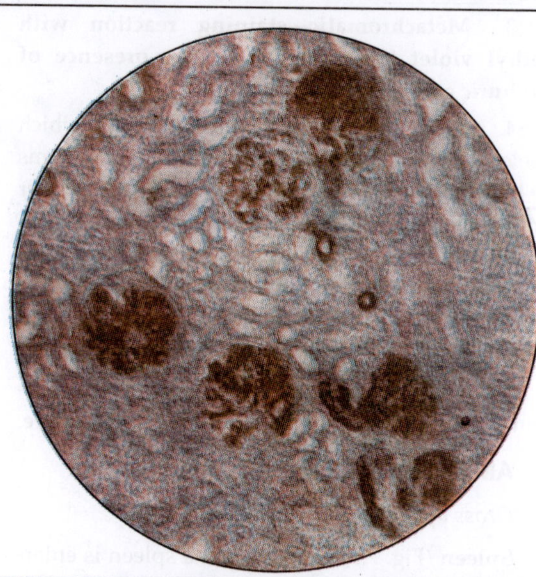

Fig. 7.8: Amyloid degeneration of Kidney—Amyloid material has been deposited in the walls of the afferent arterioles and **in the capillaries of the glomerular tufts.** The renal tissue in the neighbourhood of some of the affected glomeruli is atrophied and infiltrated with lymphocytes; Methyl violet × 60

TUMORS

***Synonym*:** Neoplasm, new growths, etc.

Definition

A neoplasm is an autonomous, uncontrollable, and irreversible new growth, i.e., it follows its own laws of growth and does not follow the law of natural growth of the normal tissue.

CONNECTIVE TISSUE TUMORS (MESENCHYMAL)

BENIGN TUMORS

FIBROMA (Fig. 7.9 & 7.10)

10. HARD FIBROMA (Fig. 7.9)

The suffix "OMA" means tumor.

Gross appearance:

1. Encapsulated tumor, firm or hard and white in color.
2. Cut section—bands of glistening white **fibrous tissue**, running in **different directions.**

Microscopic appearance (H & E):

1. Pink stained fibrous tissue of adult type (tough collagen bundles and fibrocytes) irregularly

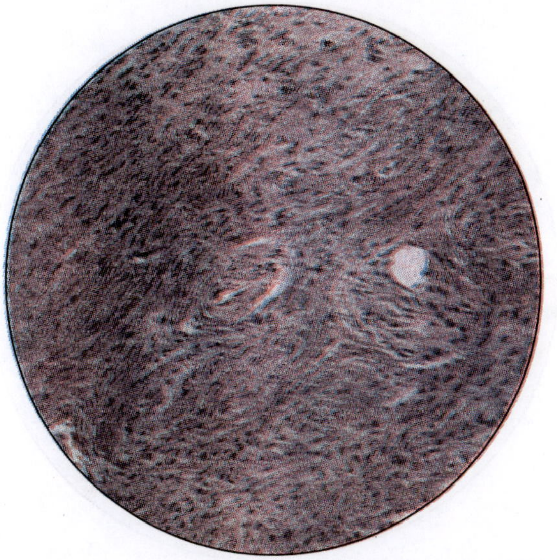

Fig. 7.9: Hard fibroma—The tissue consists of interlacing bundles of well developed fibrous (collagen) tissue. Hematoxylin and Eosin. × 60

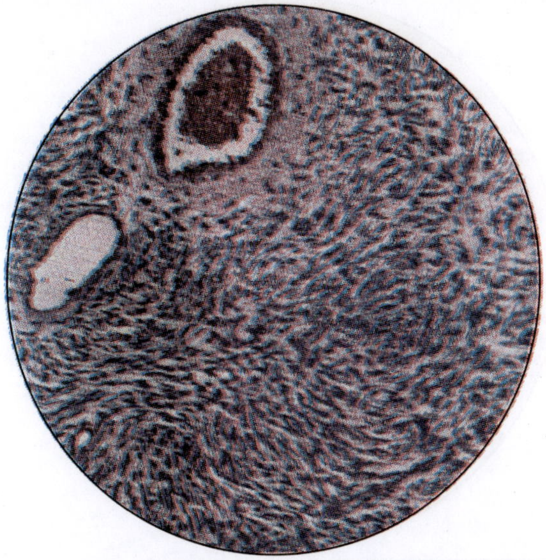

Fig. 7.10: Soft fibroma—The tissue consists of interlacing bundles of cells separated by scanty collagen. The arteriole at the top is deficient in muscle. Hematoxylin and Eosin. × 120

arranged in broad columns which runs in all directions.

2. Cellular elements are comparatively scanty with flattened and tapering nuclei showing normal mitosis in excess.

3. Cells are mature relatively less plumpy **fibroblasts cells**; nuclei are tapering, may show a **whorled appearance** in the growing part.

4. Blood vessels are well-supported and possess definite walls **lined by endothelium** (adult type).

5. Considerable proportion of **collagen** often in a state of hyaline degeneration (**hyalinization**).

11. SOFT FIBROMA (Fig. 7.10)

Gross appearance:

See earlier (pref. Hard Fibroma).

Microscopic appearance:

1. It is **more cellular** with **scanty fibrillar material and whorl formation** at places.

2. Rapidly growing **immature fibroblasts** are loosely arranged in irregular groups.

3. Vessels are **well formed** (lined with endothelium). Cells are more numerous round the vascular channels.

4. Nuclei show abundance of **normal mitosis**.

In modern concept, however, there is nothing like Hard fibroma and Soft fibroma. They are only Fibroma.

COLLAGEN IS THE SECRETORY PRODUCT OF MATURE FIBROBLASTS. **HYPERMATURE** FIBROBLASTS ARE FIBROCYTES (VERY SLENDER).

12. NEUROFIBROMA

Clinical types

Nodular, diffuse or plexiform.

Molluscum fibrosum is a condition of multiple neurofibromatosis; **runs in families** and called **von Recklinghausen's disease**. The condition is usually benign, but neurofibrosarcoma (malignant) may develop. The tumor grows either from the **endoneurium or perineurium**.

Microscopic appearance (H & E):

1. New growth of fibrous tissue consisting of a network of cellular fibrils—**whorled, feathery** or **irregular**. This is **cellular** in the earlier phase but relatively **acellular** and later **collagenous**.

2. Individual **nerve fibrils** are separated by connective tissue but in the advanced stage, nodules may show **fibrous elements or mixture of both** neurofibrils and fibroconnective tissue.

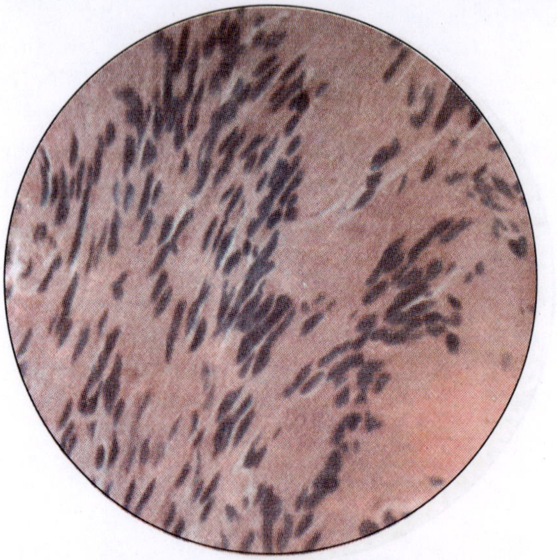

Fig. 7.11: Neurilemmoma—The tissue consists of spindle cells disposed in interlacing bundles. The nuclei show characteristic "**Regimentation**". Hematoxylin and Eosin. × 400

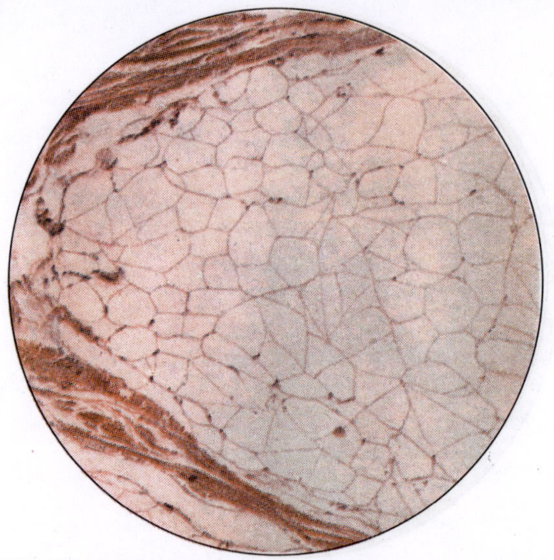

Fig. 7.12: Lipoma—The growth is made up of adult fat cells enclosed by a fibrous capsule on left. Hematoxylin and Eosin. × 80

3. **Pallisation** (alike regimentation) of the nuclei when present is characteristic. Pallisation is obliquely parallel.

13. SCHWANNOMA (Fig. 7.11)

Synonym: **Neurilemmoma**.

It resembles neurofibroma, but it is usually a **solitary tumor** and **does not run in families**. It arises from the **Sheath of Schwann** (neurilemmal sheath).

Microscopically, the feature resembles neurofibroma. Pallisation is not characteristic, **Regimentation** of cells and nuclei are **specific and characteristic, meaning prominent nuclei scattered in a bigger focus**, as if watching from there, like the regiment of an army.

14. LIPOMA (Fig. 7.12)

Gross appearance:

1. The tumor is **soft, elastic, well-circumscribed, encapsulated** and easily shelled out.
2. Skin is often **dimpled**, owing to fibrous bands passing between skin and the tumor.
3. On **cut section**—it is pale yellow in color; the knife is smeared with fat.

Microscopic appearance (H & E):

1. Fat cells showing unstained empty areas with nuclei pushed to one side of the **cells**. **Signet** or marriage **ring appearance**. The cells are often irregular in size.
2. Bands of fibrous tissue crossing the tumor.
3. Well-formed blood vessels present.
4. Areas of **calcareous and myxomatous (myxoid) degeneration** may be present.
5. Signs of inflammation with infiltration of inflammatory cells occur sometimes.

15. MYXOMA (Fig. 7.13)

Gross appearance:

Myxomata are soft, lobulated, encapsulated growths.

Microscopic appearance (H & E):

1. **Branching stellate**, myxomatous **cells** present which are scanty, large and irregular with deeply stained nuclei. These cells have long branching processes which radiate and fade away in the surrounding matrix to form a network. **Cells** and their nuclei **are uniform** as to size, shape and staining.
2. Bluish homogeneous materials fill up the interstices.
3. Strands of delicate fibroconnective tissue divides the tumor.
4. Blood vessels are well formed with imperfectly supported capillaries.

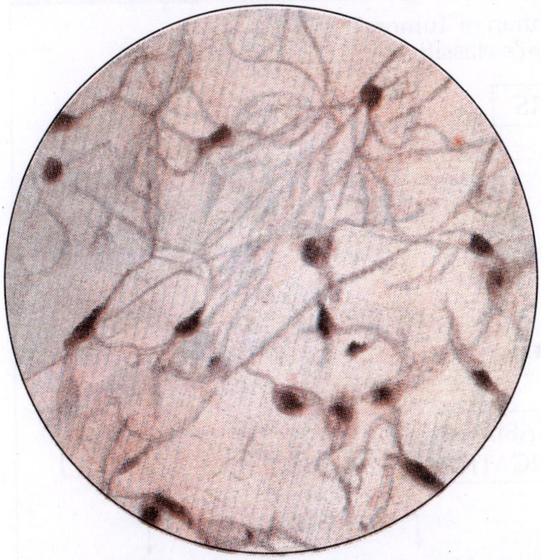

Fig. 7.13: Myxoma—The tissue consists of scanty, branching cells irregularly distributed in an abundant, clear matrix. Hematoxylin and Eosin. × 340

16. CHONDROMA (Fig. 7.14)

Gross appearance:

The tumor is ***firm, elastic, lobulated,*** and well **encapsulated**.

Cut surface—bluish grey, translucent and homogeneous.

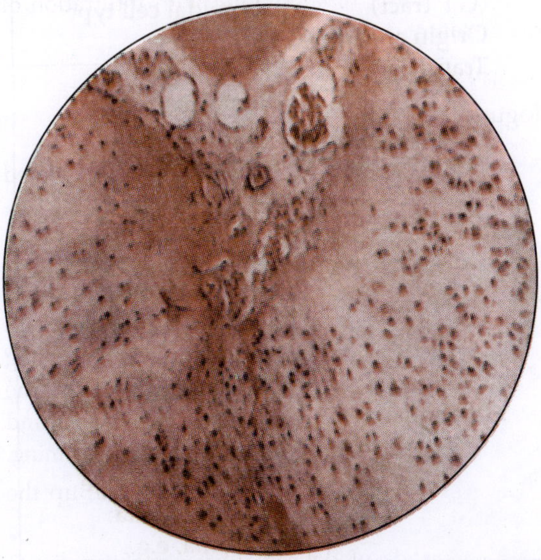

Fig. 7.14: Chondroma—Two islets of irregular hyaline cartilage are separated by a vascular, fibroblastic septum which is acting as a perichondrium. Hematoxylin and Eosin. × 100

Microscopic appearance (H & E):

1. Irregularly stained hyaline matrix containing a variable number of **cartilage cells** lying **singly, in pair** or **in tetrads**.
2. Some **empty spaces** are seen wherefrom cells have dislocated.
3. Arrangement of **cells** is irregular with considerable variation in size and shape, e.g., stellate or fusiform.
4. Strands of **fibrous tissue**.
5. The matrix may be myxomatous with **large, branching stellate myxoid cells** when the tumor is called **myxochondroma**.

17. OSTEOMA (Fig. 7.15)

Gross appearance:

The tumors are exceedingly hard, well encapsulated, rounded, sessile.

Microscopic appearance (H & E):

1. Bony structure with **canaliculi** which **are few** (in case of **ivory exostosis**).
2. Periosteal **fibrous membrane covering** the layer of **osteoblasts**.
3. Bony lamellae show **formed Haversian canal**.
4. **Spongy osteoma** shows **irregular trabeculae with islands of bone** and normal mitoses and **large spaces containing spherical fat cells**.

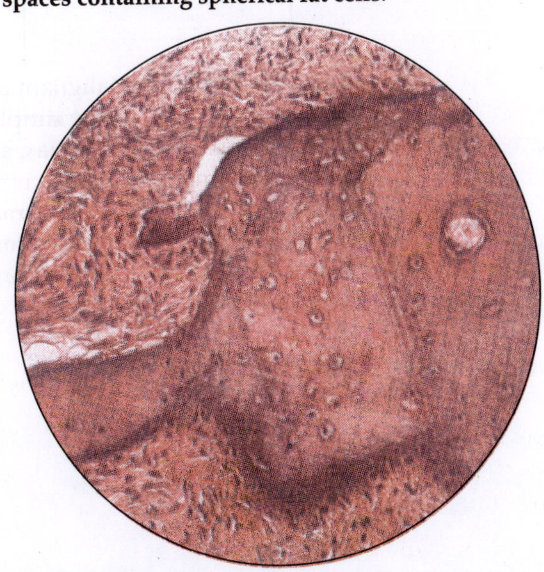

Fig. 7.15: Osteoma—Spongy-osteoma. Hematoxylin and Eosin. × 100 diam.

Histogenetic Classification of Tumors*
(Chiefly based on Adami's classification)

TUMORS

- Blastoma **(body tumors)**
  - Hyaloma (Pulp tumors) (**CONNECTIVE TISSUE**)
  - Lepidoma (Rind tumors) (**EPITHELIAL TISSUE**)
- Teratoma **(extrabody tumors)**
  - Dermoid of ovaries and testis

HISTOGENETIC BASIS OF MODERN CLASSIFICATION

CONNECTIVE TISSUE

- **Benign (Typical)**
  - Fibroma
  - Lipoma
  - Myoma
  - Chondroma
  - Angioma
  - Neurinoma (Neurile-*mnoma*, Neurofibroma, etc.)
  - Myxoma
  - Osteoma
- **Malignant (Atypical)**
  - **Sarcomas**
    - Primary (de novo)
      - Round-cell Sarcoma
        1. Lymphoma (Lymphosarcoma)
        2. Spindle-cell Sarcoma (Fibrosarcoma)
        3. Mixed cell Sarcoma (Fibroleiomyosarcoma), etc.
        4. Steosarcoma Rhabdomyosarcoma
    - Secondary
      - Malignant analogue of the simple hyalomas; e.g., Fibrosarcoma, Liposarcoma, Myosarcoma, Chondrosarcoma

EPITHELIAL TISSUE

- **Benign** (Typical) **(Adenoma)**
  - **Adenoma**
  - Cystadenoma
  - Fibroadenoma
  - **Papilloma** and Polyp:
    - Squamous cell
    - Columnar cell (G.I. tract)
    - Origin and Transitional cell
  - **Melanoma**
- **Malignant** (Atypical) **(Carcinoma)**
  - Basal cell type
    - Basal cell carcinoma
  - Squamous cell (epidermoid) type (epithelioma) **SCCA**
  - Columnar cell type **(Adenocarcinoma)**
  - Spheroidal cell type:
    - (a) Scirrhous carcinoma
    - (b) Encephaloid (Medullary) carcinoma
  - Malignant analogue of benign lepidomata, e.g.,
    - Malignant adenoma (Adenoma malignum)
    - **Cystadenocarcinoma** (Malignant fibroadenoma)
  - Melanocarcinoma columnar or cuboidal cell type
  - **Mixed hyaloma**: Lepidoma, e.g.,
    - Adenolymphoma,
    - Adenosarcoma(Wirr's)
    - Lymphoepithelioma

18. MYOMAS

Benign tumors of muscles are of two types:

1. Leiomyoma—tumor originating from **non-striped (unstriated, involuntary, smooth) muscle tissue.**

2. Rhabdomyoma—tumor originating from **striped (striated, voluntary) muscle tissue.**

19. LEIOMYOMA (Fibroid) (Fig. 7.16)

Synonyms:

Fibromyoma, fibroleiomyoma, fibroid uterus, etc.

Gross appearance:

The size varies from a pea upto a voluminous growth of more than 5 kg.

1. Leiomyoma may be **single** or **multiple**, of various size, **dense, solid growth**, often becoming **soft due to cystic** or retrogressive **changes.**

2. They are well **encapsulated**, well **circumscribed**, occasionally **pedunculated.**

3. **Cut surface** presents a characteristically **whorled appearance** due to **interlacing bundles of collagen and muscle fibres** cut in various planes.

Microscopic appearance:

1. Unstriped muscle fibres running as irregular and interlacing bundles **cut in various planes.**

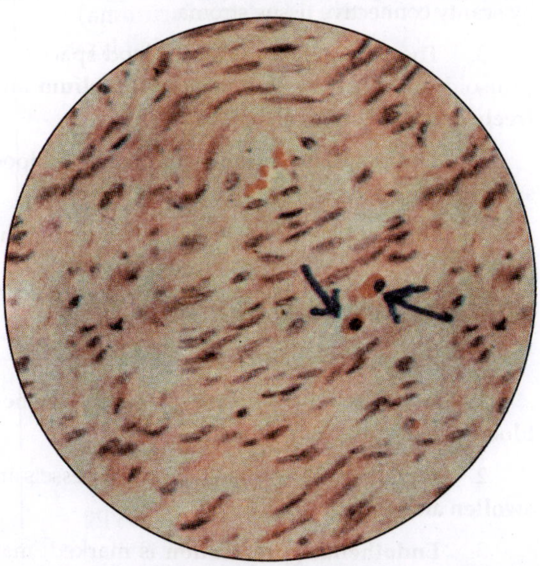

Fig. 7.16: Leiomyoma—showing proliferation of both collagen tissue bundle and smooth muscle tissue bundle (which should interlace and cut in various planes during processing and should form **whorl formations**). Hematoxylin and Eosin. × 240

2. The muscle fibres possess long rod-shaped **nuclei devoid of mitosis,** and look **yellow** with **van Gieson's (special) stain.**

3. The muscle fibres are intermingled intimately with fibrous tissue.

4. The fibrous tissue, unlike muscle cells, possesses nuclei with tapering extremities showing high (normal) **mitotic figures;** fibrocollagenous tissue takes **red stain with van Gieson's special stain.**

5. Hyalinized areas are seen round the blood vessels which is a **complication.** Other complicaitons are **red degeneration (hemorrhage and necrosis), malignant change (leiomyosarcoma).**

RHABDOMYOMA

It is a rare soft tissue tumor of the tongue, pharynx and larynx, and ***grossly*** represented by small, soft swelling.

Microscopic appearance:

1. Large spherical and oval cells.

2. Cytoplasmic content is glycogen and hence looks vacuolated.

3. **Special stain PTAH (Phospho-Tungstic Acid Hematoxylin)** stains the **cross striations** of skeletal **muscles.**

MYOBLASTOMA

The variety called **granular cell myoblastoma** occurs in striated muslces with appearance of **granular cells;** with **PAS positive** medium sized **granules** scattered all over the cytoplasm. They are sometimes malignant. It is believed that **they arise from Schwann's sheath** and **not from muscle fibres.**

It is called GRANULAR CELL MYOBLASTOMA but it appears to **arise from nerve (Schwann) sheath.** It has also been called **a tumor of uncertain histogenesis.**

HAMARTOMAS
(Fault, or Misfire)

Hamartomas are congenital abnormalities giving rise to **tumor-like manifestations, e.g., angiomas.**

ANGIOMAS

Tumor is composed of vascular tissue and may arise from: (a) blood vessels (**hemangioma**); (b) Lymphatics (**lymphangioma**).

HEMANGIOMA

A hemangioma is the new formation of blood vessels; often congenital. Chiefly, there are **four or five types**:

1. **Cavernous** hemangioma: It consists of irregular, **inter-communicating caverns** or cavity-like spaces **containing blood**.

2. **Capillary** hemangioma: It is composed of a tuft of proliferating thin-walled capillaries.

Other three types are:

3. **Plexiform** hemangioma.

4. **Glomangioma**—In nail beds and glans penis of Glomus tissue origin.

5. **Sclerosing hemangioma**.

SCLEROSING HEMANGIOMA

Microscopic appearance:

1. There is overgrowth of collagen (connective) tissue around blood vessels.

2. The blood vessels are prominently lined by endothelial cells and endothelial cells protrude into the lumen.

3. The blood vessels are narrow or compressed by (peripheral) proliferation of fibroconnective tissue.

4. The vessels may be **occluded** due to the compression by peripheral collagen tissue with hanging effect of endothelial cells towards lumens of blood vessels.

5. There is **extravasation of red cells** (due to narrowing and occlusion resulting in local high pressure of blood).

6. **Hemosiderin** pigment from damaged red cells containing lipids are all engulfed by macrophages that shows **Prussian blue reaction positive**.

7. A few **giant cells** may also be present.

20. CAVERNOUS HAEMANGIOMA—LIVER

Gross appearance (Fig. 7.17):

Forms a dark red or purple, circumscribed, slightly elevated growth; often single.

Microscopic appearance:

1. It has the structure of **erectile tissue**, being composed of **large blood spaces**.

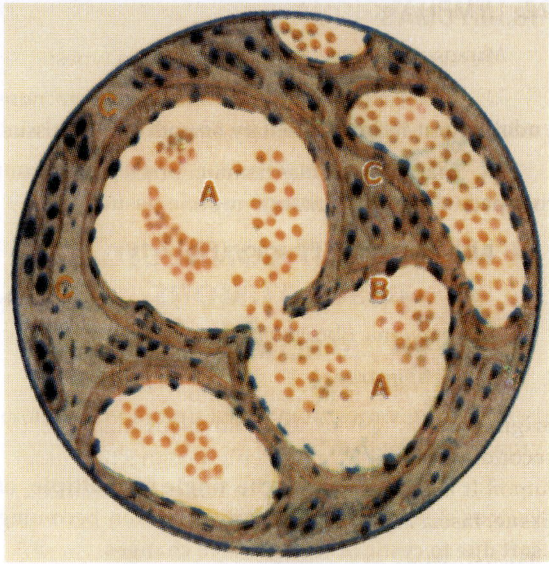

Fig. 7.17: Cavernous Hemangioma of the Liver—A. Two caverns (big dilated hollow spaces) are seen communicating with each other and they are partly filled with red cells; B. Endothelial cells lining the cavernous spaces characterized by plumpy nuclei; C. Partly compressed liver cell cords are seen as syncytium with 2 to 5 nuclei in the common cytoplasmic mass. Hematoxylin and Eosin. × 320

2. Blood spaces are separated from one another by scanty connective tissue stroma.

3. The thin-walled **caverns** (blood spaces) or sinusoids are lined by **flattened endothelium** and **freely communicate** with one **another**.

4. Thrombosis is fairly common in the blood spaces.

5. Normal liver tissue is seen surrounding the tumor.

21. CAPILLARY HEMANGIOMA

Microscopic appearance:

1. It consists of **network** of newly formed **blood vessels** filled with blood.

2. **Endothelial cells** lining the blood vessels are **swollen and enlarged.**

3. **Endothelial proliferation** is marked; may produce **solid buds** of cells that become several layers deep **occluding the lumen.**

4. **Supporting connective tissue** may also **hypertrophy**, but it is usually scanty.

22. LYMPHANGIOMA

Microscopic appearance:

1. It consists of well formed **spaces lined by endothelium** and supported by fibrous tissue matrix.

2. Closely resembles hemangiomas except that the space or vessels **contain** lymph.

MALIGNANT CONNECTIVE TISSUE TUMORS

SARCOMAS

Sarcoma is a malignant tumor of **mesoblastic origin**. They might arise **de novo (primary)** or as **secondary** change from a benign connective tissue tumor. It is commonly **seen in bone, subcutaneous tissue, fascia and muscle.**

Classification of Sarcoma

1. **Cytological:** According to the form of cell which predominates; e.g., **lymphocytic** (or **round cell**) **sarcoma, fibro** (or **spindle-cell**) **sarcoma**, etc.

2. **Histological:** According to the type of connective tissue from which it arises, e.g., **fibrosarcoma, chondrosarcoma,** etc.

USUALLY BLOOD VESSELS (or sinuses or spaces) are of EMBRYONIC TYPE (without ENDOTHELIAL LINING).

23. FIBROSARCOMA (Fig. 7.18) (Spindle-cell Sarcoma)

Microscopic appearance:

1. Spindle-shaped cells; nuclei stain deep blue and show abnormal or atypical mitosis.

2. The cells run in different directions and when cut transversely they may appear round.

3. Fibrils are numerous in intercellular (or extracellular) matrix.

4. The **blood vessels** are wide and thin-walled; they are **embryonic** type in the form of **thin-walled** blood spaces **without endothelial lining**, and which may contain malignant cells (metastatic) in their lumina.

5. **Tumor giant cells** are conspicuous.

In spindle-cell sarcomas, cells are fibroblastic, uniform and large. Cells also possess a relatively large amount of cytoplasm.

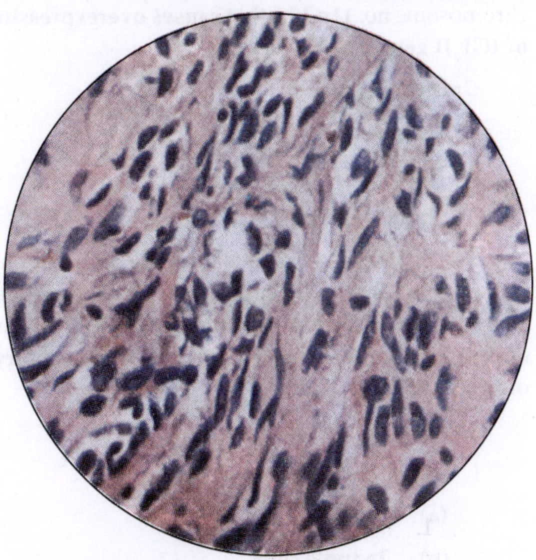

Fig. 7.18: Fibrosarcoma—The tissue consists of large spindle cells and a moderate amount of collagenous matrix, and tumor giant cells. Hematoxylin and Eosin. × 320

24. RHABDOMYOSARCOMA

Occurrence: It is the most common soft tissue sarcomatous tumor of **childhood** that may occur usually **within 20 years of age.** They usually occur in the **extremities** and **neck region**. It also occurs in **genitourinary (urinary bladder)** and **head region (nasopharynx)** where there is **minimum amount of skeletal muscles**. It also occurs in the hollow organ, i.e., **common bile duct**. When it **occurs in the vagina it is called sarcoma botryoides** or botryoid sarcoma.

Histologically they are of 3 types:

1. **Embryonal rhabdomyosarcoma** (including sarcoma botryoides in the vaginal muscle).

2. **Alveolar rhabdomyosarcoma.**

3. **Pleomorphic variant.**

Histological **diagnostic cells** are **round** and **elongated rhabdomyoblasts** with eosinophilic granules at the periphery of the cell. Rhabdomyoblasts are also called **strap and tadpole cells.** The cells possess cross striations. Sarcomeres (containing antigen) are seen by electron microscope, and **immunohistochemically** they are **detected (stained) by antibodies (to myogenic markers** e.g., 1. **Myogenin**, 2. **Desmin**, and 3. **Myod**[1]).

Embryonal rhabdomyosarcoma (including sarcoma botryoides) has parental isodisomy of the chromosome no. **11p 15.5 that causes overexpression of IGF II gene.**

Gross appearance:

1. Greyish tan
2. Soft
3. Infiltrative mass
4. Submucosal zone of hollow and tubular organs (nasopharynx, vagina, urinary bladder and common bile duct) form the **cambium layer** by virtue of hypercellularity in the **subtype**, i.e., **sarcoma botryoides** occurring in vagina.

Microscopic appearance:

1. **Rhabdomyoblasts**: They are
   (a) **Strap cells**
   (b) **Tadpole cells**

   Rhabdomyoblasts mimic striped voluntary muscle cells (**rectangular**) with **cross striations.**

2. **Rhabdomyosarcomatous tumor cells** are arranged in sheets of:
   (a) **Round cells**
   (b) **Spindle cells**
3. Stroma: It is a **myxoid stroma.**
4. Presence of conspicuous **tumor giant cells.**

25. CHONDROSARCOMA

There is swelling in relation to cartilage, which is fixed to the bone.

Grossly, it is a firm to **hard, globular round mass.**

Cut surface shows areas of hemorrhage.

Microscopic appearance:

1. **Numerous cartilage cells** that vary in size, shape and nuclear configuration and lie **in a bluish hyaline matrix** with formation of imperfectly-developed hyaline cartilage.
2. **Cells are polyhedral** and **widely separated.**
3. Band of **spindle cells separated** by scanty **fibrillary matrix.**
4. **Atypical mitoses** are numerous.
5. **Embryonic** blood **vessels** are **eroded** by tumor cells **with areas of hemorrhages.**

26. OSTEOSARCOMA

It may be **sclerosing** or **osteogenic** (or osteoblastic) osteosarcoma indicating more bone formation; or **osteolytic** (osteoclastic) osteosarcoma with destruction of bone, more than its formation. For further classification see authors' Text book of Pathology.

OSTEOGENIC SARCOMA (Fig. 7.19)

Synonym:

Sclerosing osteosarcoma.

Gross appearance:

1. The tumor appears as a **fusiform swelling** at the **end of the bone**, fading away on to the shaft.
2. It invades the surrounding soft tissues and may **involve the shaft, medulla and the periosteum.**
3. Fine spicules of bones are found radiating outward from the central mass, (X-ray—**sun-ray appearance** due to **periosteal reaction,** and **Codman's triangle formation**).
4. Consistency of the tumor varies with the amount of **bone formed by periosteal reaction.**

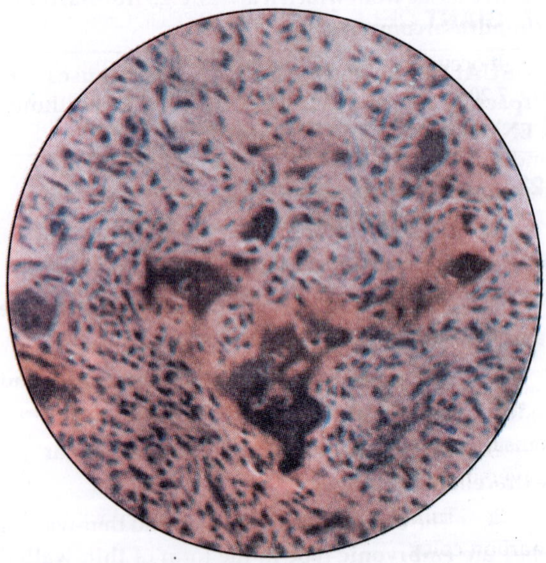

Fig. 7.19: Osteosarcoma—Several islets of imperfectly formed bone have been produced by differentiation from the surrounding spindle-cell tissue. Tumor giant cells are present. Hematoxylin and Eosin. × 320

5. The tumor is **highly vascular,** and **hemorrhages** inside any tumor may present **cysts filled**

with blood; necrosis; softening and degeneration occurs which are common.

Cut surface is variegated.

Microscopic appearance:

Features are extraordinarily variable, and complex; **pleomorphism** of cells occur; stroma is present. Some bony matrix is usually recognized at places.

1. The tumor consists of **small, oblong** or elongated **spindle cells**, but **large polyhedral** and **round cells** may occur with abnormal or **atypical mitoses.**

2. **Tumor giant cells** are characteristically conspicuous and specific; being irregular and atypical in size and shape, and contain **2-4 irregular, large nuclei** which are **oval, indented,** highly hyperchromatic and indistinct.

3. **Embryonic type blood vessels are numerous** and lie in close relation to the tumor cells. Endothelial lining of **vascular spaces** is lacking (i.e., embryonic type). They are often **lined by tumor cells.**

4. **Hemorrhage, necrosis** and **myxomatous** degenerative **changes** are very common.

27. GIANT CELL TUMOR (OSTEOCLASTOMA)

It occurs principally at the **end of the long bones Fig. 7.20** (metaphysis or epiphysis; **Fig. 7.20**). Common location is the **knee (lower end of the femur, upper end of the tibia)**, but may occur in any **bone developed from cartilage.**

Pathological fractures with "egg shell crackling teel" are characteristic. Soap bubble appearance occurs in X-ray.

Gross appearance:

1. The bone is greatly expanded; cortex is reduced to a thin shell. Surface gives **crackling sensation** when handled. Bony trabeculae are seen traversing the cavity.

2. Tumor mass has a **soft** consistency and a **maroon color.**

3. It is sharply limited (lineated) from the **healthy medullary cavity,** and **infiltration** of the **surrounding healthy tissue is unusual** (cf. Osteogenic sarcoma).

Microscopic appearance:

1. The tumor consists of **spindle cells; numerous rounded cells** during active growth.

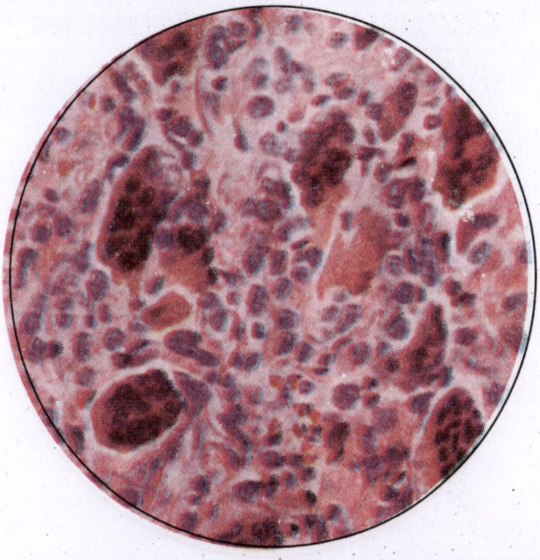

Fig. 7.20: Giant-cell tumor of Bone (Osteoclastoma)—The tissue consists of two cell types—Giant cells with basophilic cytoplasm and multiple irregularly distributed nuclei, and small, spindle shaped or oval cells with vesicular nucleus constituting stroma. Hematoxylin and Eosin. × 320

2. Numerous **large multinucleated giant cells of osteoclastoma type**; number of nuclei vary from 12 to 15, situated towards the centre of giant cells.

3. **Blood vessels are** comparatively **rudimentary** and in places supported by adventitia. Strands of fibrous tissue support them.

4. Areas of **myxoid** and **fatty change.**

N.B. The tumor is locally malignant and does not usually give rise to distant metastasis. It may recur after removal and may rarely cause metastasis.

HODGKIN'S DISEASE—LYMPH NODE

(VARIANT OF LYMPHOMA)—(HODGKIN LYMPHOMA)

Definition

Hodgkin's disease is a type of lymphoma **characterized by the proliferation of malignant reticulum cells, which may be monomorphic or polymorphic. RS cells, may or may not be** associated with **pleomorphic cellular infiltration.**

For classification, see authors' Textbook of Pathology.

Gross appearance:

Aggregated lymph nodes rendering **India rubber-like feel.** It may occur in any lymph node, or organ rich in RE cells, e.g., liver, spleen, etc.

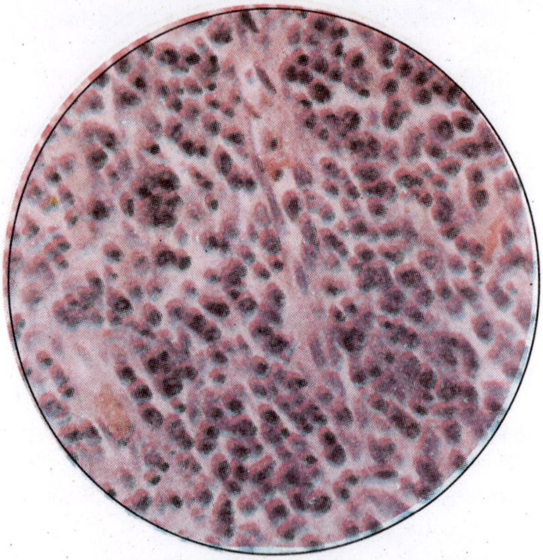

Fig. 7.21: NHL-Non Hodgkin Lymphoma—The cells which are small and round are uniformly and closely arranged and supplied by vessels lined by a single layer of endothelium. Hematoxylin and Eosin. × 305

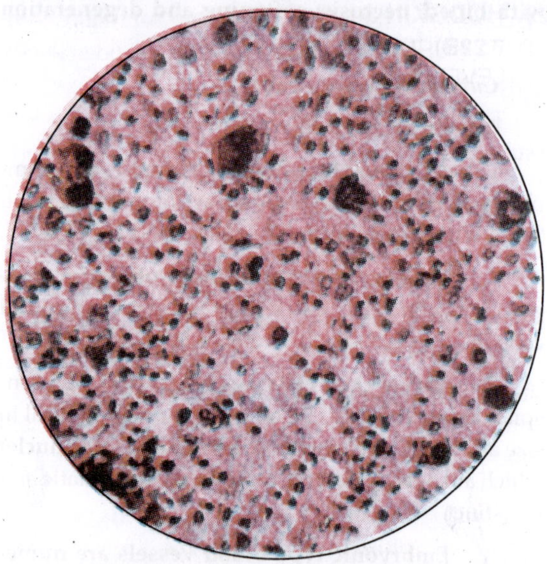

Fig. 7.22A: Hodgkin's Lymphoma—Lymph gland: The original lymphoid tissue has for the most part been replaced by medium sized cells with pale cytoplasm and vesicular nucleus amongst which are several larger cells (**Hodgkin giant cells**, or mirror image, or RS giant cells) with either several nuclei, or a single lobulated, or ring-shaped nucleus. Hematoxylin and Eosin. × 240. Hodgkin's Lymphoma of histologic Lymphocyte predominance type showing a prominent "POPCORN" cell with prominent large nucleolus which appear to look like an inclusion

Microscopical appearance:

1. Reticulum cells are present.
2. **Reed-Sternberg (RS) giant cells** [also known as Dorothy-Reed or Sternberg-Reed or **mirror image type** of giant cells]. It is a malignant endothelial cell, nucleus of which may be monomorphus or polymorphus.
3. Lymphocytes.
4. Histiocytes.
5. Eosinophilic leukocytes.
6. Neutrophilic leukocytes.
7. Plasma cells.

Of these, the most important element is the **proliferation of reticulum cells** which occurs primarily before the pleomorphism of cells have occurred.

28. NON-HODGKIN LYMPHOMA (NHL)

(LARGE ROUND CELL SARCOMA; LYMPHOBLASTOMA) (**Fig. 7.21, 7.22**)

This lesion starts in the follicles of a lymph node or Malpighian bodies (in the spleen) around the central artery; or in Peyer's patches, oropharynx, bone marrow and the skin.

Later, the lesion may involve the spleen, liver, bone marrow; peripheral blood may show the picture of leukemia.

Gross appearance:

The lymph nodes are **indolent, at first firm** and **then hard** due to proliferation of lymphocytes, but **later on** may become **soft** and **jelly-like due to degeneration.**

Microscopic appearance:

1. The cells are **round and large** in size.
2. **Intercellular substance shows** more **fibrillary structure**; fibrils being more abundant and greater in thickness.
3. **Nucleus** is stained deeply (**hyperchromatic**) and may show abnormal mitosis.
4. Blood vessels are embryonic in nature (without endothelial lining) and often lined by tumor cells.

29. HODGKIN'S LYMPHOMAS (HL) (Fig. 7.22A, 7.22B) CLASSIFICATION (AT MOLECULAR LEVEL)

This is a malignant tumor of lymph nodes. It has 5 subtypes:

1. **Nodular Sclerosis Type (Fig. 7.22A):**

   This type is a **lacunar variant of RS cells:**

   ***IMMUNOPHENOTYPE* (IPT):**

   RS cells are present as: **CD15+, CD30+, EBV-ve.**

   ***Morphology* (i.e. MPL)**

   i) **Lacunar cells** are present
   ii) Occasional **RS cells (DIAGNOSTIC)**
   iii) **T lymphocytes, plasma cells, eosinophils** and **macrophages**, fibrous bands dividing the cellular areas are present.
   iv) **EBV is negative.**

2. **Mixed Cellularity Type (Fig. 7.22A):**

   This type is a **mononuclear cells variant:**

   ***IMMUNOPHENOTYPE* (IPT):**

   i) **Mononuclear cells** (lymphocytes, plasma cells and macrophages).
   ii) **RS cells** (which are **DIAGNOSTIC**) are **CD15+, CD30+.**
   iii) **EBV present** it is +ve in 70% cases.

   ***Morphology* (i.e. MPL): T lymphocytes, plasma cells, eosinophils, macrophages** present.

3. **Lymphocyte Rich Type (Fig. 7.22A):**

   This type is a **mononuclear cell variant:**

   ***IMMUNOPHENOTYPE* (IPT):**

   i) **Mononuclear cells** (lymphocytes, plasma cells and macrophages).
   ii) **RS cells** (which are **DIAGNOSTIC**) are **CD15+, CD30+.**
   iii) **EBV positivity** occurs in 40% of cases.

   ***Morphology* (MPL):** Exclusively **T lymphocyte cells** are found in the background.

4. **Lymphocyte Depletion Type (Fig. 7.22A):**

   This type is a **reticular variant:**

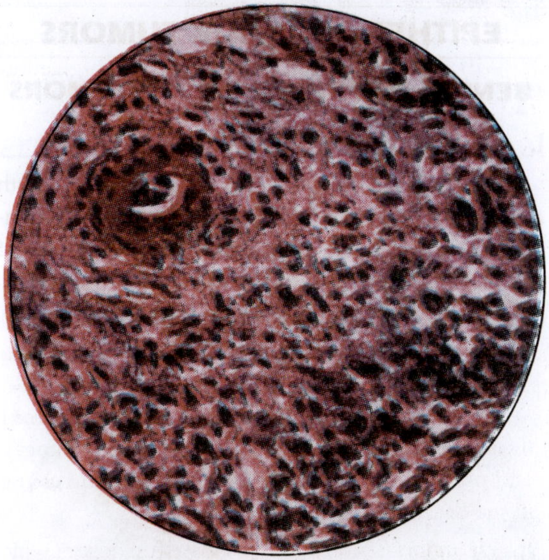

Fig. 7.22B: Hodgkin's Lymphoma—Spleen—Around artery of Malpighian corpuscle (above and to the left of centre), the lymphoid elements have been replaced by fibrous tissue, while at margin (right) the tissue consists of lymphocytes and reticulo-endothelial cells. Some eosinophilic leukocytes are present in both zones. R-S giant cells are conspicuous. Hematoxylin and Eosin. × 240

   ***IMMUNOPHENOTYPE* (IPT):**

   i) Diagnostic **RS cells** are frequent. RS cells are **CD15+, CD30+.**
   iii) EBV is present in most of the cases.

   ***Morphology* (MPL):** Background is made of scanty **reactive** cells (chiefly **T cells**).

5. **Lymphocyte Predominance Type:**

   This is a **lymphocytic (L)** and **histiocytic cells (H) variant type, i.e., popcorn cell** variant type. **POPCORN CELLS ARE DIAGNOSTIC.**

   ***IMMUNOPHENOTYPE* (IPT):**

   i) **Diagnostic popcorn (L & H) cells.**
   ii) **RS cells are CD20+, CD15–, CD30–.**
   iii) **EBV is negative.**

   ***Morphology* (i.e. MPL):** Presence of:

   iv) Background of lymphoid **follicular dendritic cells.**
   v) **Reactive B cells.**

EPITHELIAL TISSUE TUMORS

BENIGN EPITHELIAL TISSUE TUMORS

I. PAPILLOMAS (Squamous & Villous)

A papilloma is a benign epithelial, polypoid growth arising from the cells lining the skin, mucous membrane and ducts, and composed of a **central core of** connective tissue (a **capillary**) covered by epithelium.

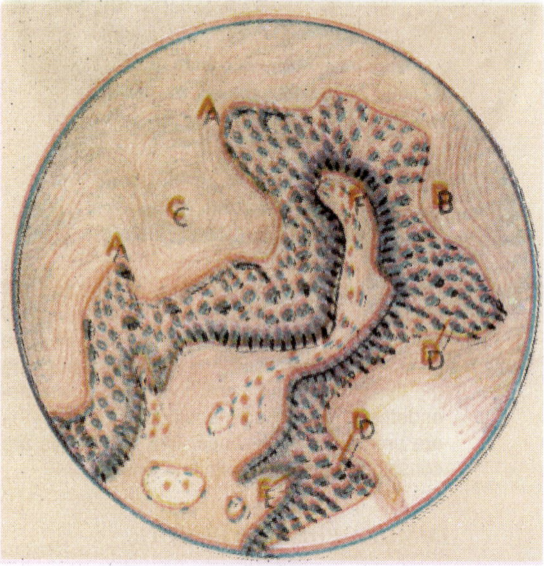

Fig. 7.23: Squamous (Cell) Papilloma—A. **Papillomatosis** (elevations) showing proliferated, raised cornified epithelium at the surface; B. Depression of the (cornified) epithelial cell layer; C. **Hyperkeratosis** showing marked, compact keratinization at the surface by keratinized epithelial layers; D. Showing **acanthosis**, meaning marked proliferation of the rete malpighii (prickle cell or squamous cell layer); E. Showing stratum basale (basal cell layer). By the two sides of 'E', **elongation of rete malpighii** is seen which is also characteristic of squamous (cell) papilloma; F. The **central core of blood vessel** (capillary) running from the deeper subepithelial tissue upto superficial subepithelial layer beneath the upper (or epidermal) papillomatous area

30. SQUAMOUS PAPILLOMA (SKIN) (Fig. 7.23)

Microscopic appearance:

1. The tumor consists of a **central core of** connective tissue, containing **blood vessel** reacting near about the surface and **covered by stratified squamous epithelium**.

2. The epithelial (prickle cell, i.e. acanthotic) layers covering the squamous papilloma are frequently much thickened (a. **acanthotic**), and contain a dense layer of keratin (b. **hyperkeratotic**).

3. **Elongated rete pegs** (blunt dermal interpapillary processes of epithelium) extending downward in the subepithelial connective tissue (**papillomatosis**).

4. Demarcation between the epidermis and the connective tissue of the dermis, i.e., the **basement membrane** is regular, distinct, and **intact**; there is no sign of invasion or breakthrough.

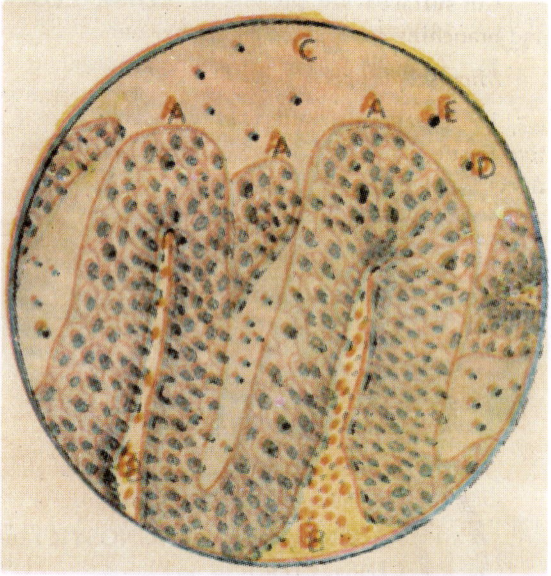

Fig. 7.24: Villous Papilloma—A. **Papillomatosis of** the **proliferated transitional cells**; B. **Central core of blood vessels** (capillaries) filled with red cells that track in the subepithelial tissue beneath the papillomatous area; C. Stroma; D. Lymphocyte; E. Plasma cell

31. VILLOUS PAPILLOMA—URINARY BLADDER (Fig. 7.24)

Microscopic appearance:

1. Numerous, long, delicate, branching **villous processes**, with thin vascularized connective tissue core.

2. The **central vascular core** is covered by proliferated **transitional epithelium** (resembling that of the normal bladder; superficial flattened cells are absent).

3. The **core or the central stalk** is distinct from the overlying mucous membrane. It consists of **scanty, well-formed connective tissue containing thin-walled blood vessels and large capillary loops**.

4. Cells are regularly arranged and there is no sign of invasion; **basement membrane is intact**.

II. FIBROADENOMAS (Breast)

32. INTRACANALICULAR FIBROADENOMA

Gross appearance (see Fig. 7.25, Fig. 7.59 also):

This is usually a nodular piece of tissue measuring about 4 to 10 cm in its diameter, which may be a round or oval mass covered by a relatively thin, glistening capsule rendering a greyish white or greyish pink hue (color).

Cut surface resembles soft fibroma with curved and **branching clefts lined by epithelium.**

Microscopic appearance:

1. Great **proliferation of loose diffuse connective tissue** which **invaginates** into the **wall of the ducts.**

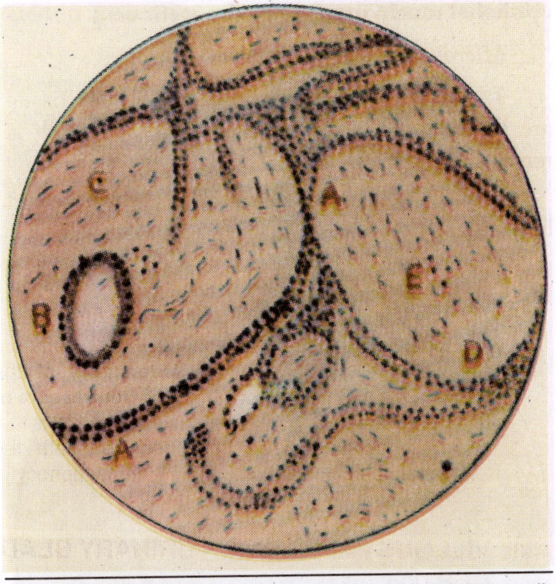

Fig. 7.25: Fibroadenoma of Breast—It is chiefly intracanalicular, but pericanalicular type of change is also seen at places in some acini. A. Intracanalicular type of compressed acini. The glandular acini at first become huge and dilated. Later, they are compressed by proliferating fibrous tissue and narrowed, being converted into chinks (chink-like spaces); B. Pericanalicular fibroadenoma where the round and oval glandular acini maintain their morphology, except for regular proliferation and hyperplasia of the lining cuboidal epithelium of the acini; C. There is mild infiltration of the collagenic stroma (wherefrom the word 'fibro' of Fibroadenoma appears). D. Fibrocytes are seen in the stroma; E. There is mild infiltration of the stroma with plasma cells

2. This growth of the **fibrous tissue contracts** to form **elongation and distortion** of the lumen of the ducts. In spite of huge **dilatation of the ducts,** they are converted into **chinks** (compressed **narrow spaces**).

3. The lumina of the **ducts** are still obviously patent and **lined by cubical epithelium** with **intact basement membrane.**

33. PERICANALICULAR FIBROADENOMA

Gross appearance:

Same as that of Intracanalicular type.

Cut surface is **white,** dry and **homogeneous.**

Microscopic appearance **(Fig. 7.26):**

1. **Proliferation of fibrous** and **glandular tissue** is characteristic.

2. **Distended acini** of **variable sizes** are seen lined with cubical epithelium. The **basement membrane is intact.**

3. Marked **proliferation of connective tissue and blood vessels** is seen around the newly formed acini **without invaginating the ducts.**

4. There is **no cellular infiltration.**

5. Fibrous tissue may show **myxomatous change.**

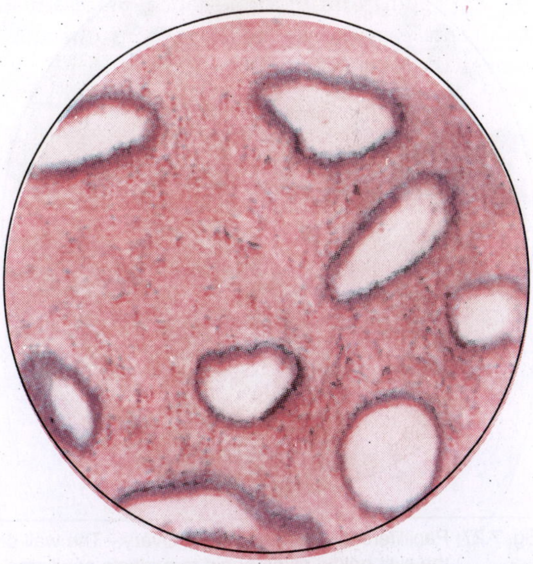

Fig. 7.26: Fibroadenoma of Breast—Pericanalicular type: The glands are regular and embedded in abundant fibrous tissue. Hematoxylin and Eosin. × 90

CYSTADENOMAS (OVARY)

34. [PAPILLIFEROUS (PAPILLARY)] SEROUS CYSTADENOMA (Fig. 7.27)

It is less common than the mucinous variety; slowly growing with papillary processes.

Gross Pathology:

The cyst is of variable size and of **round shape**. Markings of a few blood vessels are prominent.

On cutting open, serous or slightly straw-colored fluid comes out of the cyst. The wall of the cyst is thin and greyish white in appearance.

Microscopic appearance (Fig. 7.27):

1. The wall of the tumor consists of a layer of **dense fibrous tissue** supplied with numerous thin walled arteries and veins.

2. The papillary processes consist of fibrous tissue which are edematous and show infiltration with **lymphocytes and eosinophils**. The cyst also contains vessels supplying the papillary elements.

3. Intracystic projections are lined by **cubical or flat type of epithelial cells.**

4. The cells are more acidophilic and more granular than in the case of mucinous type. There is absence of mucin-secreting columnar cells.

5. Signs of malignancy may be present in the solid part of the tumor.

Malignant analogue is **papillary cystadenocarcinoma.**

In non-papillary variety, papillary (epithelial) structures (papillae) are absent.

35. MUCINOUS CYSTADENOMA (Fig. 7.28)

Gross appearance:

Size. Big football like.

Cut surface. Multiloculated cystic spaces containing **mucin** (viscid fluid), separated by thin, fibrous septa. Papillary projections are usually absent. This is **epithelial mucin precipitated by acetic acid.**

Microscopic appearance:

1. **Cystic spaces** supported by fibrous tissue are **lined by tall columnar epithelium**, which is remarkably uniform.

2. The cells contain the **nucleus at the base** and have clear cytoplasm.

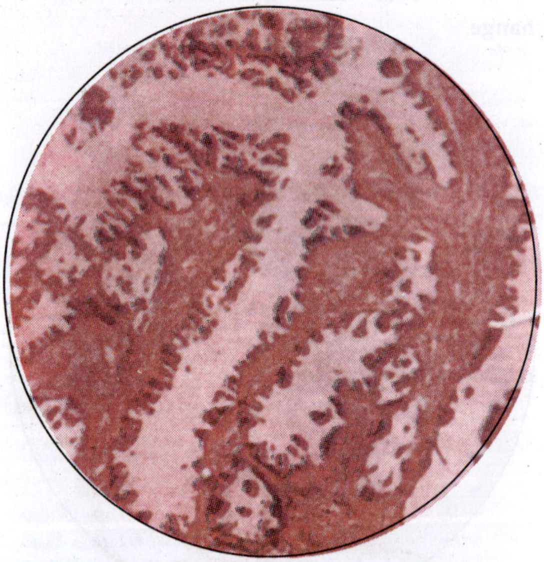

Fig. 7.27: Papilliferous cystadenoma of Ovary—The wall of the cyst below gives origin to multiple papilloma. These consist of a fibrous core covered by columnar epithelium and sometimes show a honeycomb structure due to the secretion of penetrating glands. Hematoxylin and Eosin. × 55

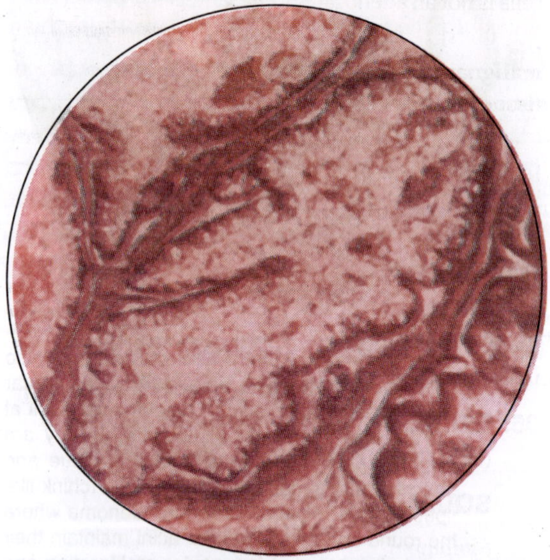

Fig. 7.28: Mucinous cystadenoma of Ovary—The tissue consists of glands. These are lined by a single row of strikingly tall columnar cells which have sometimes proliferated into papillomatous processes. The cells are distended with mucin and further amount of acidophilic secretion are present in the lumina. Hematoxylin and Eosin. × 60

3. Mucoid secretion (**Mucin**) present in **the cells** shows **goblet cell appearance.**

4. **Malignant changes** are rare; if at all, give rise to mucinous cystadenocarcinoma.

MALIGNANT EPITHELIAL TISSUE TUMORS (CARCINOMAS)

Carcinomas are malignant tumors which originate from the epithelium of the skin or mucous membrane of stomach, colon, gall-bladder, bronchi, etc. When they arise from glandular epithelium, they are known as adenocarcinoma.

HISTOLOGICAL (HISTOGENETIC) CLASSIFICATION OF CARCINOMAS BASED ON CELL TYPES

A. **Epidermoid carcinoma** (English), **Squamous cell carcinoma** (American), or **Epithelioma**: Arising from **squamous cell** of the **skin and mucous membrane.**

B. **Basal cell carcinoma (columnar cell origin).**

C. **Adenocarcinoma**: Arising from **columnar or cubical cells** from glandular elements (**Fig. 7.30**). Basal cell carcinoma though arises from columnar cells is not an adenocarcinoma, and is a separate entity.

1. **Scirrhous carcinoma (Fig. 7.31)**: Islets of **malignant cells** in preponderant **(ocean of) fibrous tissue**; in spite of this **prognosis** is **worse.**

2. **Encephaloid** (brain-like huge), or **Medullary carcinoma (Fig. 7.32)**: This is a spheroidal cell carcinoma. Highly cellular; practically insignificant fibrous tissue. **Prognosis** is much **better** than the scirrhous type.

C. **Anaplastic carcinoma**: It is often called spindle cell carcinoma, composed of **de-differentiated** or undifferentiated **anaplastic** cells. It is highly malignant.

36. EPIDERMOID CARCINOMA (SCC) (Squamous cell origin) (Fig. 7.29)

SQUAMOUS CELL CARCINOMA (SCC)

Synonym:

Epithelioma (from skin and mucous membrane), or Epidermoid carcinoma.

Gross Pathology:

A (i) **proliferative,** or (ii) **ulcerative,** or (iii) **diffuse infiltrative** growth in the skin and mucous surfaces. The growth in the mucous surfaces may occur as **diffuse infiltrative type.**

Microscopic appearance:

1. Masses of **proliferating squamous cells** of the dermal interpapillary processes, i.e. of 'rete malpighii which invade the lymph spaces of the underlying connective tissue: Nuclei are hyperchromatic and show abnormal or atypical mitoses.

2. **Hyperkeratosis**

3. **Acanthosis**

4. **ATYPICAL MITOSES** are of following types: (a) **Irregular,** (b) **rosette,** (c) **polyploid,** (d) **bizarre,** (e) **aneuploid.**

5. The **basement membrane is broken through** by the infiltrating malignant cells.

6. Formation of **cell-nests** (Epithelial pearls or epithelial horns or Keratin plugs) consist of the following:

The **cells in the centre become compressed, flattened** and undergo **keratinization,** and are strongly **eosinophilic,** often without any nucleus; basal cells and koilocytes (invading malignant prickle cells having **cytoplasmic basophilia**) undergo hyperplasia.

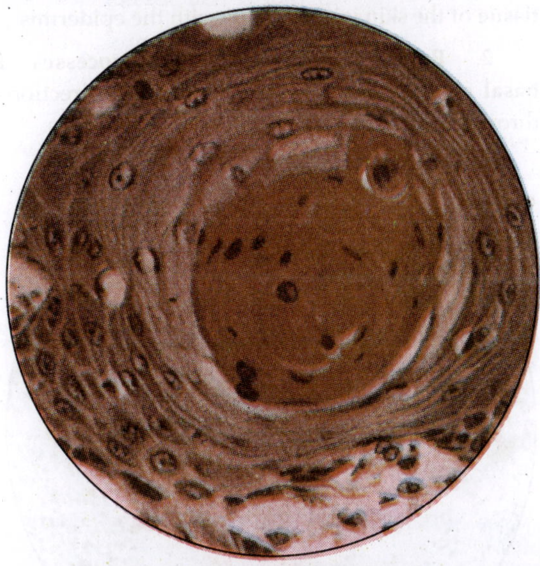

Fig. 7.29: Squamous carcinoma of Tongue—Typical "Cell nest"—The "Nest" is composed of several layers of flattened and compressed "Prickle cells" concentrically arranged about a core of homogeneous, strongly acidophilic hyaline likely to be keratin. Hematoxylin and Eosin. × 360

7. There is **individual cell keratinization.**

8. Prominence of **intercytoplasmic bridges.**

9. Peripheral cells correspond to the deeper and more actively proliferating layers of epithelium and **show whorl formation (epithelial pearl)**, which is a characteristic of epidermoid carcinoma in grades I and II.

10. **Proliferation of koilocytes** (partly vacuolated cells).

11. The connective tissue between the cellular masses is fibro-cellular and shows a **zone of lymphocytic infiltration** at margins of the invading column.

37. BASAL CELL EPITHELIOMA OR CARCINOMA (Basal cell origin) (RODENT ULCER)

Site of the lesion is above the **line joining the ear lobule** and **the angle of the mouth usually**.

***Gross Pathology*:**

Ulcerated piece of tissue may be sometimes **fungating** (Basi-squamous; mixed).

Microscopic appearance **(Fig. 7.30):**

1. The **growth** which **infiltrates the deeper tissue** of the skin is continuous with the epidermis.

2. **Papilliform** or club-shaped **processes of basal cells pass downwards** in various directions through the subcutaneous tissues, or the dermis.

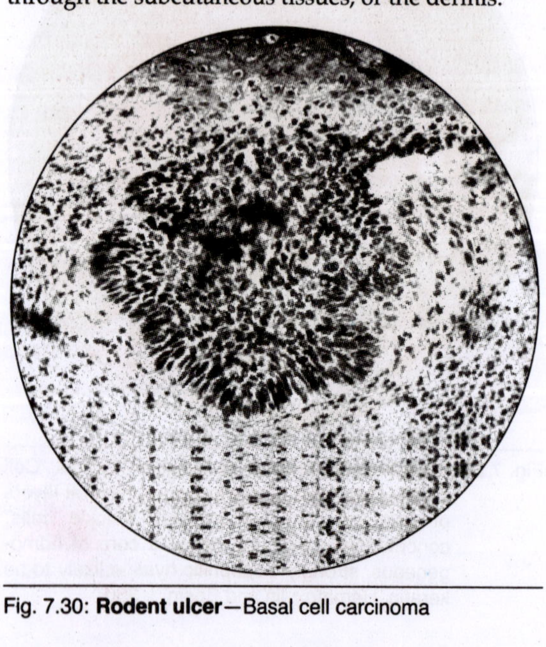

Fig. 7.30: **Rodent ulcer**—Basal cell carcinoma

3. The **cells** characteristically **show palisading arrangement** (palisation); they stain deep **basophilic** and are of **columnar cell** type.

4. Diffuse **lymphocytic infiltration** round the area of invasion is seen.

Sometimes there may be mixed entity of both **basal cells and the squamous cells.** This entity is better called **Basisquamous** or **Squamo-basal carcinoma.**

38. BREAST CANCERS OF SPHEROIDAL CELL ORIGIN (Fig. 7.31)

I. SCIRRHOUS CARCINOMA—BREAST

Microscopic appearance:

1. Scattered and **scanty solid masses of round or polyhedral epithelial cells,** varying in size and shape **in a dense fibrous tissue stroma.** Descriptively, solitary or **small island of cells in an ocean of fibrous tissue stroma.**

2. **Cells are spheroidal (round) or polyhedral** with granular cytoplasm, deeply stained nuclei showing infrequent **atypical mitotic figures** (see previous page).

3. In the fibrous tissue stroma, comparatively **well-formed blood vessels** are seen.

4. **Stroma** may be **infiltrated with lymphocytes.**

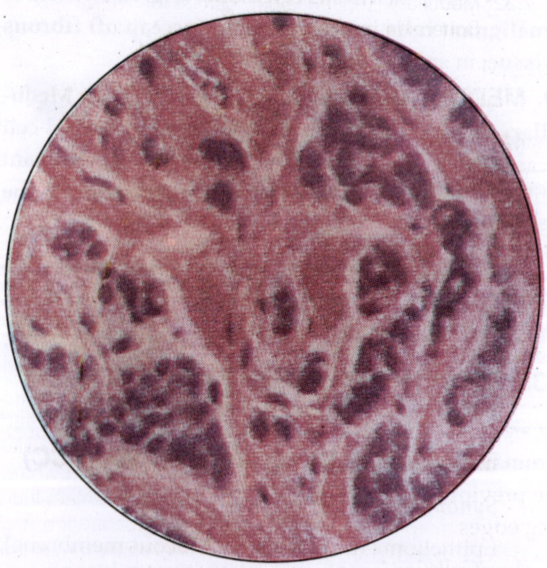

Fig. 7.31: Spheroidal-cell Carcinoma of Breast—Scirrhous type—The growth consists of small masses of spheroidal cells enclosed by bands of dense, hyaline fibrous tissue. Hematoxylin and Eosin. × 200

This tumor metastasizes more frequently than the encephaloid variety and prognosis is, therefore, ***worse.***

II. ENCEPHALOID (MEDULLARY)

History: 30 years old lady came with a huge lump in the right breast fixed to the deeper structures.

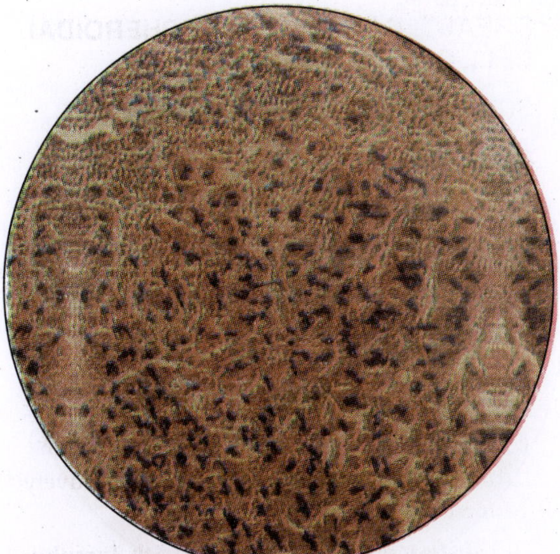

Fig. 7.32: Medullary (encephaloid carcinoma of breast; Spheroidal cell origin)

39. MEDULLARY CARCINOMA—BREAST

Microscopic appearance (Fig. 7.32):

1. **Epithelial cell groups are** considerably **large** and abundant in sheets, embedded in a **scanty delicate stroma** (cf. scirrhous).

2. Solid **alveoli are formed by** epithelial masses (due to pressure) composed of **round, oval or polyhedral cells.**

3. **Nuclei** are variable in shape according to the size and shape of cell. They **contain excess of chromatin** with numerous **atypical mitotic figures** (see previous page). Mitosis is common at the spreading edges.

4. Cellular connective tissue near advancing epithelial masses are seen.

5. **Cells** may **show** a tendency towards **degenerative changes.**

ADENOCARCINOMA (Columnar cell origin)

40. ADENOCARCINOMA (STOMACH) (Fig. 7.33)

Microscopic appearance:

1. Distinctly **aberrant glandular tissue lined by columnar cells.**

2. Cells are either **columnar or high cubical** with **hyperchromatic nuclei** and possess **numerous atypical mitoses** (see before; Page 103) showing evidence of increased activity of cell division.

3. Cells show extreme variation in size and shape and are often **arranged in solid masses. Lining cells are several layers deep.**

4. **Mucoid materials** stain **red with mucicarmine**; this reaction is specific (see mucicarmine stain, Chapter 1).

5. **Growth invades the muscular layer, breaking through the basement membrane.** Lymphocyte and occasional plasma-cell infiltration is present near the invading epithelium.

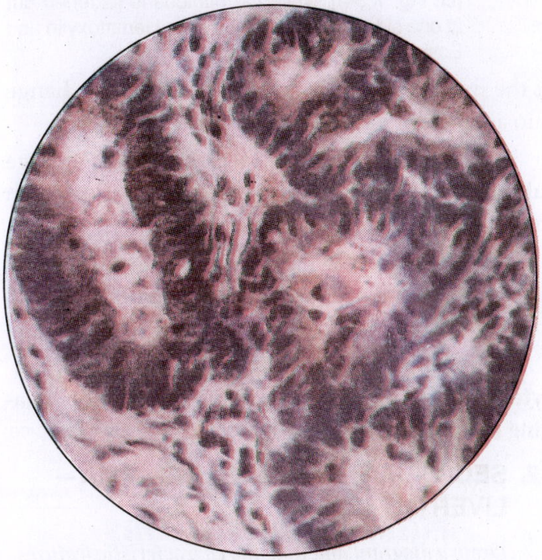

Fig. 7.33: Adenocarcinoma of Stomach—Glands are plentiful, but irregular in being lined by two or three rows of cells with hyperchromatic nuclei. Hematoxylin and Eosin. × 280

41. COLORECTAL CARCINOMA (Fig. 7.34)

Microscopic appearance:

1. Normal mucous membrane may be present

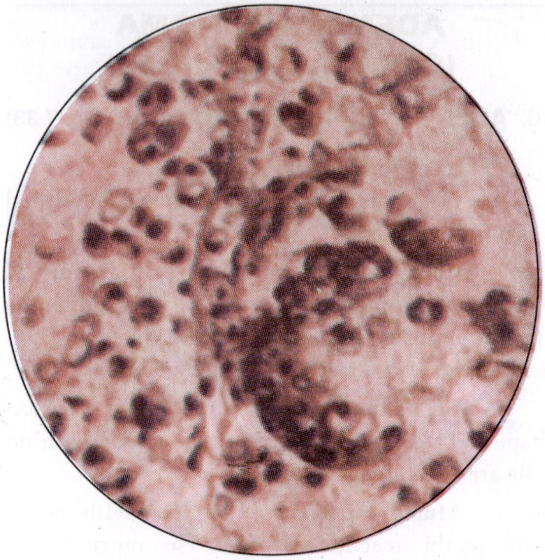

Fig. 7.34: Carcinoma of Colon showing mucoid degeneration —Numerous cells, isolated and also in masses, are separated by abundant, feebly stained mucin. Many cells are distended by a large globule of mucin [forming punched out fenestrations (windows) forming cribriform type of adenocarcinoma (cf. Fig. 7.34)], while the nucleus is flattened out at one side—"Signet-ring" forms. Hematoxylin and Eosin. × 360

at the time of malignant change. Malignant change into adenocarcinoma is often dramatically sharp.

2. **Irregular** and **atypical arrangement of large tube-like acini lined by columnar epithelium** with many **abnormal mitoses are seen.**

3. They are seen invading the **deeper structures through muscularis mucosae** and may extend to the muscular coat.

4. **Cellular infiltration is present; lymphocytes** are present in the neighbourhood of the invading epithelium.

42. SECONDARY ADENOCARCINOMA—LIVER (Fig. 7.35)

Draw a diagram and note the characteristic features.

Microscopically, malignant glandular formations in the liver are seen in lobules, which are distorted.

43. SECONDARY ADENOCARCINOMA—LYMPH NODE

Draw a diagram and note the characteristic features.

Gross pathology:

Lymph **nodes are enlarged** and hard to feel.

Cut surface. Capsule may be adherent. Patchy appearance of **cancerous deposits** at places.

Microscopic appearance:

1. **Malignant** epithelial **cells in glandular** or pseudoglandular **formations.**

2. Cancerous cells infiltrate at first (a) the **subcapsular region**, and (b) later on the **follicular region** and other parts.

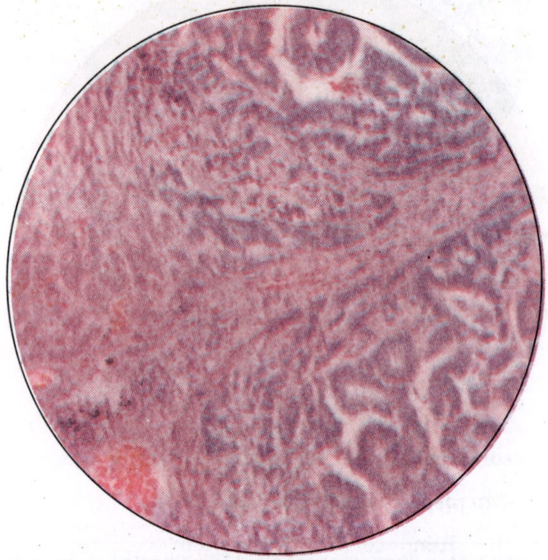

Fig. 7.35: Adenocarcinoma of Stomach secondary in Liver—The highly glandular nature of the malignant tissue is apparent. A portal lymphatic (bottom left) is plugged with new growth. The adjacent liver tissue (top left) is compressed into a pseudocapsule. Hematoxylin and Eosin. × 75

In case of secondary epidermoid (squamous cell) carcinoma (SCC) of the lymph node, features of the tumor are evident, may be **with cell nest or keratin plug formation** in the lymph node.

In case of metastatic spheroidal cell type of carcinoma in the lymph node, sheets of cells with fibrosis are seen (**scirrhous type**).

44. KRUKENBERG TUMOR—OVARY (Fig. 7.36)

History of carcinoma of stomach mentioned previously. It is a secondary tumor of the ovary, usually the primary being in the stomach. **Tumor cells drop down** from stomach on the ovary along anatomical (peritoneal pathway) and grow there.

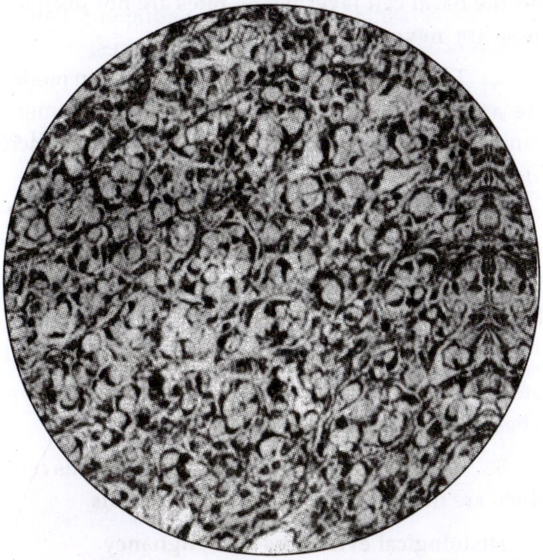

Fig. 7.36: **Krukenberg tumour** of the ovary. The tumor cells (T) are scattered, have mucin-rich cytoplasm, and are embedded in a reactive ovarian stroma

Gross appearance:

Unilateral or bilateral — often **kidney-shaped**. It is a **solid, hard irregular, tumor**.

Microscopic appearance (Fig. 7.36):

1. Tumor cells are arranged in **solid masses**.
2. **Cytoplasm is scanty**.
3. **Nuclei are flattened and pushed into the margin** giving a characteristic **signet ring appearance of cell.**
4. Stroma is cellular but variable.

45. TERATOMA—OVARY

[Benign: Dermoid Cyst; (Fig. 7.37)]

The tumor is often cystic and called dermoid cyst containing skin, hair, nail, etc. It may occur in many common sites due to the presence of totipotent(ial) cell rests, e.g., **sacrococcygeal region**, the **testis, ovaries, mediastinum**, etc.

Microscopic appearance:

1. The wall of the cyst which is lined by cubical epithelium shows at one place, a **nipple-shaped process** covered by stratified epithelium and it is known as the '**dermoid process**' shown by arrows.
2. **Mesoderm** is represented by cartilage, plain (smooth) muscle, lymphoid- and connective-tissue.

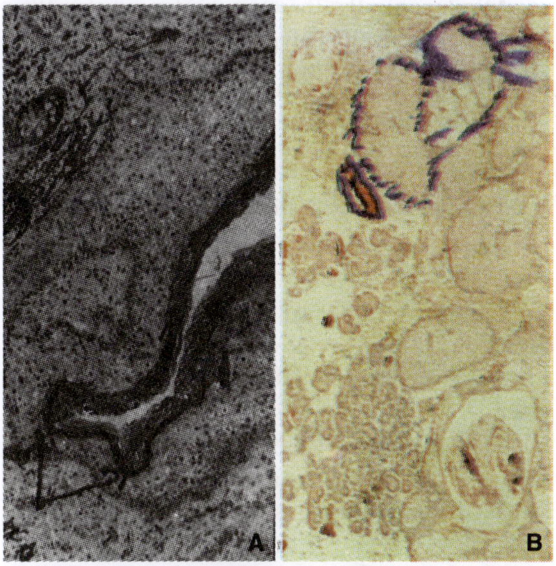

Fig. 7.37: **Ovary teratoma**

3. **Entoderm** is represented by glandular epithelium, and the **ectoderm** by skin and its appendages. Meticulous care should be taken during its surgical excision not to damage any nerve fibre.

46. PAPILLIFEROUS SEROUS CYSTADENO-CARCINOMA—OVARY (Fig. 7.38)

Grossly, it is same as the benign analogue, i.e. Papillary serous cystadenoma.

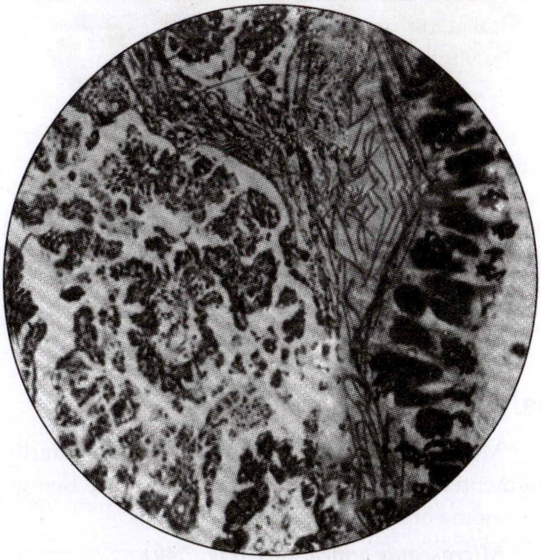

Fig. 7.38: Serous cystadenocarcinoma showing malignant acini and lining malignant columnar epithelial cells of more than a single layer, Hematoxylin and Eosin. × 400

Microscopically, there are evidences of malignancy (**adenocarcinoma type**).

47. MUCINOUS CYSTADENOCARCINOMA—OVARY (Fig. 7.39)

Gross pathology:

This is a **partially cystic tumor** of the ovary.

Engorgement of blood vessels are seen in the serous sac. It is of **bluish** and **pinkish** color at places.

Cut surface. Multilocular cystic spaces containing viscid mucin; papillary projections may be seen, and when present, offers **partially solid and cystic appearance**.

Microscopically (**Fig. 7.39**), the cellular features of malignancy (**adenocarcinoma**) are present (malignant analogue of mucinous cystadenoma).

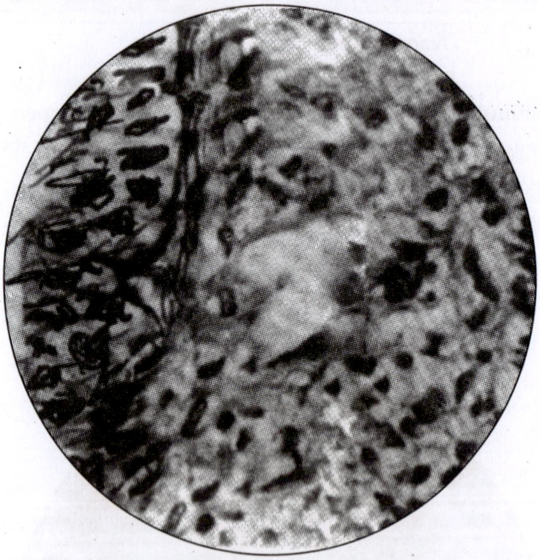

Fig. 7.39: Mucinous cystadenocarcinoma—Mucus secreting cells in more than one layer showing atypical mitoses. Hematoxylin and Eosin. × 400

PIGMENTED TUMORS

48. NEVUS—(Nevocellular Nevus)

Melanoma may be (a) **hard** or secondarily pigmented or (b) **soft** or nevus cell type. Benign Melanoma of skin is **Nevocellular nevus**.

Microscopic appearance (Fig. 7.40):

1. Sheets and **columns of clear, rounded or polyhedral cells** in the dermis (corium) often situated between the **downgrowths (rete pegs) of epidermis, and the basal cell layer** where **retes are not present**. These are '**nevus**' **cells**.

2. The cells are closely packed and contain **moderate amount of cytoplasm with melanin** pigment granules. They often form **alveoli (cell-nests)** separated from one another by collagen of the normal skin.

3. At the **margin**, these cells are often **fusiform, pigmented** (contain melanin granules) and are **called melanoblasts**; they are **dopa positive**. **Dopa is Di-Hydroxy Phenyl-Alanine.**

4. There are other cells in the dermis with elongated branching cytoplasm '**melanophores**', (phore = to bear) which are **dopa negative**.

5. **Malignant changes** take place in nevus cells which are **transformed into melanoma cells.**

Histological evidences of malignancy

(a) **Loss** of architectural **arrangement** of the **nevus cells.**

(b) **Increased vascularity.**

(c) **Deeper infiltration.**

(d) Often **cytological changes** of **malignant tumors** occur.

(e) **Inflammatory** reaction occurs in the stroma.

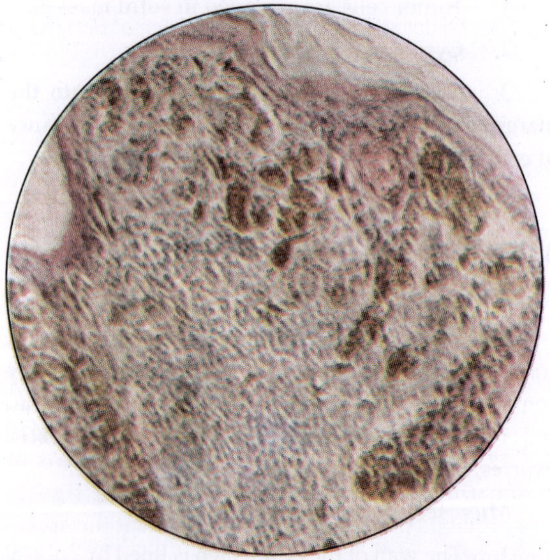

Fig. 7.40: Nevocellular Nevus (Simple Benign Melanoma)—Papillary type—The corium contains masses of closely set nevus cells, peripheral groups of which are filled with melanin. The overlying epidermis is thin and covered with a thick layer of keratin. Hematoxylin and Eosin. × 150

49. MALIGNANT MELANOMA—LIVER (Fig. 7.41)

This is a secondary growth.

Gross appearance:

Liver is enlarged, abnormally firm and numerous **subcapsular melanomatous deposits** are present.

Cut section shows innumerable areas of metastasis—usually black but may be greyish brown or yellowish white.

Microscopic appearance (Fig. 7.41):

1. **Spheroidal or spindle cells** or a mixture of both cell types.
2. Extensive areas of pigmentation alternate with equally **large patches, devoid of pigment** (non-pigmented melanoma) i.e. Amelanotic melanoma.
3. Large quantities of extracellular melanin in the process of removal by swollen **melanophores** (melano = melanin; phore = to bear), i.e. **Kupffer's cells** which are **very active (fixed) histiocytes** that line the liver sinusoids.
4. **Abnormal mitotic figures** (see page 103) are present.

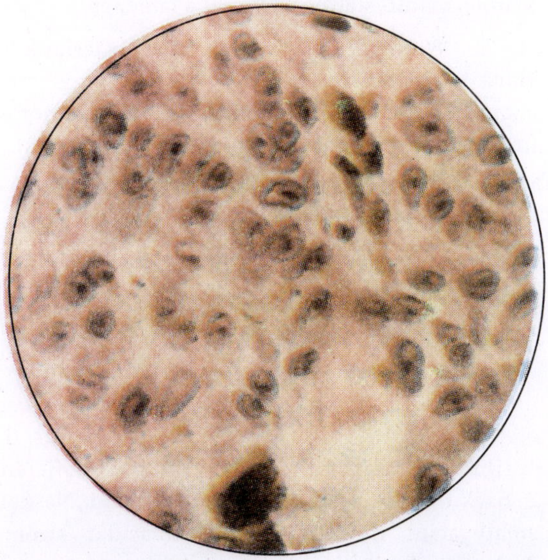

Fig. 7.41: (Malignant) Melanoma showing mixture of Spheroidal and spindle cells. Large patches devoid of pigment (amelanotic melanoma) may be present. Extracellular melanin is removed by melanophore (cells) which are swollen. Atypical mitoses are present. Hematoxylin and Eosin. × 400

5. The tissue is supplied with thin-walled, poorly supported blood vessels.
6. **Areas of necrosis** are present.
7. Hepatic trabeculae elsewhere may be flattened round the nodules into a **pseudocapsule**.

TUMORS OF THE TROPHOBLASTIC TISSUE

50. HYDATIDIFORM MOLE—(UTERUS)

This is a benign condition.

History:

25 years married female complains of passage of grape-like materials per vagina at several weeks after the last menstruation.

Gross appearance:

Clusters of vesicular bodies are passed through the vagina, giving the appearance of bunch of small grapes. They are colorless or just **greyish tan, somewhat round, shiny, glistening, soft and wet**. Each of them measures approximately 1 cm in diameter.

On cutting open, some clear, colorless fluid escapes and they become completely shrunken.

The fluid accumulates in them as a result of **hydropic or vesicular degeneration**.

Microscopic appearance:

Low power:

Large number of circular areas each outlined by a thin dark strand.

Dry High power:

1. The circular areas are **chorionic villi**, containing myxoid (oid = like) tissue with hydropic degeneration.
2. Two layers of trophoblasts are present,

   (a) **The cytotrophoblasts**, which are somewhat large **'Langhans' cell of "bull's eye" appearance**, and which should not be confused with a malignant cell (**Langhan, 1888**).

   (b) The **syncytiotrophoblasts**, which are seen in a syncytial mass as a **thin ornamented string lining the border of each vesicle**.
3. Some large **decidual cells (endometrial stromal cells** assuming large polyhedral or somewhat smooth spheroidal edematous appearance in pregnancy, i.e., **influence of HCG**) may be seen at places.
4. The tumor does not invade the uterine muscle. This is an evidence of a benign growth.

In this tumor and also in chorio-carcinoma, chorionic gonadotropin hormone [HCG] gives a **rising titre** up to **1:250 to 1:500** as evidenced by the immunological **gravindex or similar test for pregnancy**.

5. There may be formation of **syncytial giant cells** which **should not be confused with tumor giant cells.**

51. CHORION-EPITHELIOMA OR CHORIO(N)-CARCINOMA (UTERUS)

Microscopic appearance (Fig. 7.42):

1. Chorion epithelioma consists of actively growing islets of **Langhans' cells (cytotrophoblasts)** mixed with a varying proportion of **syncytial masses,** lying in a large pool of blood inside the placenta.

2. Normal relationship of the two types of cells is lost, due to exuberant growth of Langhans' cells through the outer syncytial layer. Langhans' cells are clear, arranged in sheets and are called **"Bull's eye" appearance** of cells. The **syncytial cells** often **form giant cells** (syncytial giant cells).

3. There is no definite stroma. The blood vessels are deficient and tumor cell might lie within the sinuses.

4. **Uterine muscles are invaded by the tumor cells. This is the surest evidence of malignancy.**

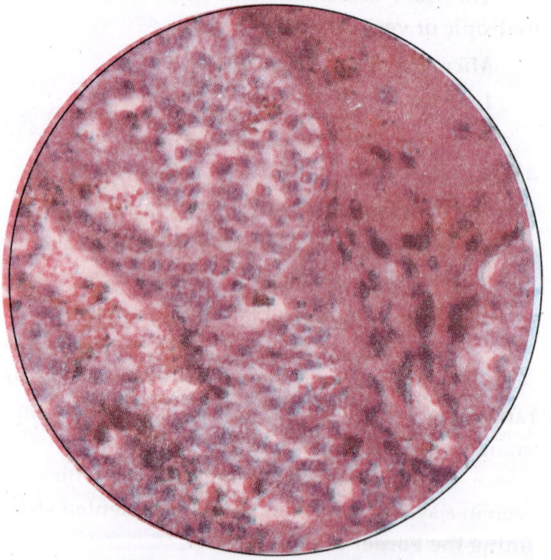

Fig. 7.42: Chorion Carcinoma—A mass of syncytium composed of acidophile cytoplasm and numerous irregularly distributed well stained nuclei are present on the right. The rest of the tissue consists of Langhans' cells with well-defined cell membrane, clear cytoplasm and relatively large nucleus. Hematoxylin and Eosin. × 150

The tumor usually metastasizes in the lung, and X-ray of the lung shows shadow of typical **cannon ball appearance**; on removal of the primary uterine tumor, the shadow in the lung disappears (hormone dependency in **hormone dependent tumor**).

MIXED PAROTID TUMOR

52. PLEOMORPHIC ADENOMA

History:

60 years old male complains of pain and swelling on the right cheek below the ear lobule (parotid region).

Microscopic appearance (Fig. 7.43):

1. Structure is diverse and pleomorphic.

2. **Cords and masses of epithelial cells** embedded **in a hyalinized connective tissue matrix,** enclosed within a well developed fibrous capsule.

3. Cuboidal epithelial cells showing glandular arrangement (**acinar structure**).

4. Mucoid **connective tissue** producing mucin (**connective tissue mucin**).

5. **Myxomatous material** simulating **cartilage cells** is homogeneous.

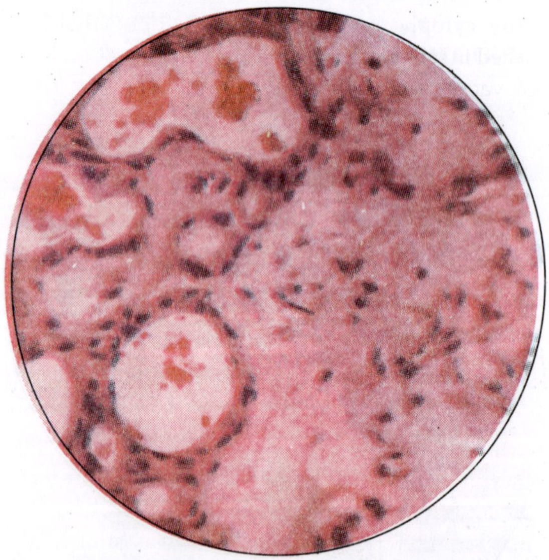

Fig. 7.43: Pleomorphic adenoma (Mixed parotid tumor)—The growth consists of two elements—(1) Glands of irregular shape and size with a lining of cubical cells and a content of acidophile secretion and (2) Myxomatous and Chondrous (cartilaginous) tissue. Hematoxylin and Eosin. × 300

6. **True cartilage cells** may also be present.

7. **Malignant changes** may be seen with hyperchromatism of nuclei and **atypical mitosis** in them.

53. CARCINOMA KIDNEY (HYPERNEPHROMA) or Renal Cell Carcinoma or Grawitz Tumor or Clear Cell Carcinoma

History:

70 years old man complained of severe back pain radiating all over the body. He was diagnosed as spondylitis; later on the pain spread all over bones and joints of the body. Kidney biopsy was submitted for histopathology.

Naked eye or gross appearance:

The tumor occupies one or both poles, usually.

It is fairly **well demarcated**. Invasion starts from the regions of origin (polar region). Later on distortion of the organ may occur.

Cut surface: It may show **variegated appearance** with hemorrhage as it invades blood vessels.

Microscopic appearance (Fig. 7.44):

1. Cells are large cylindrical polyhedral or cubical, arranged in solid sheets and columns.

2. They are stained pale, vacuolated or contain foamy cytoplasm (glycogen deposition; glycogen washed in tissue processing as it is water soluble) and look vacuolated.

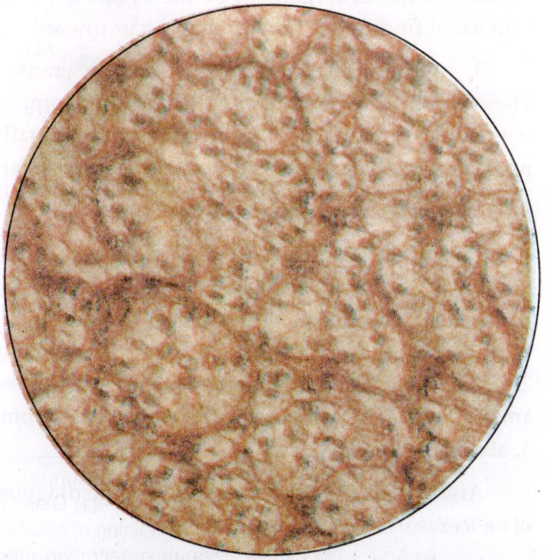

Fig. 7.44: **HYPERNEPHROMA (Renal Cell Carcinoma)**

3. The cells are supported by a delicate stroma with thin-walled blood vessels.

4. **Hemorrhagic and necrosed areas** are common.

> **N.B.** In certain areas cells are smaller, with a denser, slightly granular and eosinophilic cytoplasm, like ordinary tubular epithelium. Structures of tubules are seen.

54. WILM'S TUMOR (Fig. 7.45)

Synonyms:

NEPHROBLASTOMA, RENAL ADENOSARCOMA.

History:

10 years old boy complains of huge swelling of left side of the abdomen. He is also suffering from **dysuria**.

Naked eye or gross appearance:

It is a huge tumor, often cystic, encapsulated by a false capsule made of surrounding condensed renal cortical tissue. The tumor may destroy the whole kidney and spread to the surrounding tissue. It arises from any portion outside the renal tissue. The color is bluish white or pale-gray. There is less marked and scanty thin walled vessels. The ***cut surface*** shows wider areas of necrosis and hemorrhage and a variegated appearance.

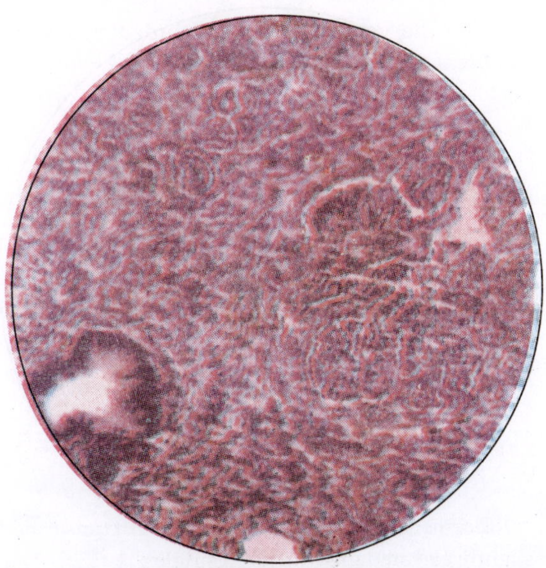

Fig. 7.45: **WILM'S TUMOUR** (Nephroblastoma)—Imperfectly formed glomeruli and tubules are embedded in a spindle-cell sarcomatous tissue—smooth muscle cell and fibrous tissue. Hematoxylin and Eosin. × 160

Microscopic appearance (Fig. 7.45):

It stimulates embryonic renal tissue with varying degrees of differentiation. The general **microscopic appearance is like that of a sarcoma**. The **cells** are either **spherical** or **fusiform**. Glandular **(tubular glandular) elements** are nearly always present and these tumors are then called **adenosarcomas**. Other elements, like the **smooth muscles, striated muscles, cartilage and bones** may also be present.

GENITAL SYSTEM

55. HYPERTROPHY (Benign hyperplasia) of the Prostate [BPH/BNH (Benign nodular hyperplasia); Fig. 7.46]

History:

60 year old male complains of dysuria, nocturia, and terminal dribbling.

The prostate may be large and soft, or relatively smaller, even harder. **Nodularity is characteristic**. The **lateral lobes** usually **are enlarged**.

Naked eye or gross appearance:

The **gland** is **enlarged**.

The **surface** of the prostate is **nodular** and may be **irregular**. The **cut surface** is reddish brown and **homogeneous**.

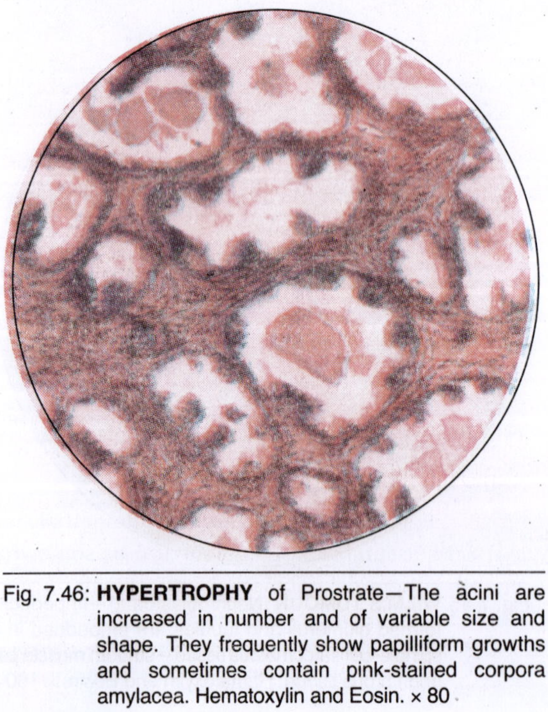

Fig. 7.46: **HYPERTROPHY** of Prostrate—The acini are increased in number and of variable size and shape. They frequently show papilliform growths and sometimes contain pink-stained corpora amylacea. Hematoxylin and Eosin. × 80

Microscopic appearance:

1. There is **glandular hyperplasia** with **overgrowth of fibromuscular tissues.**

2. The **acini are enlarged**. The **papillary process** of an epithelium may **project into the lumen**, or the **epithelium may project into the lumen of the gland**.

3. Each **acinus is lined by 2 layers of epithelial cells**, the **outer cuboidal layer**, and **inner low columnar layer of cells** which are **indistinct**.

4. Formation of **corpora amylacea** is seen in the glandular space.

56. Adenocarcinoma Prostate (Fig. 7.47)

History:

65 year old male complains of pain in the pelvic region. Serum prostate specific antigen (PSA) shows high level in blood.

Naked eye or gross appearance:

1. **BPH** or nodular hyperplasia has little relation with prostatic cancer. **Causative factor** is the **androgen** (in early age, 35 years or 30). But cancer occurs at a later age when significant androgen level is not there. That means in middle-aged subject prostatic cancer is already determined whose **carcinomatous manifestations occur at a later age**.

2. 80% of the lesion **starts at the posterior lobe**. **Hard consistency** by P/R examination is most **characteristic**. Enlargement of the organ is not an important finding (as growth may occur inwards).

3. **On cutting through**, there is a **gritty** sensation. There is no bulging out of the cut surface. The organ is not nodular nor lobulated; **yellowish islands of malignant cells** are the **positive findings on the cut surface**.

Microscopic appearance (Fig. 7.47):

Essentially the lesion is that of an adenocarcinoma with varying degrees of differentiation. Acini are well formed, but muscular element of the 1. **fibromuscular** stroma (tissue **sling**) **is deficient.** 2. **back to back arrangement of the acini**. Nests of **small acini invade the fibromuscular stroma**. 3. **abnormal mitosis** is few or absent.

Any one of the following favours the diagnosis of cancer:

(a) **Invasion of blood vessels.**

(b) **Invasion of the capsule.**

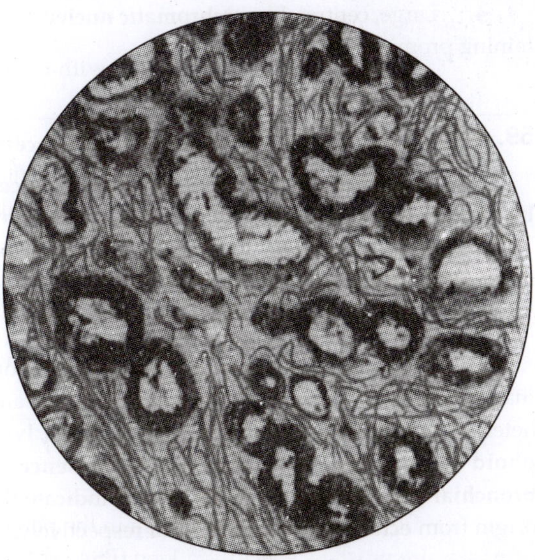

Fig. 7.47: **ADENOCARCINOMA PROSTATE**—The acini are lined by single layer of cuboidal cells as opposed to the normal double layer cells, the **inner columnar** and the **outer cuboidal cells**. Moreover immunoperoxidase staining shows **positive reaction with** the **lining tumour epithelial cells. PSA (prostate specific antigen)** level is raised in blood above 4–8 ng/ml

(c) **Invasion of perineural and perivascular lymphatics.**

(d) Instead of 2 layers, **malignant acini are lined by a single layer of cells.**

(e) Serum Acid Phosphatase above 3K-A units/dl.

In rare cases, glands and lining cells may undergo **squamous metaplastic changes** and the corresponding **carcinoma** may be **of squamous cell type**.

57. PENIS–CARCINOMA (SCC) (FIG. 7.48)

History:

35 years old male presented himself with **fungating, polypoid** and **cauliflower like growth** on the prepucial skin.

Most of the penile cancers are **epidermoid carcinomas (SCC)** and only a few cases may be adenocarcinoma (5%) arising from the **meibomian glands at the corona.**

Naked eye or gross appearance:

Grossly there are **three types** of epidermoid carcinoma.

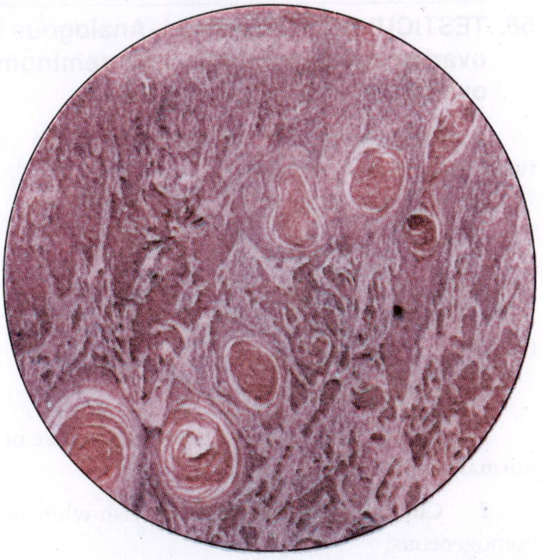

Fig. 7.48: **Squamous carcinoma** of **Penis**—The submucosa has been invaded by processes of growth of epithelial tissue; transverse section of some of which has produced several "Cell nests". Hematoxylin and Eosin. × 25

1. Proliferative **polypoid, fungating or cauliflower-like growth type.**
2. **Ulcerative type** and
3. **Diffuse infiltrative type.**

The most dangerous and invading type is diffuse infiltrative type of growth.

Microscopic appearance (Fig. 7.48):

1. They give the picture of **SCC** as elsewhere. The main features are
2. Atypical epithelial hyperplasia (**Acanthosis**).
3. **Break-through or breach in the basement membrane** of stratum germinativum.
4. (Downward) **proliferation of koilocytes** which are **infiltrating malignant** squamous epithelial **cells with perinuclear** halo.
5. **Individual cell keratinization** in **grade I** and **grade II SCC.**
6. **Epithelial cell nests** or **epithelial pearls** or **epithelial horns** or **epithelial whorls** are formed.
7. **Grade I** and **II SCC** shows marked keratinization and cell nest formations respectively.
8. **Grade III** and **IV** shows 51-100% cells undergoing de-differentiation respectively.

In case of adenocarcinoma, acini show **absence of basal cells.**

58. TESTICULAR SEMINOMA—Analogous to ovarian dysgerminoma, i.e., seminoma ovarii)

Testicular seminoma is a **testicular germ cell tumor**. There are two types:

1. **Classical seminoma** and

2. **Spermatocytic seminoma**. Typical seminoma cells are diffusely positive for the tumor markers **c-kit, OCT4**, and placental alkaline phosphatase (**PLAP**).

Naked eye or gross appearance:

1. Bulky tumor, may be **10 times the size of a normal testis.**

2. **Cut surface** is lobulated, greyish white and homogeneous.

3. Extension of the tumor may occur to the epididymis, spermatic cord and the scrotal sac.

Microscopic appearance (Fig. 7.49):

1. Sheets of uniform (and monotonous) looking **cells** which are **round to polygonal** in shape.

2. Cells have distinct membrane.

3. **Cytoplasm is clear**, watery-looking and contains glycogen.

4. Large, central, **hyperchromatic nucleus** containing prominent nucleolus.

5. Mitoses are variable.

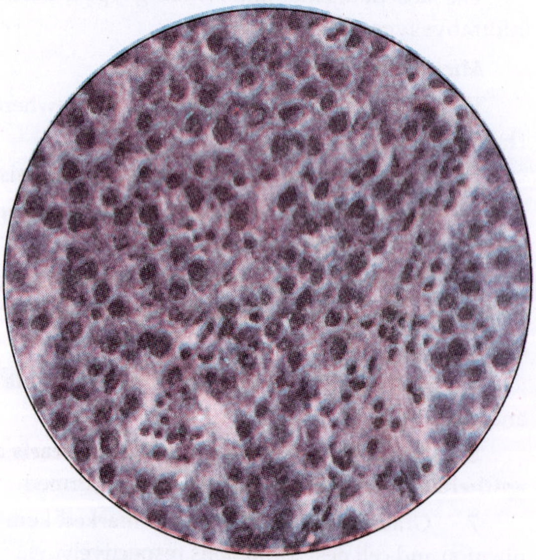

Fig. 7.49: Seminoma—The tissue consists of large, round or polyhedral cells with scanty cytoplasm and relatively large nucleus. The fibrous frame-work is characteristically infiltrated with lymphocytes. Hematoxylin and Eosin. × 350

59. Testicular teratoma (Fig. 7.50)

This tumor **arises from more than one germ cell layer**. They are large tumors of 5 to 10 cm in diameter. The **mature teratoma** that shows some **futile organ formation is benign.**

Naked eye or gross appearance:

The tumor is composed of various tissues (more than one germinal layer), hence they look solid and heterogeneous. **Cartilages, plain muscle tissue, lymphoid tissues arise from mesoderm; presence of bronchial glands** and **intestinal glands** indicate the origin from **ectoderm** and **endoderm** respectively.

Microscopic appearance (Fig. 7.50):

Collection of differentiated cells and organoid structures, like:

1. ***Mesoderm:***
   (a) Muscle bundles
   (b) Islands of cartilage
   (c) Lymphoid collections.

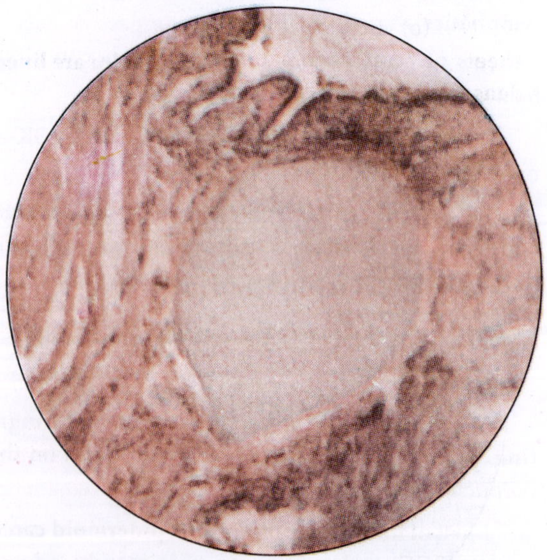

Fig. 7.50: Testicular teratoma—**The mesoderm** is represented by cartilage (centre), Plain muscle (left), Lymphoid tissue (bottom right), Ordinary connective tissue, and **The entoderm** by glandular epithelium (top right). The association of these tissues is suggestive of bronchial architecture. Hematoxylin and Eosin. × 350

2. *Ectoderm:*
   (a) Clusters of squamous epithelium
   (b) Thyroid gland structure
   (c) Respiratory epithelium
   (d) Neural tissue
   (e) Bits of brain tissue.
3. *Entoderm:*

   Bits of intestinal and bronchial wall.

All tissues are embedded in fibrous and myxoid stroma.

60. ENDOMETRIUM IN PROLIFERATIVE PHASE

Microscopic appearance (Fig. 7.51):

There are hormonal cyclical changes in the endometrial mucosa:

1. Glandular or acinar elements.
2. Stromal element.

(a) **Glandular elements:** Acini are tightly bound and compact in their outlook **lined by tall columnar epithelium with dark elongated nuclei at the bottom** (base), i.e., at the base of the cell in the cytoplasm. The acinar lumina represent empty spaces.

(b) **Stroma is dense, compact** consists of **sheets of "comma" shaped small cells containing dense dark blue nuclei**.

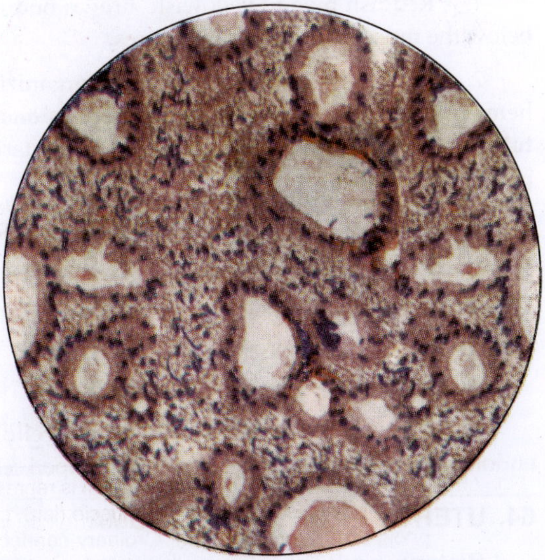

Fig. 7.51: Endometrium in Proliferative Phase—Nuclei of cuboidal cells are at the base. Hematoxylin and Eosin. × 200

61. ENDOMETRIUM—SECRETORY PHASE

There are three menstrual cyclic phases, i.e.

1. Resting phase
2. Proliferative phase and
3. Secretory phase.

Naked eye or gross appearance:

The endometrium is highly moist; juicy markedly edematous and a sort of **fishy odour; slimy, mucilaginous appearance** with prominent vascularity, and **marked vasodilation.**

Microscopic appearance:

1. **Mucous glandular change:** Outline of the glands are **tortuous**. The internal **luminal surface of the glands show "saw toothed"** or the so-called **"sea saw" arrangement**. The **glands** are **enlarged, dilated** and **tortuous**. The mucosal **columnar epithelial lining shows** somewhat soft and melted appearance. The lumina show **homogeneous, eosinophilic, pink appearance of the mucus present (in the lumen),** as well as those emerging from the secretion of the lining columnar epithelial cells. The **cells are full and turgid** due to the presence of the intracellular edematous fluid, and the mucus. The rarefied lightly stained nuclei are near the apical region of the lining columnar mucus containing cells and so to say, all the lining cells show **subnuclear vacuolation of the secretory phase** (as opposed to epinuclear vacuolation in the proliferative phase).

2. **Stromal change:** The stroma is fully edematous. The **"comma" shaped stromal cells** are set apart at a distance from one another by the presence of edematous fluid. Stroma is edematous. The **blood vessels** are **engorged, dilated and tortuous**. There are areas of **hemorrhage all through.**

62. ENDOMETRIUM—PROLIFERATIVE PHASE WITH CYSTIC DILATION OF ENDOMETRIAL GLANDS

25 year old female complains of excessive uterine bleeding and sometimes period starts long before the due date. Endometrial biopsy was submitted for Histopathological investigation.

Gross description includes the hormonal changes of endometrium at menopausal age.

This corresponds to the **endometrium of menopausal and perimenopausal women**. This is hormonal transitional senile age-associated with various

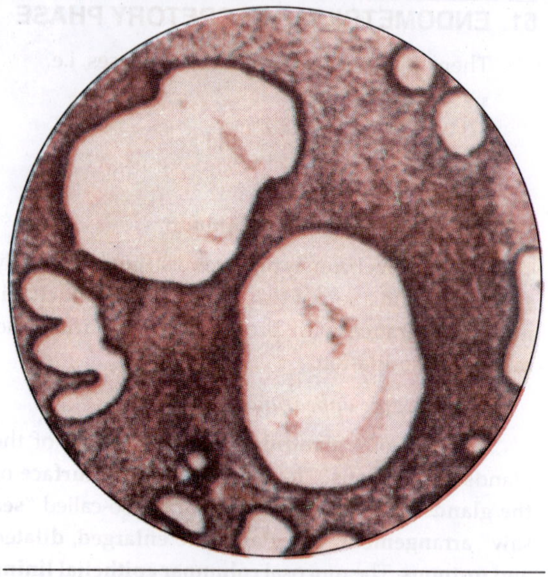

Fig. 7.52: Hyperplasia of Endometrium with cystic dilation of endometrial glands—The glands are irregular in size, shape and distribution and the largest two amount to small cysts. They are lined by well stained columnar and cubical epithelium and embedded in a highly cellular stroma. Hematoxylin and Eosin. × 50

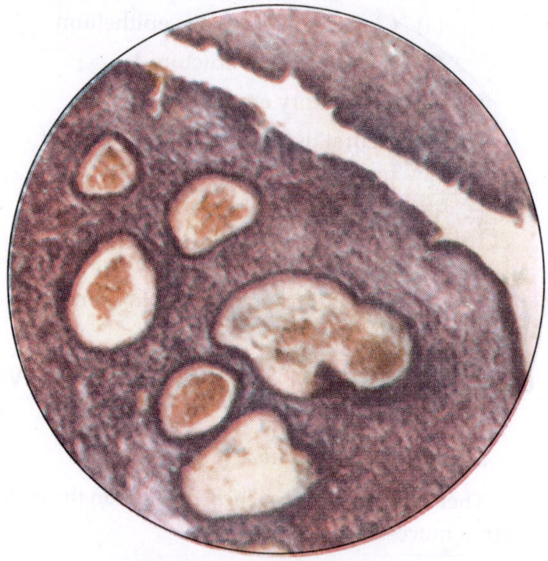

Fig. 7.53: Endometriosis ovary—From cyst above, an evagination extends downward and to left, several **glands containing blood** are present. To the right of evagination, cyst and glands are lined by columnar epithelium and embedded in a **highly cellular stroma**. Hematoxylin and Eosin. × 55

morphological changes in the endometrium. Usually there is glandular lining and **atrophy of endometrium with stromal fibrosis**. Sometimes, in this condition there is net progressive pseudohyperplasia under some type of feedback mechanism when there are morphological **"SWISS-CHEESE"** pattern of changes of endometrial **glands** comprising **inactive retrogressive non-functional lining epithelium of the glands.**

Microscopic appearance (Fig. 7.52):

1. Intermingling of 2 types of glands:

(a) Cystic dilation and enlargement of endometrial glands **simulating those in the proliferative phase.**

(b) **Small and atrophic types of glands** in the proliferative phase.

2. The **stroma** like that of **proliferative phase**.

63. ENDOMETRIOSIS (Fig. 7.53)

Endometriosis is the presence of endometrial tissue outside the endometrium. When endometrial tissue is present in the myometrium, it is called **adenomyosis**. Otherwise when present outside the uterus, it is called endometriosis, e.g., **(a) ovaries, (b) uterine ligaments, (c) rectovaginal septum, (d) cul de sac, (e) pelvic ligament, (f) large and small intestine, and the appendix, (g) mucosa of the cervix, vagina, and fallopian tubes, (h) laparotomy scars**, etc.

Naked eye or gross appearance:

1. Reddish blue to yellowish brown nodules below the mucosal and serosal surfaces.

2. In widespread involvement, organizing hemorrhage causes **extensive fibrous adhesions in tubes and the ovaries that obliterate** the recto-uterine **pouch of Douglas.**

3. **In the ovaries large cystic masses** may occur.

Microscopic appearance (Fig. 7.53):

1. Endometrial glands are lined by columnar epithelial cells.

2. Most of the glands contain blood.

3. Glands are embedded in a highly cellular endometrial stroma containing **"comma"** shaped cells.

64. UTERUS—ADENOCARCINOMA

History:

58 year old lady came with the complaints of **irregular painful bleeding, P/V off and on.** Dilation

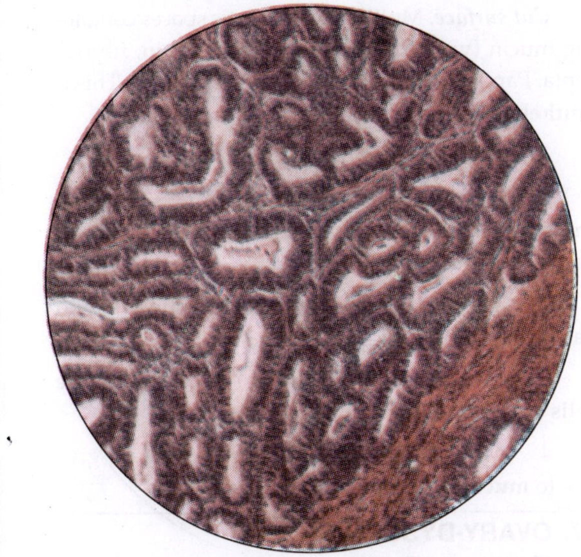

Fig. 7.54: Adenocarcinoma of Corpus uteri—The glands composing the tumor are well formed and lined by columnar epithelium, but vary in size and shape and occasionally have papilliform in the growth with back to back arrangement of glands. Hematoxylin and Eosin. × 75

and curettage (D & C) was done, and the material was submitted for histopathological examination.

The tumor has **3 stages: Stage I, II** and **III**.

Naked eye or gross appearance:

The tumor starts in the endometrium at the fundus of the uterus. It spreads diffusely on the superficial aspect of endometrium and form thick, rough, polypoid mass before its myometrial invasion. Often the tumor is of **papillary type**. The uterus is enlarged. The tumor is bulky and friable often with necrotic areas.

Microscopic appearance (Fig. 7.54):

The lesion is essentially an adenocarcinoma with well-differentiated glandular structures. The glandular arrangements are very close and is called **"back to back" arrangement** with irregular placement of glands. More than one glands invade the basement membrane of another and coalesce.

In **anaplastic form**, the glandular lining consists of malignant cells that show hyperchromatic nuclei with **atypical mitoses** of the nuclei.

There is tendency of the malignant acini to penetrate the myometrium deeply.

In rare cases, there is metaplastic change of columnar cells towards conversion to squamous form when the tumor directs to form **adenoacanthoma** and **epidermoid carcinoma (SCC)**.

65. LEIOMYOMA [(Fibroid) Fibroleiomyoma]

History:

40 year old lady complains of pain in the loin, and massive uterine bleeding. P/V examination showed a mass continuous with the uterus.

Synonyms:

Fibromyoma, fibroleiomyoma, fibroid uterus, etc.

Naked eye or gross appearance:

1. Leiomyoma may be single or multiple, of various sizes, dense, solid growth, often becoming soft due to cystic and retrogressive changes.

2. They are well encapsulated, well circumscribed, and occasionally pedunculated.

3. **Cut surface** presents a characteristically **whorled appearance due to interlacing bundles** of muscle fibres and collagen fibres cut in various plane.

Microscopic appearance (Fig. 7.55):

1. Unstriped muscle fibres running in various directions forming interlacing muscle and collagen-bundles cut in various planes.

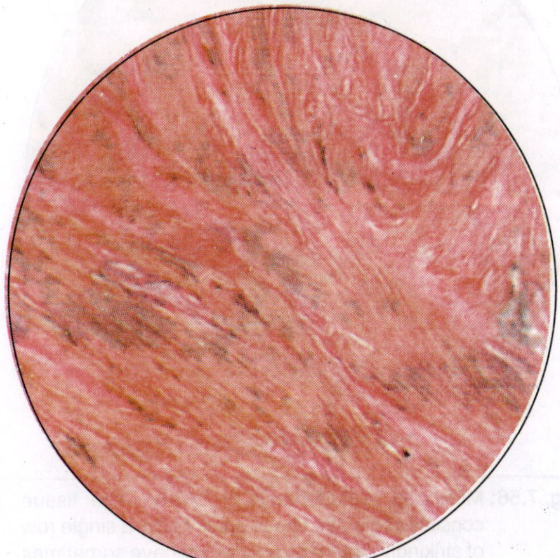

Fig. 7.55: Fibroleiomyoma—Interlacing bundles of plain muscle (yellow), and Fibrous tissue (pink) as seen by van Gieson stain. Hematoxylin and Eosin. × 75

2. The **muscle fibres** possess long **rod-shaped nuclei**, and take yellow color with van Gieson's stain (special stain).

3. The **fibrous tissue**, unlike muscle cells, possesses nuclei with **tapering extremities** showing highly increased (**normal**) **mitotic figures**; fibrous tissue takes the red color with van Gieson's stain (special stain for collagen-red, and smooth muscle-yellow).

4. Hyalinized areas are seen round the blood vessels.

5. Areas of hemorrhage and degeneration [hemorrhagic (red) degeneration] present.

66. OVARY-MUCINOUS CYSTADENOMA

History:

25 years old lady was complaining of unilateral heaviness in the pelvis. On palpation a mass was found on the right pelvic region. It was operated and submitted for histopathology.

Naked eye or gross appearance:

Size: Big soccer (football)-like.

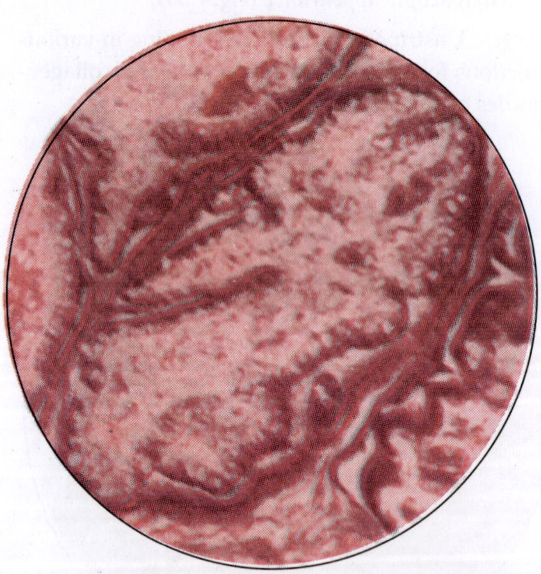

Fig. 7.56: Mucinous cystadenoma of Ovary—The tissue consists of glands. These are lined by a single row of strikingly columnar cells which have sometimes proliferated into papillomatous processes. The cells are distended with mucin and further amount of this acidophile secretion is present in the lumina. Hematoxylin and Eosin. × 60

Cut surface. Multiloculated cystic spaces containing mucin (viscid fluid), separated by thin, fibrous septa. Papillary projections are usually absent. This is **epithelial mucin precipitated by acetic acid**.

Microscopic appearance (Fig. 7.56):

1. Cystic spaces supported by fibrous tissue are **lined by tall columnar epithelium**, which is remarkably uniform.

2. The cells contain the **nucleus at the base** and have clear cytoplasm.

3. Mucoid secretion (mucin)* is present **in the cells** that show **goblet cell appearance**.

4. **Malignant changes** are rare, if at all, give rise to **mucinous cystadenocarcinoma**.

67. OVARY-DYSGERMINOMA

(Seminoma Ovarii)

See testicular seminoma see Fig. 7.25.

History:

30 years old lady complained of heaviness on the left pelvis. Operation was done. A lump was found and submitted for histopathological examination.

It arises from cell rests of undifferentiated mesenchyme in the gonad which fails to grow either to the **male or to female direction**.

It occurs before 35 years of age mostly in children and young adolescents.

Naked eye or gross appearance:

It is a huge tumor of rubbery consistency and is pinkish in colour, friable and encapsulated.

The **cut surface** is yellowish due to fatty change.

Microscopic appearance (Fig. 7.57):

The tumor cells are uniformly large, monotonous looking spherical cells with vesicular nuclei in them. The cells are **grouped in solid masses of alveoli** separated by connective tissue septa. There is a large number of **lymphocytic infiltration**.

Usually abnormal or **atypical mitoses are present** and the **number of abnormal mitoses determines the prognosis of a particular case**.

Virchow's left sided **supraclavicular** lymph node is the important site for the extrapelvic and **distant** metastasis.

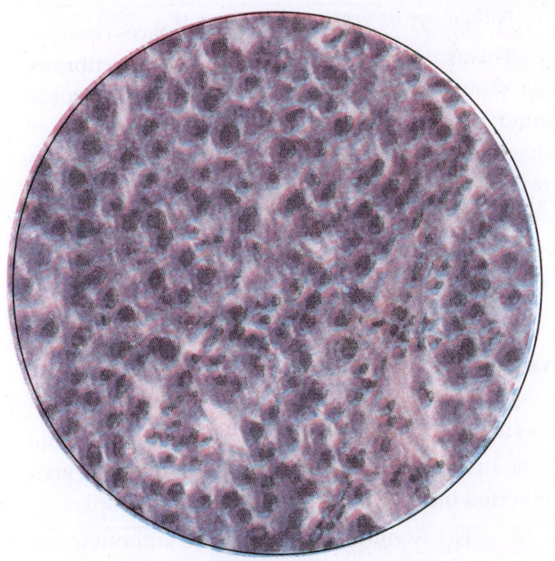

Fig. 7.57: Dysgerminoma—The tissue consists of large, round or polyhedral cells with scanty cytoplasm and relatively large nucleus. The fibrous frame-work is characteristically infiltrated with lymphocytes. Hematoxylin and Eosin. × 350

The tumor is less malignant than the granular **cell tumor.**

68. TERATOMA-OVARY

History:

25 years old lady was complaining of unilateral heaviness in the pelvis. On palpation, a mass was found on the right pelvic region. It was operated and submitted for histopathology.

Gross appearance:

The tumor is often cystic and called dermoid cyst of the ovary containing skin, hair, nail, etc. It may occur in many common sites due to the presence of **toti-potential cell rests, e.g., sacrococcygeal region,** the **testis, ovaries, mediastinum,** etc.

Microscopic appearance (Fig. 7.58A & B):

1. The wall of the cyst is lined by cubical epithelium at one place; a **nipple-shaped process** covered by stratified epithelium is seen which is known as the **dermoid process** (Fig. 7.58A).
2. **Mesoderm** is represented by **cartilage, plain muscle, lymphoid tissue** and **connective tissue**.
3. **Endoderm** is represented by **glandular epithelium**, and the **ectoderm by skin and its appendages.**

BREAST (Revision)

69. FIBROADENOMAS

A. Intracanalicular Fibroadenomas (Breast)

History:

25 years old female complained of a big breast causing heaviness for one year. On clinical examination a mobile mass (not fixed to the deeper structure)

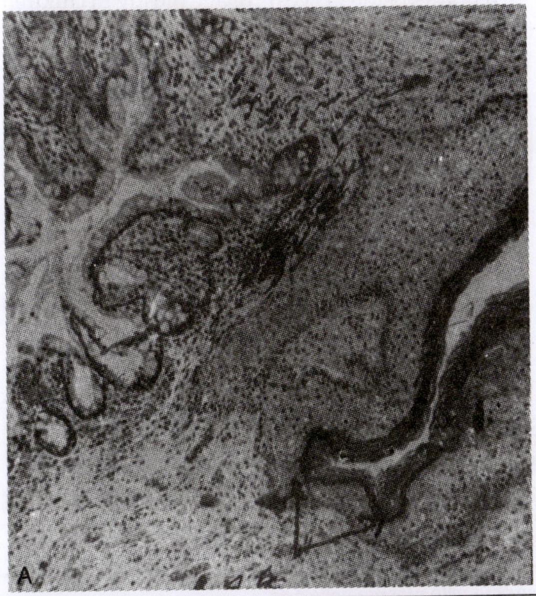

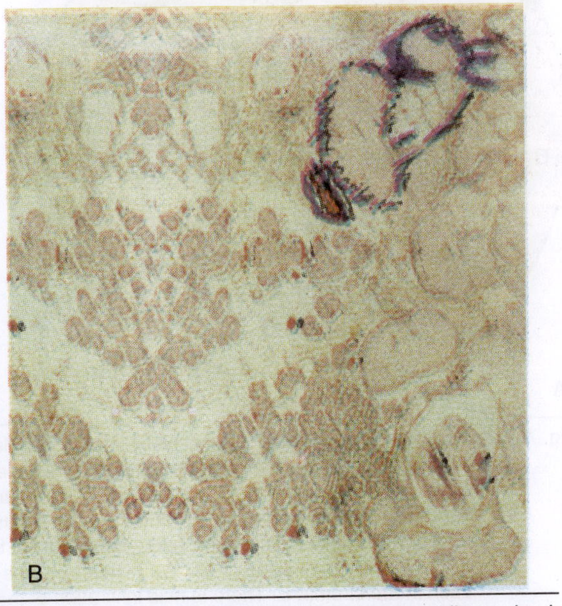

Fig. 7.58A & B: (Usually benign, i.e. Mature Teratoma of Ovary i.e., Dermoid Cyst >95%). Left half showing salivary gland; Right half showing sebaceous glands and hair follicles

was felt in the respective breast. The mass was operated and sent for histopathology.

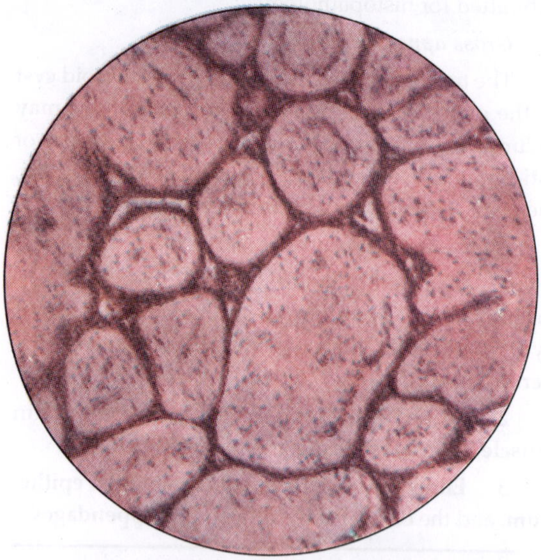

Fig. 7.59: Fibroadenoma of Breast—Intracanalicular type—The glands are stretched and distorted by an ingrowth of fibrous tissue in the form of blunt, rounded projections. Hematoxylin and Eosin. × 80

Naked eye or gross appearance (Fig. 7.59):

This is usually a nodular piece of tissue measuring about 4 to 10 cm in its diameter, which may be a round or oval mass covered by a relatively thin, glistening capsule rendering a greyish white or grayish pink or bluish gray color.

Cut surface resembles soft fibroma with curved and branching clefts lined by cubical epithelium.

Microscopic appearance (Fig. 7.60A):

1. Great **proliferation of loose diffuse connective tissue** that **invaginates** into the wall of the ducts.
2. This growth of the fibrous tissue contracts to form elongation and distortion of the lumina of the ducts. In spite of huge dilation of the ducts, they are converted into **chinks** (compressed narrow spaces).
3. The lumina of the **ducts** are still obviously **patent** and lined by cubical epithelium with **basement membrane intact**.

B. Pericanalicular Fibroadenoma

Naked eye or gross appearance:

Same as that of Intracanalicular type.

Cut surface is white, dry and homogeneous.

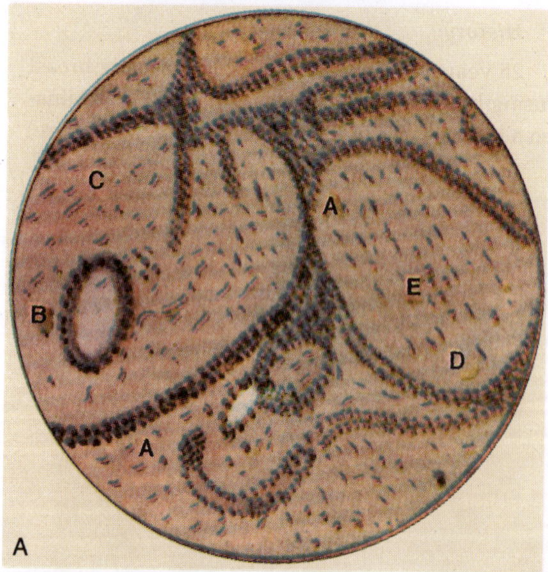

A

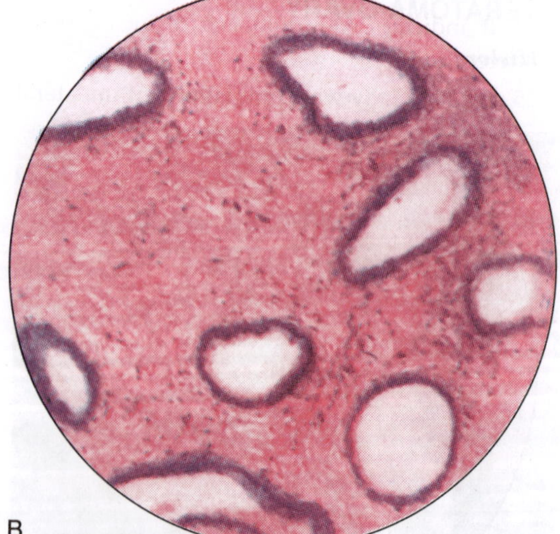

B

Fig. 7.60A: Fibroadenoma of Breast—It is chiefly intracanalicular, but pericanalicular type of change is also seen at places in some acini. A. **Intracanalicular type** of compressed acini. The glandular acini at first become huge and dilated. Later, they are compressed by proliferating fibrous tissue and narrowed, being converted into chinks (chink-like) spaces; B. **Pericanalicular fibroadenoma** where the round and oval glandular acini maintain their morphology, except for regular proliferation and hyperplasia of the lining cuboidal epithelium of the acini; C. There is mild infiltration of the collagenic stroma (wherefrom the word 'fibro' of Fibroadenoma appears). D. Fibrocytes are seen in the stroma; E. There is mild infiltration of the stroma with plasma cells and

Fig. 7.60B: Fibroadenoma of Breast—Pericanalicular type: The glands are regular and embedded in abundant fibrous tissue. Hematoxylin and Eosin. × 80.

Microscopic appearance **(Fig. 7.60B and 7.26):**

1. **Proliferation of fibrous and glandular tissue** is characteristic.
2. **Distended acini** of variable sizes are seen lined by cubical epithelium. The **basement membrane is intact.**
3. Marked proliferation of connective tissue and blood vessels is seen around the newly formed acini without invaginating the ducts.
4. There is no **cellular infiltration in pericanalicular fibroadenoma.**
5. Fibrous tissue may show **myxoid change.**

70. BREAST—ADENOCARCINOMA (Fig. 7.61)

THE NON-INVASIVE INTRADUCT(AL) CARCINOMA

Naked eye or gross appearance:

Size: 3–5 cm in diameter.

The **cut surface** shows come-down type cheesy, necrotic material in the cystic dilation of the ducts. This is called (a) **Comedocarcinomatous type,** (b) **Papillomatous** or papillary **type** that are friable and (c) **Polypoid type**—intraductal non-invasive **localized carcinoma.**

Microscopic appearance (Fig. 7.61):

It indicates four patterns of arrangement in different combinations, like

(a) **Comedo type**
(b) **Papillary type**
(c) **Solid cellular pattern type** and
(d) **Cribriform type (Fig. 7.34—Adenocarcinoma colon).**

The **comedo type** comprises central necrotic debris surrounded by tumor cells in the ducts. The papillary type has got the formation of **intraductal papillary projections of tumor cells** without any fibro-vascular stalk (Papilloma having core of connective tissue of capillary).

The **cribriform type** is indicated by **punched out** fenestrations in the intraductal tumor **(c.f. Fig. 7.34).**

71. PAGET'S DISEASE OF THE NIPPLE

Gross appearance:

Overlying dark skin of the nipple and the areola show fissures, encrustations and frank ulceration too. **Serosanguinous fluid ooze out** from the ulcerations and erosions which dry up and form crust.

Microscopic appearance (Fig. 7.62):

Presence of Paget's cells in single as well as in small clusters in the acanthotic cell (rete) layers. Paget's cells are conspicuous and stand out prominently in the thorny, i.e. acanthotic cell layer. These are bigger cells than the epidermal cells. They are **spherical cells** with

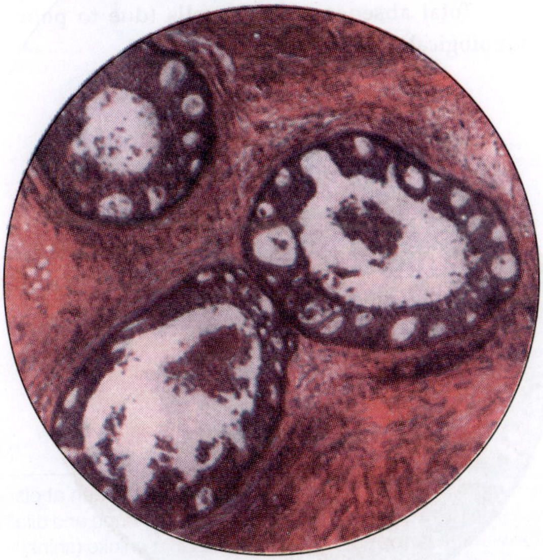

Fig. 7.61: Noninvasive Intraduct carcinoma of Breast—The three ducts in the field are distended and lined by proliferated epithelium in which local degeneration and autolysis have given rise to a cribriform appearance. Hematoxylin and Eosin. × 40

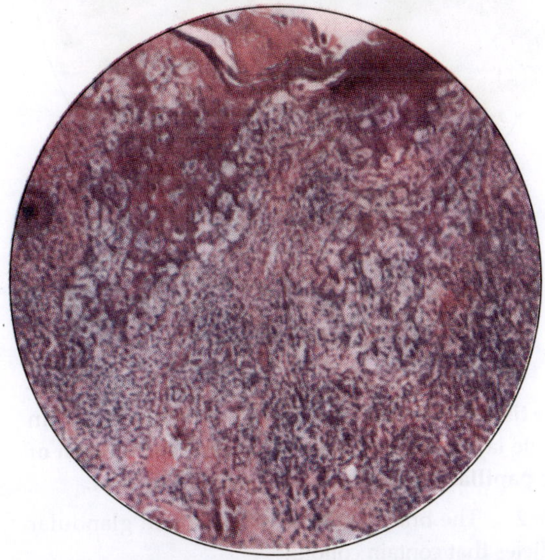

Fig. 7.62: Paget's disease of Nipple—The epidermis is hyperplastic and strikingly infiltrated with large, clear (Paget) cells. The cornified layer is thickened, while the cutis is overrun with chronic inflammatory elements. Hematoxylin and Eosin. × 50

hyperchromatic nuclei and is **mucicarmine** (stain) **positive for glycogen; cytoplasmic perinuclear halo** (empty circular space) is present around the nuclei (pronuclear in distribution). Paget's cells are adenocarcinoma type of cuboidal cells. Paget's disease is the evidence of direct dermal invasion of intraductal carcinoma and may be **invasive or non-invasive**.

72. THYROID—PAPILLARY CARCINOMA

Naked eye or gross appearance:

Size: very small upto 10 cm in diameter.

The **cut surface** is grayish white and **hard** due to the presence of **excessive collagen tissue** in the tumor; sometimes cystic change appears in the tumor as a whole and papillae or papillary processes project into the cystic space, and then the tumor is called **papillary cyst-adenocarcinoma**.

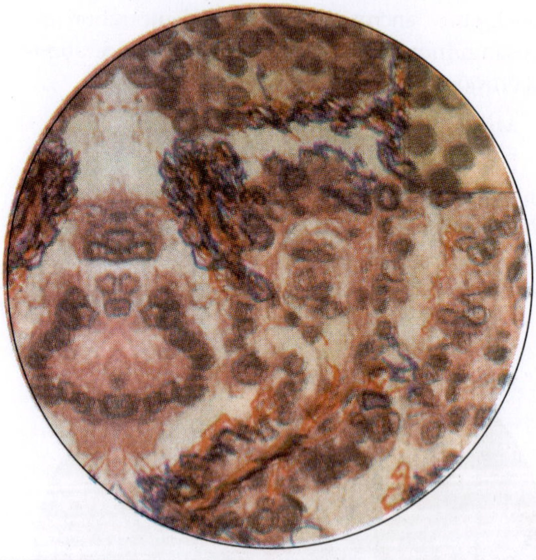

Fig. 7.63: Papillary carcinoma of the thyroid gland

Microscopic appearance (Fig. 7.63):

1. The **papillae** comprise **fibro-vascular connective tissue core** in the stalk and they (papillae) contain single layer of tumor cells which **line the margin of the papillary stalks** and their branches thereof.

2. The branches and stalks contain glandular follicles that contain colloid.

3. 50% of the cases show the presence of **psammoma** bodies in the fibro-connective tissue, which are **calcified solid spherules made of the stromal tissue-elements of the papillary stalk**.

Papillary carcinoma may be:

(a) **Pure papillary** element, or

(b) **Mixed papillary** type as well as **follicular** type (carcinoma).

73. LEPROSY (Fig. 7.64 & 7.65)

Classification:

LEPROMATOUS (POLAR) TYPE (LL)

Microscopic appearance (Fig. 7.64 & 7.65):

1. **Epidermis is thinned** and flattened out.

2. **Clear subepidermal (clear) papillary zone "GRENZ"** zone is present without any cellular infiltrate (without inflammatory cells below atrophied epidermus).

3. **Characteristic cells are histiocytes,** in which the protoplasm frequently undergoes **fatty change** with vacuoles formation (**foamy** or **Lepra cells of Virchow**) that are present in the dermis. **Fatty change** in cytoplasm of histiocytes (macrophages) that occurs by **imbibation of mycolic (fatty) acid that is present in the cell wall** of ingested lepra bacilli.

4. **Nerves stand out** in the granuloma prominently without any involvement except perineural lymphocytic infiltration of lymphocytes and occasional plasma cells.

5. **Total absence of giant cells** (due to **poor immunological status** of patients).

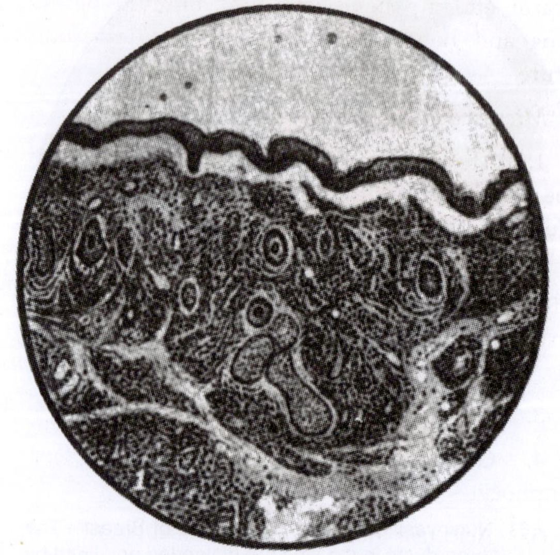

Fig. 7.64: Lepromatous Leprosy—Low power view showing well-defined clear **GRENZ** zone. Light lymphocytic infiltration in the dermis is present

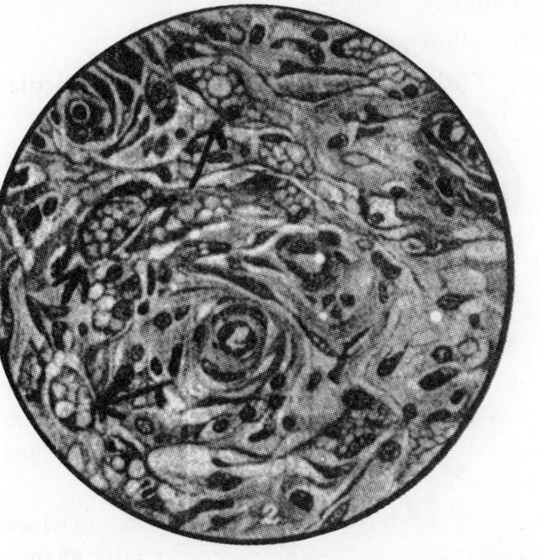

Fig. 7.65: High power view showing Virchow's (foam) cells with multiple vacuoles in histiocytes (Lepromatous)

6. **Ziehl-Neelsen (ZN) stain** shows **innumerable acid fast bacilli in smears** (not alcohol fast) and in histopathological sections present in bundles (like a **pack of cigars**). **Special stain is Fite-Faraco** (along with Giemsa stain; see Ch. on stains before).

74. TUBERCULOID LEPROSY (Polar Type 'TT')

Clinically, there develop **maculo-anesthetic** patches **on glabrous (glossy) skin** on thighs, face, forearm, etc. in patients with **high immunological status** and hence shows typical **granulomatous picture**.

Microscopic appearance **(Fig. 7.66 and 7.67):**

1. **Absence of Grenz Zone** (clear papillary zone between epidermis and dermis without any cellular infiltration).
2. Small foci and groups of epithelioid (epithelium-like) cells surrounded by dense infiltration of lymphocytes (Fig. 7.66) and occasional plasma cells.
3. Fair number of **Langhans type of giant cells**.
4. Granuloma extends upto the epidermis. Lymphocytes are found about the periphery.
5. Acid fast (not alcohol fast) bacilli (AFB) are **rarely found** in sections stained by AFS (acid fast Ziehl-Neelsen), i.e., ZN stain.

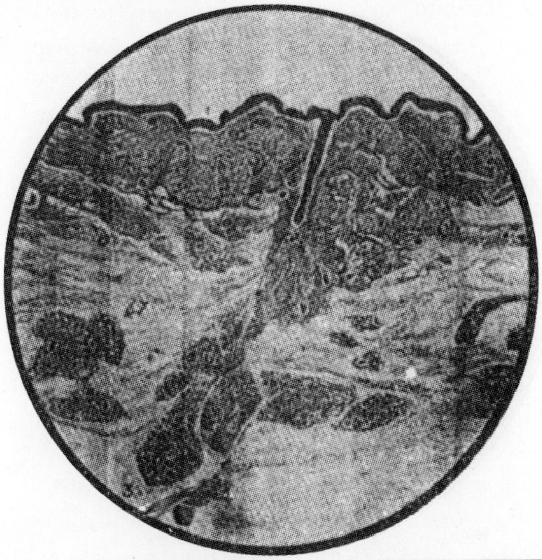

Fig. 7.66: Tuberculoid Leprosy—Low power shows focal compact lymphocytic infiltration (**Perivascular, periglandular** and **perifollicular** in distribution)

6. Nerve trunks are destroyed by the toxin.
   (a) So, there is **fibrosis** with presence of fibrocytes
   (b) There are **perineural and endoneural lymphocytic infiltrations**.
7. Total **absence of Virchow's foam cells.**

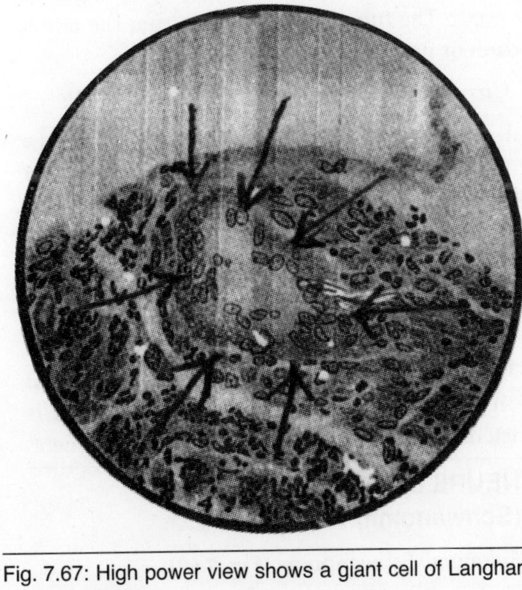

Fig. 7.67: High power view shows a giant cell of Langhans' type

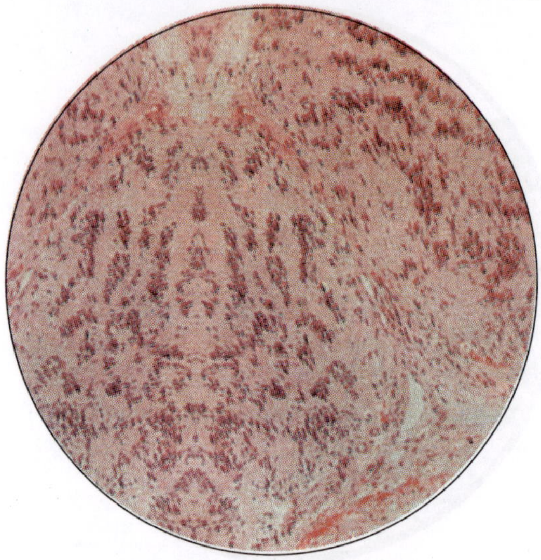

Fig. 7.68: Neurofibroma showing pallisading arrangement of cells (neuroepithelial and fibrocytes)

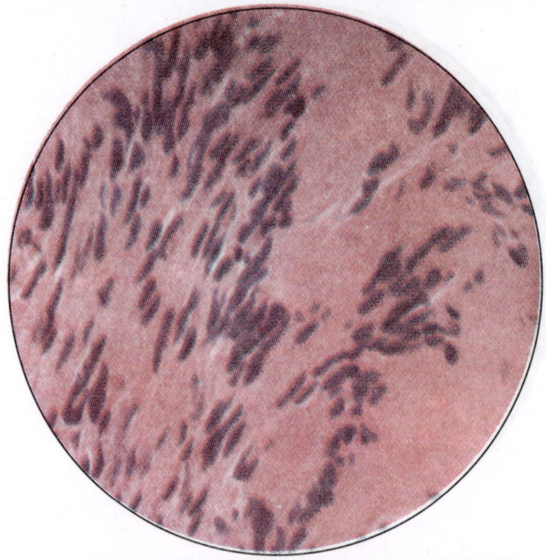

Fig. 7.69: Neurilemmoma—The tissue consists of thick and fat spindle cells disposed in interlacing bundles. The nuclei show characteristic "**regimentation.**" Hematoxylin and Eosin. × 400

75. NEUROFIBROMA (von Recklinghausen's disease)

Clinical types

Nodular, diffuse or plexiform.

Molluscum fibrosum is a condition of multiple neurofibromatosis; **runs in families** and called **von Recklinghausen's disease**. The condition is usually benign, but neurofibrosarcomatous (malignant) change may occur. The tumor grows either from the **endoneurium or perineurium.**

Microscopic appearance [(H & E); Fig. 7.68]:

1. New growth of fibrous tissue consisting of a network of cellular fibrils—**whorled, feathery** or **irregular.** This is cellular in the earlier phase but relatively acellular and later collagenous.
2. Individual **nerve fibrils** are separated by connective tissue but in the advanced stage, nodules may show **fibrous elements or mixture of both.**
3. **Pallisation** (obliquely parallel somewhat alike regimentation) of the nuclei when present is characteristic. It is also called pallisading arrangement.

76. NEURILEMMOMA (Revision) (Schwanoma)

Synonym: Schwannoma (**Fig. 7.69**).

It resembles neurofibroma, but it is usually a **solitary tumor** and **does not run in families**.

It arises from the **Sheath of Schwann** (i.e. reurilemma sheath).

Microscopically, the feature resembles neurofibroma. Pallisation is not characteristic, **Regimentation** of cells and the nuclei are specific and characteristic, meaning **prominent nuclei scattered in a bigger focus,** as if watching from there, like the regiment of an army.

77. LIPOMA (Fig. 7.70) (Revision)

Naked eye or gross appearance:

1. The tumor is **soft, elastic, well-circumscribed, encapsulated** and easily shelled out.
2. Skin is often **dimpled**, owing to fibrous bands passing between skin and the tumor.
3. Cut section—It is pale yellow in color; the knife is greasy and smeared with fat.

Microscopic appearance [(H & E); Fig. 7.70]:

1. Fat cells showing unstained empty areas with nuclei pushed to one side of the cells. Signet (marriage) ring appearance. The cells are often irregular in size.
2. Bands of fibrous tissue crossing the tumor.
3. Well-formed blood vessels present.
4. Areas of calcareous or myxomatous degeneration may be present.

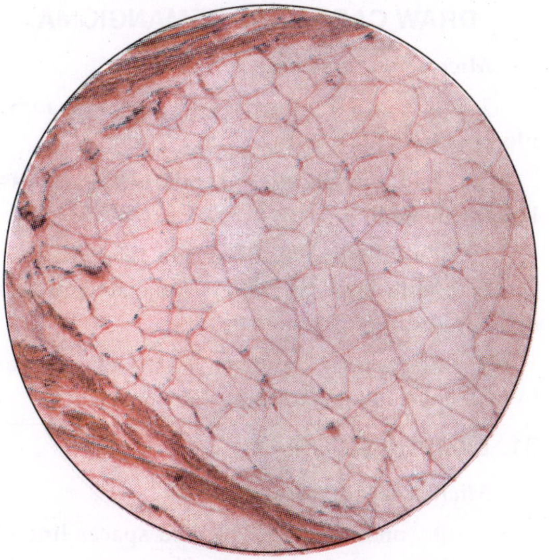

Fig. 7.70: Lipoma—The growth is made up of adult fat cells adipocytes enclosed by a fibrous capsule on left. Hematoxylin and Eosin. × 80

5. Signs of inflammation with infiltration of inflammatory cells occur sometimes.

78. CHONDROMA (Fig. 7.71) (Revision)

Naked eye or gross appearance:

The tumor is ***firm, elastic, lobulated,*** and well **encapsulated.**

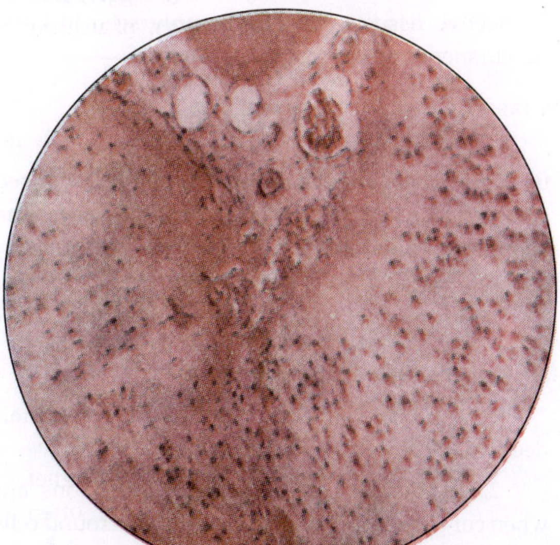

Fig. 7.71: Chondroma—Two islets of irregular hyaline cartilage are separated by a vascular, fibroblastic septum which is acting as a perichondrium. Hematoxylin and Eosin. × 100

Cut surface—bluish grey, translucent and homogeneous.

Microscopic appearance [(H & E); Fig. 7.71]:

1. Irregularly stained hyaline matrix containing a variable number of **cartilage cells** lying **singly, in pair or in tetrads.**
2. Some **empty spaces** are seen from which the cells have dislocated.
3. Arrangement of **cells** is irregular with considerable variation in size and shape, e.g., stellate or fusiform.
4. Strands of **fibrous tissue.**
5. The matrix may be myxomatous, **large, branching stellate myxomatous cells,** when the tumor is called **myxochondroma.**

79. LEIOMYOMA (FIBROID) (Fig. 7.72) (Revision)

Synonyms:

Fibromyoma, fibroleiomyoma, fibroid uterus, etc.

This is a mixed tumor of fibrous, and smooth-muscle tissue.

Naked eye or gross appearance:

1. Leiomyoma may be **single** or **multiple**, of various size, **dense, solid growth,** often becoming **soft due to cystic, hemorrhagic, and retrogressive changes.**
2. They are well **encapsulated**, well **circumscribed,** occasionally **pedunculated.**
3. **Cut surface** presents a characteristically **whorled appearance** due to **interlacing bundles of fibres** of **smooth muscle, and collagen tissue** cut in various planes.

Microscopic appearance (Fig. 7.72):

1. Nonstriped somewhat slender, fusiform muscle fibres running in irregular pattern, and interlacing bundles of collagen and smooth muscles cut in various directions showing **whorling or whorled appearance.**
2. The muscle fibres possess long rod-shaped **nuclei devoid of mitosis,** and take **yellow** color with **van Gieson's (special) stain**; collagen fibres show **pink** color.
3. The muscle fibres are intermingled intimately with fibrous tissue.

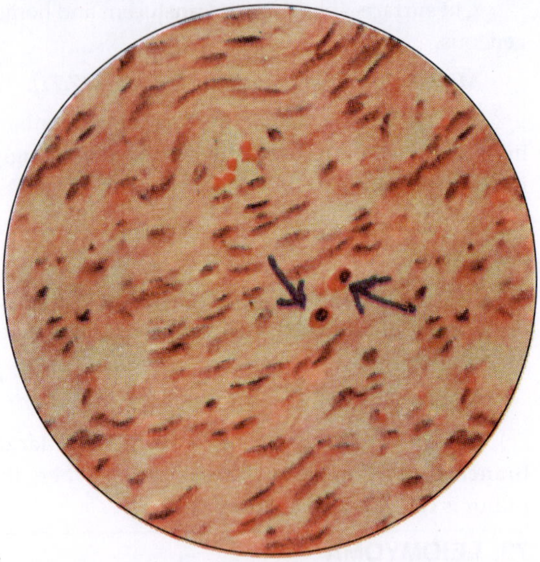

Fig. 7.72: Leiomyoma (fibroleiomyoma, i.e., fibroid) showing smooth muscle **cells** in between interlacing bundles of fibrous tissue. Hematoxylin and Eosin. × 240

4. The fibrous tissue, unlike muscle cells, possess nuclei with tapering extremities showing high normal mitotic figures; **fibrous tissue takes the red stain with van Gieson's (special) stain**.

5. Hyalinized and sometimes hemorrhagic areas are seen round the blood vessels.

80. CAVERNOUS HEMANGIOMA—LIVER

Naked eye or gross appearance:

Forms a dark red or purple, circumscribed, slightly elevated growth; often occurs in single.

Microscopic appearance
(see previous Fig. 7.17):

1. It has the structure of **erectile tissue**, being composed of **large blood spaces**.

2. Blood spaces are separated from one another by scanty connective tissue stroma.

3. The thin-walled **caverns** (blood spaces) or sinusoids are limited by **flattened endothelium** and they **freely communicate** with one **another**.

4. **Thrombosis** is fairly common **in the blood spaces**.

5. Normal liver tissue is seen surrounding the tumor.

DRAW CAPILLARY HEMANGIOMA

Microscopic appearance:

1. It consists of **network** of newly formed **blood vessels** filled with blood.

2. **Endothelial cells** lining the blood vessels are **large and swollen**.

3. **Endothelial proliferation** is marked; may produce **solid buds** of cells, become **several layers deep occluding the lumen**.

4. Supporting connective tissue may also hypertrophy, but it is usually scanty.

81. LYMPHANGIOMA

Microscopic appearance:

1. It consists of well formed **spaces lined by endothelium** and supported by fibrous tissue matrix.

2. Closely resembles hemangiomas except that the space or lumen of vessels **containing** lymph.

MALIGNANT CONNECTIVE TISSUE TUMORS

SARCOMAS (Revision)

Sarcoma is a malignant tumor i.e., mesenchymal or **mesoblastic origin**. They might **arise de novo** (primary) or **as a secondary change** from a benign connective tissue tumor; commonly seen in bone, subcutaneous tissue, fascia and muscle.

Classification of Sarcoma

It is a histogenetic classification based on the tissue of origin, i.e., according to the type of connective tissue from which it arises, e.g., **fibrosarcoma, chondrosarcoma,** etc.

82. FIBROSARCOMA (Fig. 7.73) (Revision) (Spindle-cell Sarcoma)

Microscopic appearance:

1. Spindle-shaped fibroblast cells; nuclei stain deeply and show **abnormal mitosis**.

2. The cells run in different directions and when cut transversely they may appear as round cells.

3. Fibrils are numerous in the inter-cellular matrix.

4. The **blood vessels** are wide and thin-walled; they are **embryonic** in the form of **thin-walled** blood

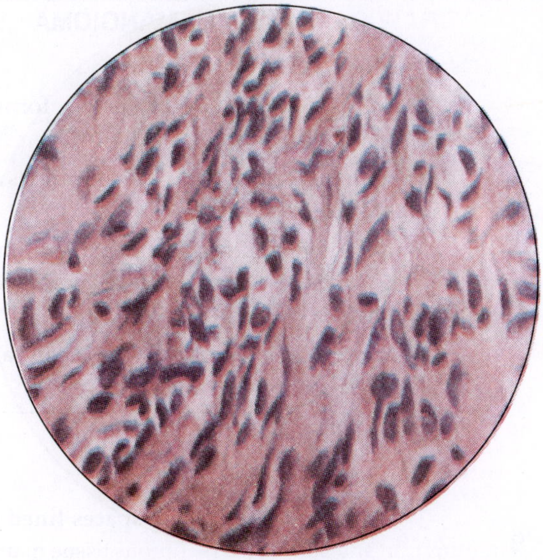

Fig. 7.73: Fibrosarcoma—The tissue consists of large malignant fibroblasts (spindle cells) and a moderate amount of collagenous matrix, and tumor giant cells. Hematoxylin and Eosin. × 360

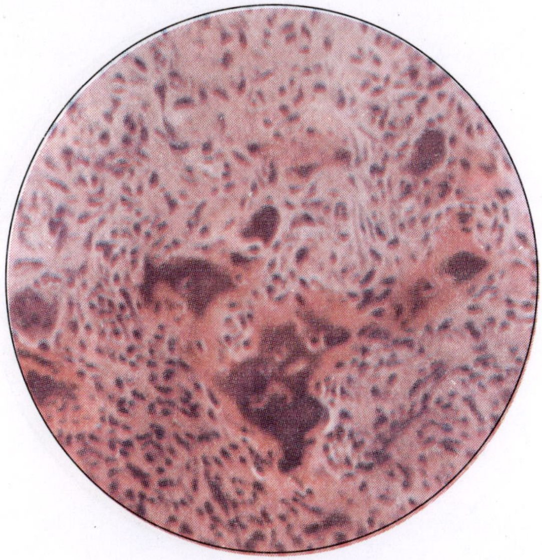

Fig. 7.74: Osteosarcoma—Several islets of imperfectly formed bone have been produced by differentiation from the surrounding spindle-cell tissue, tumor giant cells are present. Hematoxylin and Eosin. × 200 diam.

spaces frequently devoid of endothelial lining; **lumen** of which may **contain malignant cells (metastatic)**.

5. **Tumor giant cells** are conspicuous.

In the spindle-cell (fibro-)sarcomas, cells are fibroblastic, uniform and large. Cells also possess a relatively large amount of cytoplasm.

OSTEOSARCOMA (Fig. 7.74) (Revision)

It may be sclerosing or osteogenic osteosarcoma indicating more bone formation; or osteolytic osteosarcoma with destruction of bone, more than its formation. For further classification see authors' Text book of Pathology; they may be **endosteal and parosteal**.

83. OSTEOGENIC SARCOMA (Fig. 7.74)

Synonym: Sclerosing osteosarcoma.

Naked eye or gross appearance:

1. The tumor appears as a **fusiform swelling** at the **end of the bone**, fading away on to the shaft.

2. It invades the surrounding soft tissues and may **involve the shaft, medulla and the periosteum**.

3. Fine spicules of bones are found radiating outward from the central mass, (**X-ray: sun-ray appearance** due to **periosteal reaction**).

4. Consistency of the tumor varies with the amount of **bone formed by periosteal reaction**; **X-ray**: shows formation of **Codman's triangle**.

5. The tumor is **highly vascular**, and **hemorrhages** inside the tumor may present as **cysts filled with blood; necrosis, softening and degeneration** are common.

Cut surface is variegated.

Microscopic appearance (Fig. 7.74):

Features are extraordinarily variable, complex; **pleomorphism** of cells and the stroma is present. Some bony matrix is usually recognized at places.

1. The tumor consists of **small, oblong** or elongated **spindle cells**, but **large polyhedral** or **round cells** may occur with abnormal or atypical mitosis.

2. **Tumor giant cells** are characteristically conspicuous and specific; being irregular and atypical in size and shape, and contain **2-4 irregular, large nuclei** which are **oval, indented** and highly hyperchromatic and indistinct.

3. **Embryonic type of blood vessels** (i.e., absence of endothelial lining) **are numerous** and lie in close relation to the tumor cells. Endothelial lining of **vascular spaces** is lacking. They are often **lined by tumor cells**.

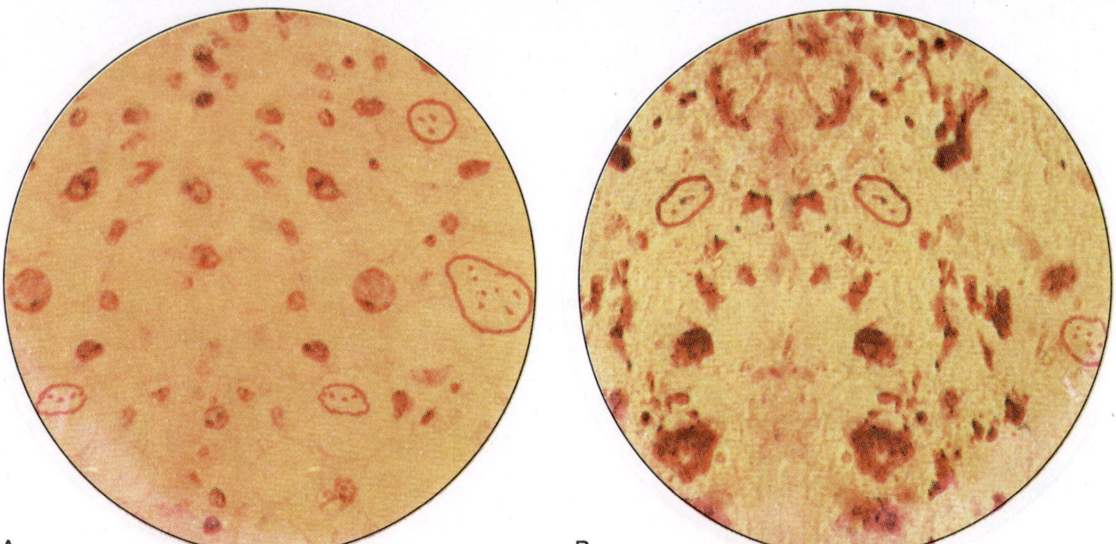

A B

Fig. 7.75: Liposarcoma—A. H & E stained microphoto; B. Sudan IV stained red areas of lipid material

4. **Hemorrhage**, **necrosis** and myxomatous changes are very common.

5. Presence of osteoid formation, osteoblasts are very characteristic.

84. LIPOSARCOMA (Fig. 7.75)

It is a common sarcoma in adults, and rare in children. There is **amplification of the region of q14 to q15 of the chromosome no. 12** and contains **MDM2 oncogene**. This oncogene inhibits the gene (protein) **P53**. This occurs in **common variant, i.e., adipogenic liposarcoma.** The **fat cells** that **undergo fatty change** with big vesicular mules are called **Lipoblast.** In variants of liposarcoma, e.g., Myxoid type, and **Round cell type** have the following chromosomal **abnormality in the region p11, q13, t12** and **t16 of the chromosome no. 12.**

Clinically, liposarcoma usually occurs in the **proximal extremities** and **retroperitoneal region.** Probably it has become a fashion to name the **retroperitoneal liposarcoma as stromal cell carcinoma** which may be a **misnomer and controversial.**

Microscopic appearance:

1. Though **lipocytes** adipocytes are the cells of the benign tumor (lipoma), in malignancy also they are the usual bulk of cells.

2. Presence of **lipoblast cells** is the **hallmark of liposarcoma.** There are **4 grades** or variants of liposarcomas:

(a) Well differentiated **Grade I**—In this variety there are presence of **sufficient lipocytes**; the tumor cells contain **supernumerary rings, and giant red chromosomes** which are the genetic or chromosomal amplifications as mentioned above.

The tumor cells are not lipogenic or adipogenic. The other variants are:

(b) **Myxoid type**

(c) **Round cell type** and

(d) **Pleomorphic, i.e., Grade-IV. In these 3 types the tumor cells are not lipogenic or adipogenic** and are called **lipoblasts**. Certain percentage of lipoblasts undergo **fatty differentiation** (change). Lipoblasts contain clear, spherical **lipid vacuoles** in the cytoplasm which **scallop the nucleus**. Lipoblasts mimic the fetal fat cells.

3. Presence of **Embryonic** (or fetal) **type of blood vessels,** i.e. blood vessels without inner endothelial lining.

85. CHONDROSARCOMA (Fig. 7.76)

Sites: There is swelling in relation to cartilage, which is **fixed to bone.**

1. Central (or intramedullary)
2. Peripheral (or juxtacortical)
3. Surface (or superficial).

This is malignant tumor of the myxoid cells and hyaline cartilage.

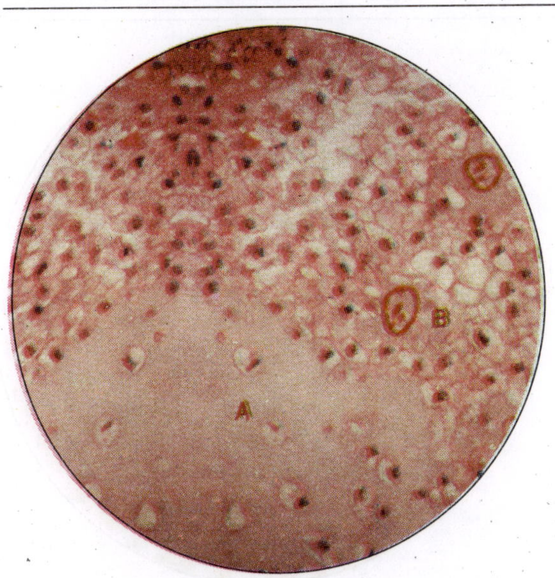

Fig. 7.76: Chondrosarcoma—A. Cartilagenous mother tissue, B. Malignant infiltrating area with degeneration, and showing embryonic type of blood vessels without endothelial lining

Histologically, the tumor may be of the following variants:

1. Conventional variant, i.e., Hyaline or Myxoid variant
2. Clear cell type
3. Dedifferentiated type
4. Mesenchymal variant.

Gross appearance:

1. **Large bulky**
2. **Greyish-white tan**
3. **Glistening**
4. **Spotty calcifications**
5. **Central necrosis causing cystic spaces (in intramedullary type).**

Microscopic appearance **(Fig. 7.76):**

1. **Hypercellularity of hyaline CARTILAGE cells, and myxoid cells**
2. **Cellular atypia**
3. **Chondrocytes**
4. **Chondroblasts (with rarely binucleate cells)**
5. **Bizarre type of tumor giant cells in higher grade (grade 3)**
6. **Presence of embryonic type of blood vessels i.e., vessels without inner endothelial lining.**

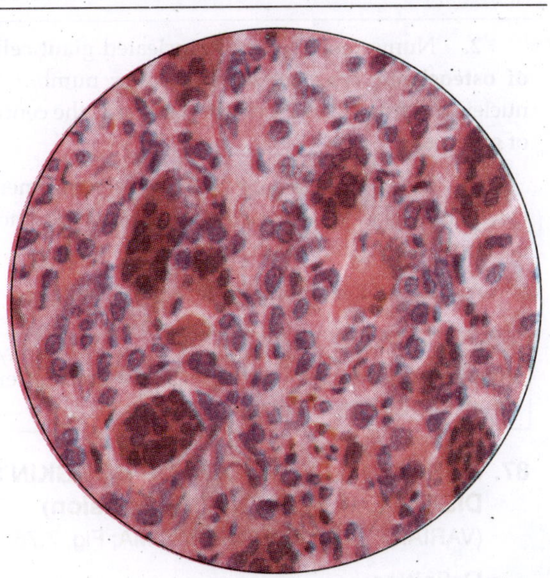

Fig. 7.77: Giant-cell tumor of Bone (Osteoclastoma)—The tissue consists of two cell types: (a) Giant cells with basophilic cytoplasm; (b) multiple irregularly distributed nuclei, and small, spindle shaped or oval cells with vesicular nucleus constituting stroma. Hematoxylin and Eosin. × 320

86. GIANT CELL TUMOR (Revision) (OSTEOCLASTOMA) (Fig. 7.77)

It occurs principally at the **end of the long bones**, metaphysis and epiphysis. Common location is the knee (lower end of the **femur**, upper end of the tibia), but may occur in many bones which develop from cartilage.

Pathological fractures with egg shell crackling-feel are characteristic. Soap bubble appearance occurs in X-ray.

Naked eye or gross appearance:

1. The bone is greatly expanded; cortex is reduced to a mere shell. Surface gives **crackling sensation** when handled. **Bony trabeculae** are seen **traversing the cavity.**

2. Tumor mass has a **soft** consistency with a **maroon color.**

3. It is sharply limited from the **healthy medullary cavity;** infiltration of the **surrounding healthy tissue** is unusual (cf. Osteogenic sarcoma).

Microscopic appearance (Fig. 7.77):

1. The tumor consists of: (a) **spindle cells;** (b) **numerous rounded cells** during active growth are also recognized.

2. Numerous large multinucleated **giant cells of osteoclastic type** are seen to occur; number of nuclei vary from 12 to 15, situated towards the centre of giant cells.

3. Blood vessels are comparatively rudimentary and in places supported by adventitia. Strands of fibrous tissue support them.

4. Area of **myxomatous** and **fatty change**.

N.B. The tumor is malignant and does not usually give rise to distant metastasis. It may recur after removal and may rarely cause metastasis.

87. HODGKIN'S LYMPHOMA OR HODGKIN'S DISEASE—LYMPH NODE (Revision)

(VARIANT OF LYMPHOSARCOMA; Fig. 7.78)

Definition

Hodgkin's disease is a type of lymphoma characterized by the proliferation of malignant reticulum cells, which may be monomorphic or polymorphic and may or may not be associated with pleomorphic cellular infiltration.

Naked or gross appearance (Fig. 7.78):

Aggregated lymph nodes rendering India rubber-like **feel**. It may occur in any lymph node or organ rich in RE cells, e.g., liver, spleen, lymph node, etc.

Microscopic appearance (Fig. 7.78):

1. Reticulum cells.
2. **Reed-Sternberg giant cells** (also known as **Dorothy-Reed, or Sternberg-reed, or mirror image type of giant cells)**. It is a malignant endothelial cell, nucleus of which may be monomorphus or polymorphus.
3. **Lymphocytes.**
4. **Histiocytes.**
5. **Eosinophilic leukocytes.**
6. **Neutrophilic leukocytes.**
7. **Plasma cells.**

Of these, the most important element is the proliferation of reticulum cells which occurs primarily before pleomorphism of cells.

88. HODGKIN'S LYMPHOMAS (HL)

This is a malignant tumor of lymph nodes. It has 5 subtypes:

1. **Nodular Sclerosis type:**

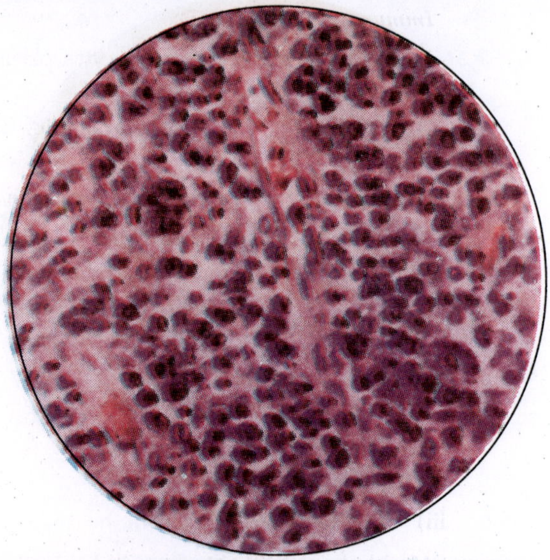

Fig. 7.78: NHL-Non Hodgkin Lymphoma—The cells which are small and round are uniformly and closely arranged and supplied by vessels consisting of a single layer of endothelium. Hematoxylin and Eosin. × 325

This type is a **lacunar variant:**

***Immunophenotype* (IPT)**: RS cells are present CD15+, CD30+; EBV-ve

***Morphology* (MPL)**

i) **LACUNAR CELLS** are present
ii) Occasional RS cells (diagnostic)
iii) T lymphocytes, plasma cells, eosinophils and macrophages fibrous bands dividing the cellular areas.
iv) **EBV is negative.**

2. **Mixed cellularity type:**

This type is a mononuclear cell variant:

***Immunophenotype* (IPT):**

i) **Mononuclear cells (lymphocytes, plasma cells and macrophages).**
ii) **RS cells** (which are **diagnostic**) are **CD15+, CD30+.**
iii) EBV present and **+ve in 70% cases.**

***Morphology* (MPL):** T lymphocytes, plasma cells, eosinophils, macrophages present.

3. **Lymphocyte rich type:**

This type is a mononuclear cell variant:

Immunophenotype **(IPT):**

i) Mononuclear cells (lymphocytes, plasma cells and macrophages).

ii) **RS cells** (which are **diagnostic**) are **CD15+, CD30+.**

iii) EBV positivity occurs in 40% of cases.

Morphology **(MPL):** Exclusively T lymphocyte cells are found in the background.

4. **Lymphocyte depletion type:**

This type is a reticular variant:

Immunophenotype **(IPT):**

i) **Diagnostic RS cells are fequent.**

ii) RS cells are **CD15+, CD30+.**

iii) EBV is present in most of the cases.

Morphology **(MPL):** Background is made of **scanty, reactive cells (chiefly T cells).**

5. **Lymphocyte predominance type:**

This is a lymphocytic and histiocytic cells variant type, i.e., **POPCORN cell** variant type. **POPCORN cells are diagnostic.**

Immunophenotype **(IPT):**

i) **Diagnostic POPCORN (L & H) cells.**

ii) **RS cells are CD20+, CD15–, CD30–.**

iii) **EBV is negative.**

Morphology **(MPL):** Presence of:

iv) **Background of lymphoid follicular dendritic cells.**

v) **Reactive B cells.**

TYPES OF LYMPHOMAS

There are 6 main types of lymphosarcomas. All are Non-Hodgkin Lymphomas (NHL) **except no. 4.** They are namely:

1. **Giant follicle lymphoma (Macrofollicular lymphoma; Brill Symmer's disease).**
2. **Lymphoblastoma (NHL).**
3. **Lymphocytoma (NHL).**
4. **Hodgkin's Lymphoma (HL); disease.**
5. **Plasmacytoma** (Plasma cell sarcoma or myeloma) in Monoclonal (Plasma cell). Gammopathy, or Multiple myeloma (Myelomatosis).
6. **Reticulum cell sarcoma.**

Microscopically, lymph node capsular infiltration by mononuclears is the foremost criterion for the evidence of lymphoma.

CENTRAL NERVOUS SYSTEM

89. MENINGIOMA (Fig. 7.79)

There are several types of meningiomas according to its variable morphology.

Naked eye or gross appearance:

Meningiomas are rounded encapsulated masses with well defined dural bases that compress the underlying brain, and which are easy to get separated from the brain. The tumor has a bosselated, or polypoid appearance. Most meningiomas have low risk of recurrences, and aggressive growth, and are graded as I/IV.

Microscopic appearance **(Fig. 7.79):**

There are various histologic patterns:

I. **Syncytial or meningothelial type.** In this, whorled clusters of tightly packed cells occur **without cell membrane.**

II. **Fibroblastic meningioma.** They consist of elongated cells with **deposit of collagen** between cells.

III. **Transitional meningioma.** This type is an admixture of both syncytial and fibroblastic types which usually contains psammoma bodies.

IV. **Psammomatous meningioma.** When psammoma bodies are present in a meningioma, it is called psammomatous meningioma. Psammoma bodies are formed from **calcification of syncytial nests of meningothelial cells.**

V. **Secretory meningioma.** When there is intracytoplasmic PAS—positive droplets. Xanthomatous degeneration, osseous metaplasia, and moderate nuclear pleomorphism commonly occurs in meningiomas.

VI. **Angioblastic meningioma.** This is characterized by the presence of angioblastic cells with tendency to form blood vessels.

VII. **Atypical meningiomas—WHO grade II/IV.**

Atypical meningiomas (WHO grade II/IV) are lesions with a **higher rate of recurrence** and more **aggressive local growth,** which requires post surgical radiation therapy. Lower grade meningiomas seldom show mitosis, but atypical one shows a higher **mitotic**

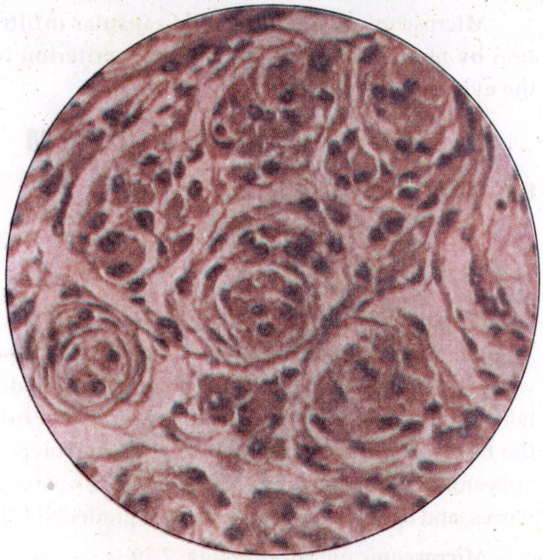

Fig. 7.79: Meningioma—The cells are oval or flattened and characteristically arranged in whorls. The cells and whorls are separated by some delicate fibres. Hematoxylin and Eosin. × 300

index of four or more mitoses per 10 high power fields or at least three atypical features [(i) increased cellularity, (ii) small cells with a high nuclear: cytoplasmic ratio, prominent nucleoli that grow without any definite pattern and (iii) evidence of necrosis]. Certain **histologic** patterns (**clear cell** and **chondroid types**) are also considered to be **grade II/IV because** of their **more aggressive behaviour.**

Anaplastic (malignant) meningioma (WHO grade III/IV) is a highly aggressive malignant tumor with the appearance of a high-grade sarcoma (but retaining histologic evidence of its meningothelial origin). Mitotic rate is high (> **20 mitoses per 10 high power fields**). (a) **Papillary meningioma** (with pleomorphic cells arranged around fibrovascular cores); (b) **Rhabdoid meningioma** (sheets of tumor cells with hyaline eosinophilic cytoplasm containing prominent intermediate filaments). Both (a) and (b) have a high recurrence rate that is considered to be **WHO grade III/IV tumors.**

Meningiomas usually are easily separable from the brain even if they displace the brain; some tumors infiltrate the brain. Brain invasion is associated with increased risk of recurrence. Meningiomas are commonly **immunoreactive** for **epithelial membrane antigen.** Presence of **keratin** occurs **with the amount** of secretory activity. These tumors are positive for the tumor marker, **carcinoembryonic antigen** (CEA).

90. ASTROCYTOMA (Fig. 7.80)

The well-differentiated low grade astrocytoma is **GFAP (Glial fibrillary acidic protein) positive** fibrillary astrocytoma. The **more malignant forms** are **anaplastic astrocytoma, gemistocytic astrocytoma, infiltrating astrocytoma** and **glioblastoma** (previously called **glioblastoma multiforme**).

FIBRILLARY (Infiltrating) ASTROCYTOMA

Naked eye or gross appearance:

1. Poorly defined, greyish, infiltrative tumor that invades brain by **diffuse infiltration.** This causes **distortion of brain.**
2. It measures from 2 cm upto a **huge size** that may replace a cerebral hemisphere.
3. The **cut surface** is soft and gelatinous, there may be **cystic degeneration.**
4. Infiltration beyond the outer margin of the well-defined tumor is almost always seen.

Microscopic appearance (**Fig. 7.80**):

1. Mild to moderate increase in cellularity with variable nuclear size.
2. **Fibrils are GFAP positive.**

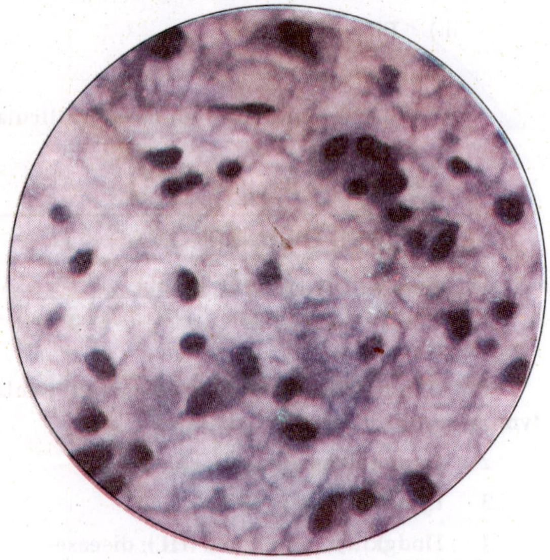

Fig. 7.80: Fibrillary astrocytoma—The cells are rather scanty and have relatively large, well stained nuclei and long, slender processes. Mallory's phosphotungstic acid Haematoxylin (PTAH). × 600

91. GLIOBLASTOMA (MULTIFORME) (Fig. 7.81)

Naked eye or gross appearance:

1. This tumor varies from region to region, e.g., grayish and white areas which are characteristic; other areas are soft and yellow (**due to necrosis**).

2. The **cut surface** is variegated due to

   (i) **Cystic degeneration**

   (ii) **Necrosis** and

   (iii) **Hemorrhage**.

Microscopic appearance (Fig. 7.81):

This resembles anaplastic astrocytoma (but with some additional features)

1. **Hypercellularity**.
2. **Nuclear pleomorphism is more**.
3. **Mitotic figures** are observed frequently.
4. **Area of necrosis and hemorrhage** may be seen.
5. **Pseudopallisation** occurs by the tumor cells that aggregate **at the edge of necrotic areas**.
6. **Vascular, and endothelial cell proliferation**.
7. Endothelial cell proliferation causes **bulging of cells inward** and encroach the lumen showing **double layer of endothelial cells** lining the vessels.
8. **The tuft formed by the cells form glomeruloid bodies. VEGF** (Vascular endothelial growth factor) is **produced by the malignant cells in response to relative hypoxia** (on demand by the malignant cells). VEGF contributes to (the already mentioned) vascular (proliferative) changes.

92. MEDULLOBLASTOMA (Fig. 7.82)

Naked eye or Gross appearance:

This tumor occurs mainly in **children** exclusively in the **cerebellum**. Though neuronal and glial markers are expressed, the tumor is often **undifferentiated**.

Morphology

In children, medulloblastomas are located in the **midline of the cerebellum**, but **lateral locations** are more often found in **adults**. Rapid growth may occlude the flow of CSF, leading to **hydrocephalus**.

Gross appearance:

The tumor is often **well circumscribed, gray, and friable**, may extend to the surface of the cerebellar folia and also involve the leptomeninges.

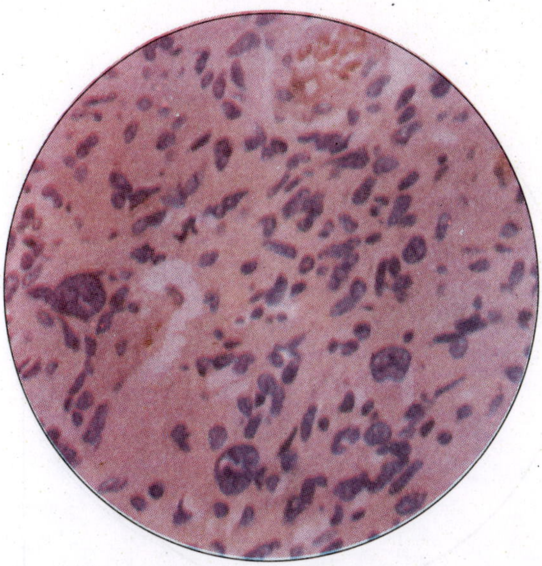

Fig. 7.81: Glioblastoma multiforme—The tissue consists of numerous glial cells which vary considerably in size, shape and nuclear configuration and which in a few cases amounts to giant cells. Blood vessels are plentiful. Hematoxylin and Eosin. × 300

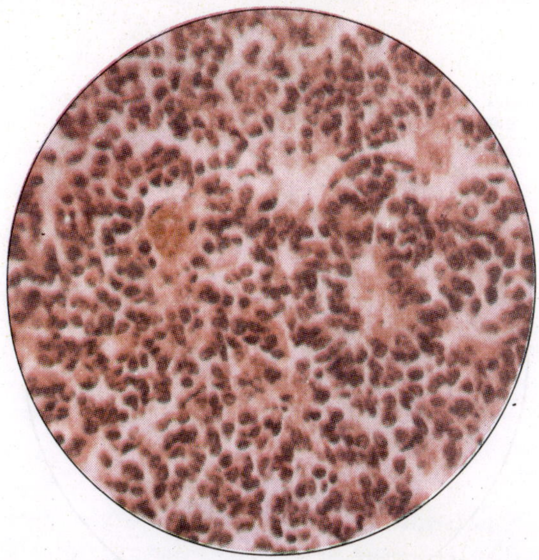

Fig. 7.82: Medulloblastoma—The tissue consists of small, oval cells with relatively large, well stained nucleus. The cells are for the most part indiscriminately arranged, but on the right the cells form incomplete circles or **pseudorosettes**. Hematoxylin and Eosin. × 30

Microscopic appearance (Fig. 7.82):

1. Medulloblastoma is extremely **cellular, with sheets of anaplastic cells (Fig. 7.82)**.
2. **Tumor cells are small** with **scanty cytoplasm**.
3. **Nuclei are hyperchromatic** which are mostly elongated and **crescent shaped**.
4. **Mitoses are abundant**.
5. **Markers of cellular proliferation, i.e., Ki-67,** are detected **in high percentage of cells**.

The tumor may express the following:

6. Neuronal (i.e., **neurosecretory) granules**.
7. **Homer-Wright rosettes**.
8. **Glial (GFAP+ve) phenotypes**.
9. In the desmoplastic variant there are areas of Stromal response, marked by collagen and reticulin deposition.
10. **Lobules or nodules** of cells forming "**pale islands**".

Complication:

Dissemination via CSF is common, presenting as nodular masses elsewhere in the CNS, including **metastases to the cauda equina** which are called **drop metastases** (alike Krukenberg's tumor).

Diagrams/Notes

Diagrams/Notes

Diagrams/Notes

Diagrams/Notes

Diagrams/Notes

Diagrams/Notes

Diagrams/Notes

Diagrams/Notes

Diagrams/Notes

Diagrams/Notes

Diagrams/Notes

Diagrams/Notes

Diagrams/Notes

Diagrams/Notes

Diagrams/Notes

Diagrams/Notes

Diagrams/Notes

Diagrams/Notes

Diagrams/Notes

Diagrams/Notes

Diagrams/Notes

PART THREE

Cytology

CHAPTER 8

EXFOLIATIVE CYTOLOGY

The importance of exfoliative cytology in cancer diagnosis has been greatly emphasised since 1950s. The main usefulness of it lies in the diagnosis of cancers. Exfoliative cytology means, cytological examination of stained smears of the cells, which have exfoliated, or fallen, or appeared in the body fluid from the mother tissue. Suppose, cancer of the stomach causes exfoliation of the malignant gastric cells. So centrifugation of the gastric juice, and smear prepared from it and stained by Papanicolaou's method, or H & E method may reveal the malignant cells. Similarly, cytological examination for malignant cells of the peritoneal fluid in cancer of the liver, or the ovaries in females; urine in cancer of the urinary bladder or elsewhere in the urinary tract; cerebrospinal fluid (CSF) in cancers of the brain; sputum in cancers of the lung; scraping material of the buccal or vaginal and cervical mucosa, and also of the tongue; in case of cancer of the cheek, the cervix, or the tongue respectively has become very useful diagnostic aid for the detection of malignant cells. **The place of cytology is much more earlier than that of histology** which appears later than the cytological changes in the diagnosis of cancer.

Moreover, certain precancerous lesions can be successfully diagnosed by cytological studies and proper precautions can be taken, say the **precancerous dysplasias** in the cervix uteri, or the **leucoplakias** of the buccal mucosa, etc.; thus, many warranted lives may be saved.

THE CHIEF TECHNIQUE OF CYTOLOGY

COLLECTION AND OBTAINING OF CELLS:

The samples may be obtained as follows:

I. **By collection of body fluids:**
   (a) **Mouth washings** or gargle — for oral cavity lesions.
   (b) **Gastric juice** collection by a **Ryle's tube** and a syringe — for stomach lesions.
   (c) **Urine collection** in a clean bottle — for urinary tract lesions.
   (d) Collection of sputum or **bronchial washings** —for lesions in the lungs or the bronchus.
   (e) **Peritoneal fluid** collection obtained by **paracentesis or tapping of ascitic fluid**; also for lesions chiefly in the liver or the ovaries, or in the peritoneum itself.
   (f) Pleural fluid collection in **pleural effusion** — for lesions in the lung or the pleura itself.
   (g) **Cerebrospinal fluid** obtained by **lumbar puncture** — for lesions in the brain or the spinal cord.
   (h) **Joint effusions** — for lesions in the joint cavity.

All body fluid obtained as above is centrifuged. The centrifuged deposit is studied in the following manners:

A. Cytological smear technique by staining with PAPANICOLAOU STAIN.

B. Centrifuged deposit in a small pack is processed as in histological procedure. This is called the **CELL BLOCK TECHNIQUE** (H & E method).

II. **The other method of obtaining cells** is by making a smear by direct scraping of the wall of the tissue by means of a wooden or bakelite spatula, wherever and whenever it is possible.

III. **Collecting cells** after endoscopic brushings.

Fixation. Once the smear is made, it is fixed in **Ether-alcohol mixture** (see below).

Ether-Alcohol Fixative

It is a cytological fixative for diagnostic exfoliative cytology for the preservation of wet smears.

Solution:

Ethyl alcohol, 95%	...	50 ml
Ether technical or anesthetic	...	50 ml

Mix well, label and put date. This should be kept in a **screw-capped vertical Coplin jar** or bottle to prevent relative evaporation, and kept chilled in a refrigerator.

Acetone may be used in place of ether.

Mode of use

Fix smears for ½ to 1 hour.

Stain by Papanicolaou's technique (see below).

I. PAPANICOLAOU'S STAIN (Fig. 8.1, Pg. 158)

Papanicolaou, G. N. (1942), Science 95, 438

Preparation

Solution (1):

Harris' Alum-Haematoxylin:

Ammonium (or potassium) alum*	...	20 g
Hematoxylin	...	1 g
Mercuric oxide	...	0.5 g
Distilled water	...	200 ml
Ethyl alcohol (absolute)	...	10 ml

Dissolve hematoxylin in alcohol.

Dissolve alum in distilled water with gentle heat.

Combine both these solutions in a 500 ml boiling flask and heat vigorously to bring rapidly to the boiling point.

Add mercuric oxide and cool immediately (or after sometime) by immersing the flask in cold water.

The solution should be dark purple after adding mercuric oxide. Put in an amber bottle; label; put date.

Preserve at room temperature in dark. This is stable for years.

Solution (2) 'OG' 6 Solution:

Orange G	...	0.50 g
Ethyl alcohol (95%)	...	100 ml
Phosphotungstic acid (PTA)	...	0.015 g

Dissolve Orange G in alcohol. Dissolve Phosphotungstic acid. Label in a bottle. Record date.

Solution (3) 'EA 36' Solution:

(a) Light green (SF yellowsih), 0.5% solution in 95% Ethanol ... 45 ml

(b) Bismarck brown, 0.5% solution in 95% Ethanol ... 10 ml

(c) Eosin (yellowish), 0.5% solution in 95% Ethanol ... 45 ml

Mix **(a), (b)** and **(c)**

(d) Phosphotungstic acid ... 0.200 g (200 mg)

Dissolve **(d)** in the above mixture

(e) Lithium carbonate (Saturated aqueous solution) ... 1 drop

Mix well, label and put date.
Filter the solution before use

Procedure

(1) Fix wet smears in ether-alcohol mixture for 30 minutes.
(2) Hydrate and stain with solution (1) for 4 minutes.
(3) Wash in tap water and blue (blueing).
(4) Dehydrate up to 95 per cent alcohol.
(5) Stain with solution (2) ('OG' 6) for 1 minute.
(6) Rinse 5-10 times in 2 jars containing 95 per cent alcohol.
(7) Stain with solution (3) ('EA' 36) for 2 minutes.
(8) Rinse 5-10 times in 3 jars containing 95 per cent alcohol. This should be a different rinse to that used after solution (2).
(9) Dehydrate, clear and mount.

Results

Basophilic cells — green to **greenish blue**;
Acidophilic cells — red to **orange**.

Cells in fragments of tissue penetrated by blood — orange to orange–green.

The following stains are useful for determining the types of nucleic acid, the DNA or the RNA of the cells. They may also be used in histopathology for the same purpose. The cytoplasm and the nucleolus takes the **red pyronin stain for RNA**; while, the **nucleus** takes up the **green color of methyl green stain for DNA** (see the stains below).

* Alum is the mixture of 2 salts of 2 different radical where Aluminium must be compulsorily present. Usually Potassium-Aluminium Chloride is used.

IIA. METHYL GREEN– PYRONIN STAIN

Kurnick, N. B. (1952), Stain Tech. 27, 233

This is a widely used method for differentiating between deoxyribonucleic acid and ribonucleic acid.

Solution (1):

Methyl green	...	0.2 g
Distilled water	...	100 ml

Solution (2):

Pyronin B	...	as required
Acetone	...	100 ml

Mode of Preparation

Solution (1) — Chloroform extraction of Methyl green.

Dissolve methyl green in distilled water. Transfer to **separating funnel** and **shake with successive changes of chloroform until no more color** is extracted. Usually 3 to 4 or 5 extractions are good enough. The extract is discarded. Record date and label.

Solution (2):

Saturate acetone with Pyronin B. Record date and label. **Chloroform extraction** of the dyes always gives best results.

Procedure

(1) Bring sections to water.

(2) Stain in solution (1) for 6 minutes.

(3) Blot dry.

(4) Rinse with 2 changes of N-butyl alcohol.

(5) Stain in solution (2) for 30-90 seconds.

(6) Clear in cedar wood oil.

(7) Rinse in xylene and mount in terpene resin (Permount or HSR).

Results

(1) Bone — **purplish-pink**.

(2) Cartilage — **green**.

(3) Cytoplasm (RNA) — **pink**.

(4) Chromatin (DNA) — **blue-green**.

(5) Nucleoli (RNA) — **red**.

(6) Erythrocytes — **brown**.

IIB. METHYL GREEN–PYRONIN STAIN

After Culling C. F. A. (1957),

Handbook of Histopathological Technique, p. 198,

Butterworth, London.

For identification of deoxyribonucleic acid (**DNA**) and ribonucleic acid (**RNA**).

Trevan, D. J. and Sharrock, A. (1951), J. Path. Bact. 63, 326.

Trevan and Sharrock's Methyl green-Pyronin (preferred for **formalin-fixed tissues**)

Solution (1a):

Pyronin Y, 5% aqueous soln.	...	17.5 ml
Methyl green, 2% aqueous soln.	...	10 ml
Distilled water	...	250 ml
Acetate buffer, pH 4.8	...	277.5 ml

Chloroform extraction of methyl green is advisable (see mode of preparation above; Solution (1), Kurnick's Methyl green-Pyronin stain).

In the original formula, Trevan and Sharrock included 65 mg of Orange G.

Final concentration of stain (per cent):

Pyronin	...	0.16 g (160 mg)
Methyl green	...	0.036 g (36 mg)

Or

Jordan and Baker's Methyl green-Pyronin

Solution (1b):

Pyronin Y, 0.5% aqueous soln.	...	37 ml
Methyl green, 0.5% aqueous soln.	...	13 ml
Acetate buffer, pH 4.8	...	50 ml

Final concentration of stain (per cent):

Pyronin	...	0.185 g (185 mg)
Methyl green	...	0.065 g (65 mg)

Solution (2):

Acetone	...	1 volume
Xylene	...	1 volume

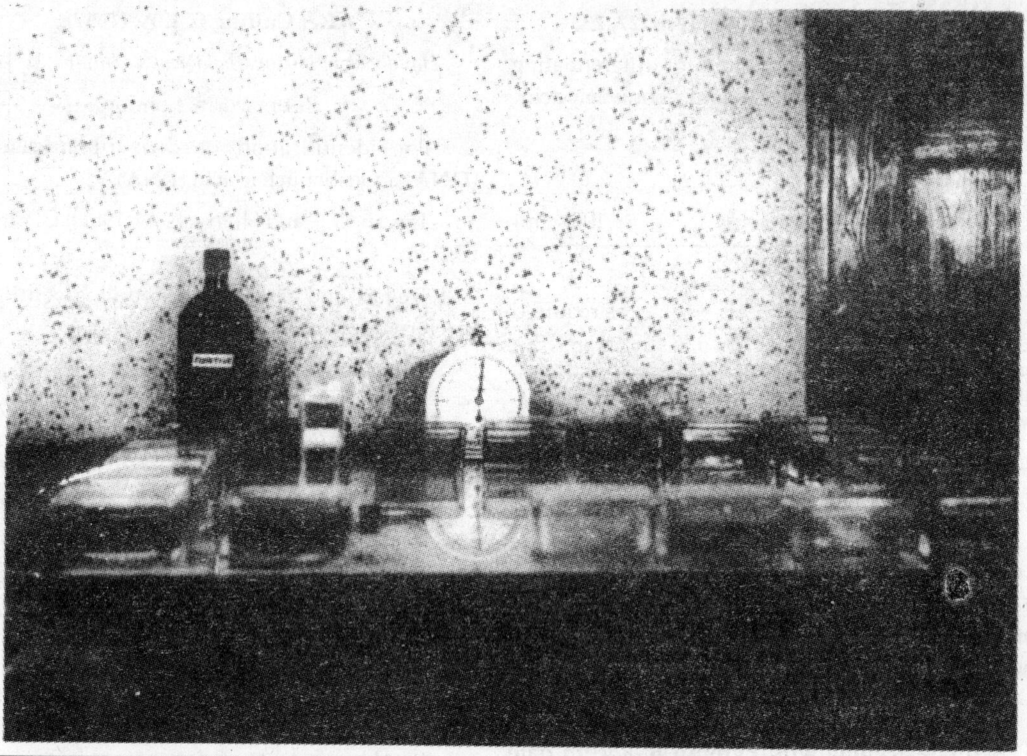

Fig. 8.1: Arrangement of Papanicolaou staining equipments for the study of exfoliative cytology

Mode of Preparation

Solution (1a):

Add Pyronin Y and Methyl green solutions to distilled water. Dilute with an equal quantity of the acetate buffer. Record date and label. The solution is best prepared just before use but it should remain **stable for 2-3 hours** or more.

Solution (1b):

Add Pyronin Y and Methyl green solution to acetate buffer. Record date and label. The solution is best prepared just before use but it should remain **stable for 2-3 months.**

Chloroform extraction of both Pyronin and Methyl green always gives best results.

Solution (2):

Mix acetone with xylene and label.

Procedure

(1) Bring sections to water.

(2) Stain in either solution (1a) or (1b) for 15-60 minutes.

(3) Rinse quickly in distilled water.

(4) Blot with non-fluffy (smooth) filter paper.

(5) Flood with 2 changes of acetone.

(6) Flood with solution (2).

(7) Clear in xylene and mount in neutral balsam or DPX.

Results

Deoxyribonucleic acid (**DNA**) — green

Ribonucleic acid (**RNA**) — red.

UNNA-PAPPENHEIM'S METHYL GREEN-PYRONIN STAIN

After White J. C. (1947). Cited by J. V. Dacie (1956). In Practical Haematology, 2nd ed., p. 73, London; Churchill

For the demonstration of RIBONUCLEIC ACID.

Heidenhain's "Susa" Fixative

Heidenhain, M. (1916), Z. wiss, Mikr. 33, 232

Solution (1):

Sodium chloride	...	5	g
Mercuric chloride	...	45	g
Trichloracetic acid	...	20	g
Acetic acid, glacial	...	40	ml
Concentrated formaldehyde solution (40%)	...	200	ml
Distilled water	...	800	ml

Solution (2):

Pyronin (G.T. Gurr)	...	0.3	g
Methyl Green (G.T. Gurr)	...	0.7	g
Glycerol	...	20	ml
Ethyl alcohol, absolute (pure)	...	2.5	ml
Phenol, 0.5% aqueous solution	...	100	ml

B.D.H. Methyl green available in India has proved to be hopeless even after chloroform extraction of the dye. So **try with Gurr's or any other German products**.

Solution (3): Tertiary N-Butanol.

Mode of Preparation

Solution (1):

Dissolve sequentially in distilled water, the sodium chloride, mercuric chloride and trichloracetic acid. Mix formalin with this, and then mix acetic acid. Store in a rubber-bung **stoppered bottle**. Record date and label.

Solution (2):

Extractions of methyl green and pyronin separately with chloroform, 3-5 times each, should stain better, (For details, see before mode of preparation of Kurnick's Methyl green-Pyronin Stain, solution 1).

Preparation of Stain

Grind the dyes in a mortar with glycerol and ethyl alcohol; add phenol. Boil the mixture for 2 minutes; filter; store in a glass-stoppered bottle and label.

Procedure

(1) Prepare thin films of peripheral blood or aspirated bone marrow and fix in **solution (1)** for 60 minutes.

(2) Remove the mercuric chloride pigment with iodine; add sodium thiosulphate.

(3) Stain with **solution (2)** for 60 minutes.

(4) Rinse in distilled water.

(5) Dehydrate in solution (3), i.e. Tertiary N-Butanol.

(6) Clear in xylene and mount in **neutral balsam**.

Results

Cell components containing **RNA; Red**

DNA; Greenish black.

Diagrams/Notes

Diagrams/Notes

PART FOUR

Clinical Pathology

CHAPTER 9

CLINICAL PATHOLOGY

EXAMINATION OF SPUTUM

COLLECTION OF SAMPLE

To obtain a good sample of sputum, an effective expectoration is necessary. The so-called sample of sputum is often extrapulmonary in nature, namely, nasopharyngeal secretion and saliva. Morning cough provides a good material for examination. **Disposal container is boiled in caustic soda or autoclaved before disposal.**

1. Macroscopic Examination

Take the sample in a sterilized Petri dish. Study: **quantity, consistency, color** (red, yellow, green, rusty, black, etc.). **Odour** fetid (or putrid), presence of **blood**, etc. Examination also for **Curshmann spirals** (yellowish-white twisted masses) and **Charcot-Leyden (C–L) crystals** (microscopic rhomboid slender crystals). **Ditrich's plugs** (yellowish–white small bodies), **concretions, casts,** etc., under the microscope.

2. Microscopic Examination (under coverslip preparation) for

Epithelium, red cell, eosinophilic leucocytes, Curshmann spirals, C-L crystals in **asthma**, and **heart failure cells** (macrophages) in **brown induration (CVC) of the lung**. Pus cells, elastic fibres (indicate **destruction of lung tissue**) seen **in phthisis, gangrene and abscess of the lung**. Parasites, like Ecchinococcus (**hydatid cyst**) can be identified by the presence of hooklets, and **E. histolytica** of liver abscess bursting into the lung can be identified by its **anchovy sauce** or chocolate **appearance** of pus and finding out of the protozoa (trophozoite form).

Asbestos bodies—**in asbestosis and pneumokoniosis, golden yellow bulbous swollen bodies** appear **at the extremities** resembling dumb-bells, or they are **beaded** like a necklace.

3. Cytology for Malignant Cells

Fix in ether-alcohol (50%-50%) mixture for ½ hour (Wet Fixation) and stain by H & E and Papanicolaou methods.

4. Bacteriological Examination

Make smears **and**

(a) Stain by **Gram's method** for Gram positive and Gram negative cocci and bacilli (for detail, see big Table on availability of bacterial flora in Practical Microbiology and Medical Bacteriology) in pathological samples; (in Practical Microbiology).

(b) Stain by Ziehl-Neelsen's **(Z-N) method for** Acid-fast Bacilli (**AFB**) (see authors' Practical Microbiology).

Smear

Stain by 1% methylene blue for 2 minutes. Determine the percentage of lymphocytes, pus cells and bacterial flora. Leishman's stain should be done for finding out eosinophils.

Culture

(a) (i) Culture on a **blood agar plate for streptococcus, Friedlander's pneumobacillus** (*Kl. pneumoniae*) and other nonspecific **pyogenic organisms**;

(ii) For **Hemophilus** group, use a **chocolate agar** and incubate in a **candle jar** under **10% CO_2 tension**;

(iii) For **Bordetella pertussis** use **Bordet Gengou plate** (media) with penicillin, preferably by the **cough plate inoculation method.**

(b) For culture of **tubercle bacilli**, after concentration method inoculate in **Loewenstein-Jensen's (L-J) medium** or **Glycerinated Dorset's egg medium** in **MacCartney vials** (30 ml) or **Bijou bottles** (5–15 ml).

Observe at least **for 3-4 weeks**, preferably **6–8 weeks** and maximum upto 12 weeks before a negative culture report is given.

Animals inoculation

Inoculate **guinea-pig** for ***Myco. tuberculosis*** preferably **intramuscularly in the thigh. Observe** for at least **6 weeks.** (For differentiation of **Bovine from human type,** inoculation of a **rabbit is necessary**; see authors' book on Medical Bacteriology and Practical Microbiology).

Culture in L-J medium that shows differential character between M. Tb and M. bovis.

Sputum may be examined for parasites (for details, see section of Practical Parasitology in Practical Microbiology Book).

EXAMINATION OF CEREBROSPINAL FLUID (CSF)

[CSF obtained by **Lumbar Puncture** done by LP Needle (See Fig. 9.1 – Pg. 164 and Fig. 9.2 – Pg. 165) for the technic for handling the needle].

I. PHYSICAL EXAMINATION

Note the quantity or volume, color, appearance, pressure, rate of flow, and specific gravity.

Appearance

Normally it is **clear, colourless;** if mixed with blood, may be pinkish or red. It may be opalescent or **turbid** in case of purulent (**pyogenic**) **meningitis.**

There may be formation of **cobweb coagulum** on standing for an hour in case of **tuberculous meningitis.**

Rate of CSF flow

It is usually **1 drop per second** (60 drops/mt).

Specific gravity: It is **1006** in normal cases.

II. BIO-CHEMICAL EXAMINATION

Usually **sugar, protein and chloride** estimations are routinely done.

A. SUGAR

Normal sugar level is 40 to 80 mg per cent (per dl).

To 1 ml of CSF add 1 ml of qualitative Benedict's solution. Briskly boil and allow it to cool. A brick red precipitate, whatsoever small it may be, indicates presence of glucose. The glucose of CSF may be estimated colorimetrically as in the case of blood sugar (see chapter on Chemical Pathology). Glucose is **absent** or **slightly present** in **pyogenic meningitis.** It is also slightly **lowered** (ignorable) **in tuberculous meningitis.**

B. PROTEIN

Normal CSF contains 12 mg to 36 mg or 40 mg protein per 100 ml.

1B. TEST (TOTAL PROTEIN)

(a) Take 0.5 ml of CSF in an empty test tube supplied in a proteinometer set. Add 1.5 ml. of **sulphosalicylic acid solution**; mix well; allow to stand for 5 minutes. Compare with the opacity tubes and match the unknown. The matching tube expresses the result in mg per 100 ml (or dl). If necessary dilute the fluid with normal saline appropriately and consider the dilution factor in the final calculation. Always consider the cell count along with the protein estimation. **Protein is variably increased in meningitis** — either **meningococcal, tubercular, syphilitic** and **fungal (cryptococcal).**

(b) Protein can be **estimated by Biuret reaction** quantitatively (see under section on **Chemical Pathology**).

2B. GLOBULIN

1. **Pandy's test for Globulin**: To 1 ml clear solution of carbolic acid, add 0.5 ml of CSF. A bluish cloudy precipitation indicates presence of globulin.

2. **None-Apelt reaction (Ross-Jones' test)**: 1 ml of saturated **ammonium sulphate** is carefully layered with 0.5 ml of clear CSF. An **increase in globulin** is indicated by **formation of a white ring** within a few seconds (A ring may form with normal CSF after 5 minutes). **Globulin is increased** specially in neurosyphilis [**tabes dorsalis, meningo (i.e. transverse) myelitis**].

C. CHLORIDE

To 2 ml CSF add a drop of potassium chromate solution as an indicator. Titrate with 0.5214 per cent $AgNO_3$, mixing the solution all the time till a permanent **salmon-pink color appears; < 600 mg%** is diagnostic **in Koch's (Tb.) meningitis,** and **cryptococcal meningitis.**

Calculation

2 ml of the $AgNO_3$ solution is equal to 0.00583 mg of NaCl. Therefore, the result is

$$\frac{\text{No. of ml of } AgNO_3 \text{ used}}{2} \times 100 \times 0.00583 \text{ mg}$$

chloride per cent. Figure **above normal** (i.e., **750 mg per cent) is seen in renal failure**. It is reduced in **tuberculous meningitis (critical low in Tb. and cryptococcal meningitis; level < 600 mg %)**.

III. CYTOLOGICAL (MICROSCOPICAL) EXAMINATION

Normally 0 to 13 lymphocytes/cmm (never more than **300 cells/cu. mm. or μl**, plus occasional Meningothelial, i.e., mesothelial cells) are present. In **pyogenic meningitis; several hundred to several thousand pus cells may be present**. In **tuberculous meningitis**, about **50–500 lymphocytes/cmm (μl)** may be present. In case of **syphilitic meningitis**, and **viral meningitis**, there may be **mild rise of lymphocytes**; less than that in **tuberculous meningitis**.

In Tb. meningitis maximum cells are 300 lymphocytes/μl but usually it is upto 100 lymphocytes/μl.

Method of TOTAL and DIFFERENTIAL COUNT
(See Figs. 13 – 16, counting chamber; later)
(see below: **REPORTING OF CYTOLOGY)**

Leukocyte Count: For total leukocyte count, use **Turk's (WBC diluting) fluid**. Take the Turk's fluid up to 0.5 marks in a WBC pipette and CSF up to mark 11 (opposite to what is done for blood leukocyte count; **dilution of CSF is thus 19 in 20** (in **improved Neubauer rulling chamber**). Count all 9 big squares of a Neubauer rulling type of chamber. Multiply the count by $^{20}/_{19}$, i.e., number of cells counted × $^{20}/_{19}$. Turk fluid helps to dissolve red cells if present in CSF.

Whether red cells are actually present in CSF (Subarachnoid Hemorrhage), or they appear from trauma due to faulty technique, can be determined by collecting the sample in different test tubes or vials. **In case of trauma due to bad technique**, it is likely that red cells will be **present only in the** first part (first 1 or **2 samples**).

Differential Leukocyte Count is done in the same way as in blood by **smearing centrifuge deposits** and **staining by Leishman's stain**.

IV. BACTERIOLOGICAL EXAMINATION

A. SMEAR EXAMINATION:
(Direct finding of organisms)

Normally CSF is sterile. In pyogenic meningitis when the **centrifuge deposit is stained with Gram's stain**, Gram positive or Gram negative cocci, or Gram positive or Gram negative bacilli (Escherichia or Hemophilus, etc.) are seen under a microscope depending on the type of infection.

In tuberculous meningitis, smears are made from the **cobweb coagulum**, (if it is formed at all), or from the centrifuged deposit. The **smear is stained by Z-N method**.

B. CULTURAL EXAMINATION (indirect findings):

Different types of cultural examination may be done, when CSF is collected aseptically. Isolation of organism is possible in different **basic** and **selective** or differential or enriched or enrichment media. If **N. meningitidis** is suspected, the **collection tube is covered by black paper to avoid diffuse sunlight exposure. Otherwise organisms die in diffuse sunlight**.

TOTAL LEUKOCYTE COUNT

It is done similar to WBC count but the dilution is 1:10 in a WBC pipette.

1. **Pyogenic Organisms:** Culture on **blood agar or chocolate agar** is done under 10% CO_2 tension in a candle jar; **N. meningitidis** and **H. influenzae** should grow in it. **Other pyogenic organisms should grow on blood agar as such (without CO_2 tension)**.

2. For **acid-fast bacilli**, culture **in Loewenstein-Jensen's medium** is essential. If the culture is positive, the material (organisms) should be inoculated intraperitoneally into two guinea-pigs, and is **observed up to 6 weeks** for evidence of any tuberculous lesion (tubercles, i.e., follicles, tubercles, ulcers or induration).

V. SEROLOGICAL EXAMINATION

CFT (Complement Fixation Test) Wassermann Reaction (W.R.), and **VDRL Microflocculation Tests** are positive, specially in neurosyphilis (see under section on Serology). CFT is done in gonococcal and tubercular infection also.

Lange's Colloidal Gold Test (when positive) shows: (a) **paretic curve in GPI;** (b) **luetic (or tabetic) curve in tabes dorsalis**, and (c) **meningitic curve in pyogenic meningitis**. (For detail, see under Spirochetes; in Practical Microbiology, Medical Bacteriology); **tabes means destruction**.

Pandy's test is positive in any type of meningitis. Wassermann test is positive in **85%** cases of syphilis irrespective of its type (probably except the early chancre or primary stage where enough of anti-

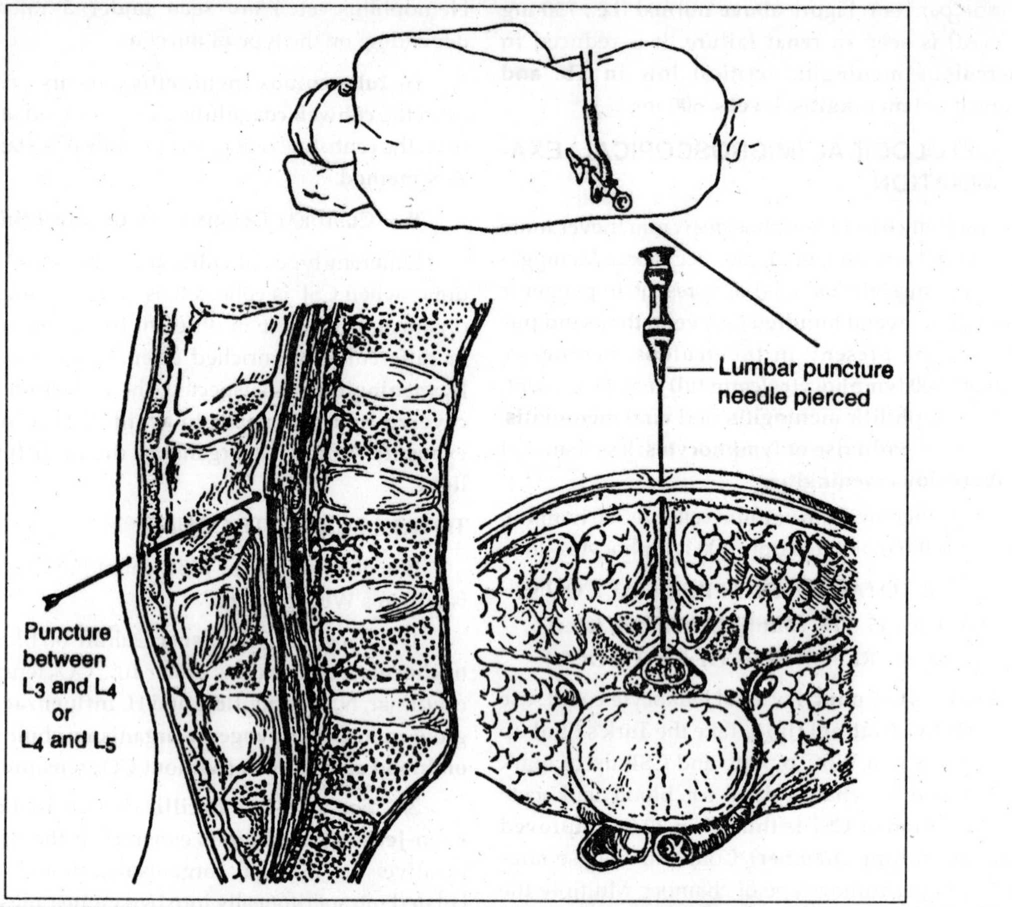

Fig. 9.1: Patient in left lateral position with knees drawn up, back, flexed. Lumbar puncture needle inserted in flexed left lateral position in between L_3 and L_4, or L_4 and L_5 intervertebral space.

body has not formed). It is 97-100% positive in **GPI** and 75% positive in **Tabes Dorsalis.**

TECHNIQUE AND REPORTING OF CYTOLOGY OF BODY FLUIDS

(DILUTION MAKING CAN BE AVOIDED ALSO)

Step 1: A total count is made by counting 2 Big squares (side by side), i.e., Left and Right **Lower** squares only or Left and Right **Upper** squares only.

Of the 4 WBC counting big squares, if counted diagonally, the counts would be same (homogeneous); purpose is to **obtain a mean count from a Heterogenous Count**. The **total number of cells of 2 big squares** multiplied by ($^9/_2$) in an undiluted sample. If 3 big squares are counted then the number of cells counted in 3 big squares are multiplied by $^9/_3$ or **3**. (See Fig. 12.3 to 12.5, and calculation thereof).

Total number of cells include both anucleated (Red) cells, and nucleated (WBCs) plus **mesothelial Meningothelial,** i.e., (endothelium-like) **cells**. In **peritoneal and pericardial fluid, it is mesothelial (endothelial) and in pleural fluid it is mesothelial cell**.

As report is given for total cells, it includes Red cells also.

Step 2: To find out **Total Nucleated Cells**, red cells are lysed in **Glacial Acetic Acid** (put **equal volumes of the sample and Acid** in a separate vial. Keep for 5 minutes, then shake) and **charge in the counting chamber**. Count cells as before and **multiply by Dilution (Acid) Factor** (i.e., 2). The expressed count gives the total number of nucleated cells.

Total **nucleated cells** when subtracted from total **number of cells (including Red cells) gives the number of only Red cells present in the sample**.

Report (Cytology):

(i) Total number of cells ... cells/cmm i.e., μl (including red cells)

(ii) **Total Nucleated cells** ... cells/cmm i.e., μl

(iii) Total Red cells ... (i - ii) = (iii) ... cells/cmm i.e., μl

(iv) **Differential count of Nucleated cells**

This can be done:

(a) By making a smear from the sample on a slide (when cell population is more) and then stained by **Leishman's Stain.**

(b) By making a smear from centrifuged deposit of the sample (when cell population is less).

(c) By directly counting the individual cell types (in the counting chamber itself; but there is a risk of error). This requires more experience.

Neutrophils	....	%
Lymphocytes	....	%
Mesothelial (meningothelial) cells	....	%

N.B. When cells are more and the count is numerous, a few small square counting of cells, should serve the purpose and multiply the number of cells with proportionate area of 9 Big squares.

Example:

When cells of 2 small squares are counted in two separate Big squares (of Left and Right sides), it is **multiplied by 8** to get the number of cells in **one big square**. Then again multiply that number (of 1 big square) by 9 to get the number of total cells.

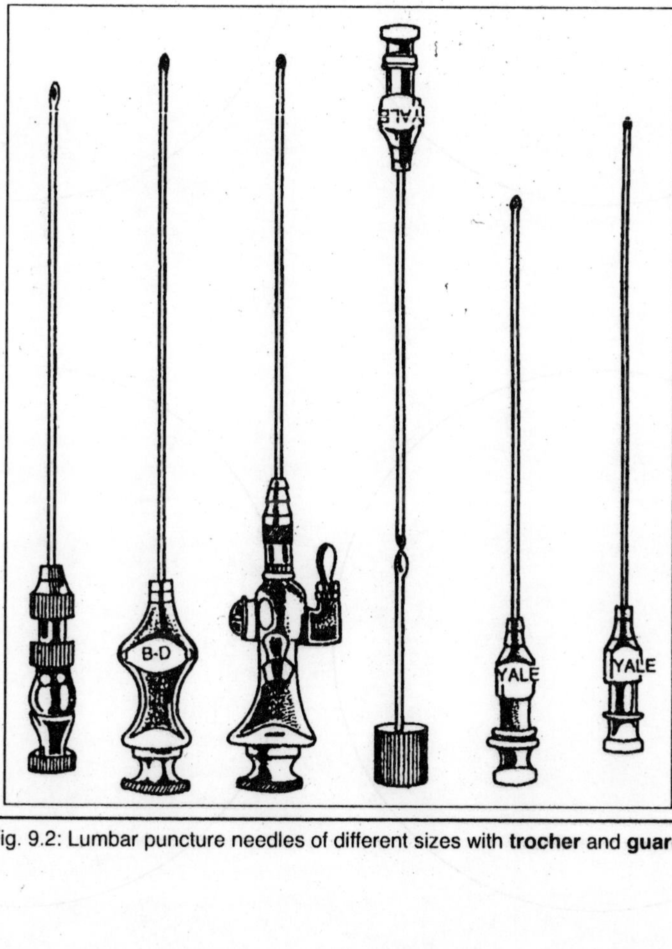

Fig. 9.2: Lumbar puncture needles of different sizes with **trocher** and **guard**

Diagrams/Notes

CHAPTER 10

EXAMINATION OF URINE

COLLECTION OF SAMPLE

The composition of urine varies with diet, intake of fluid etc. So 24 hours' sample may be representative but it is not absolutely essential. In that case, use **toluene as preservative**. For bacteriological examination, theoretically catheter specimen should be collected aseptically in a sterile container. In males, **mid-stream urine** may be collected aseptically. For all practical purposes, any sample of urine or a **morning sample** shall do. **Catheter specimen has a risk** of developing infection. So collection from direct mid-stream is fare enough.

I. PHYSICAL EXAMINATION

Determine **quantity, color, odour, appearance** and **specific gravity (sp. gr.)**.

Quantity: About **1,500 ml in 24 hours**;

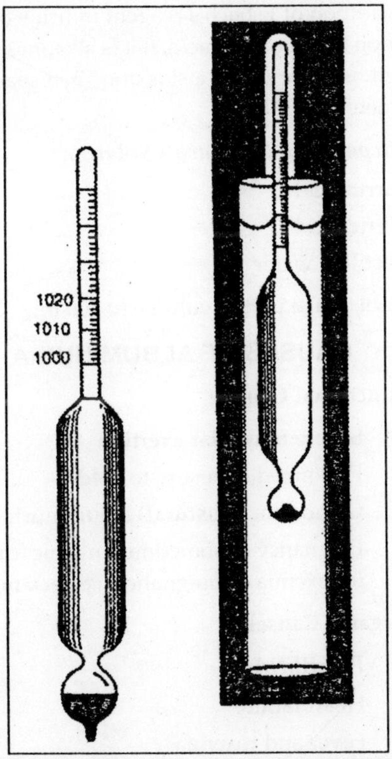

Fig. 10.1: Urinometer (A Specific Gravity Meter) with a measuring container

Color: When freshly voided may be amber or straw-colored;

Odour: Significant only in fresh urine; it is not always essential; **Acetone smell** occurs in diabetes.

Specific gravity (See **Fig. 10.1**). Specific gravity meter): Take sufficient urine in a cylinder (upto the mark of 0%). Determine specific gravity with **genuine** urinometer floating in it. Avoid foam in urine and do not let the urinometer touch the side of the container; read graduation at the lower meniscus. Dilute urine, (if necessary, to obtain enough quantity to float the urinometer, consider the dilution by multiplying the last 2 figures of specific gravity by the number of times diluted). Normally it is 1010 to 1014 but it has a wide range.

Causes of High specific gravity

1. **Concentrated urine** — due to excessive sweating, fever, diarrhoea, vomiting, dehydration etc.
2. **Uncontrolled diabetes** mellitus (Crystalloids are responsible; not the colloids).
3. **Acute nephritis.**

Causes of Low specific gravity

1. After **intake** of large quantity of **fluid—Dilution.**
2. **Chronic nephritis** (Sp. gr. is **low and fixed** at 1010).
3. Hypertension with **renal involvement.**
4. **Diabetes insipidus** (180 litres maximum output recorded).
5. After **diuretic intake** (when vol. is increased).

Causes of Low and Fixed specific gravity (1006 to 1008):

1. **Late stage of chronic nephritis** (end stage kidney).

Normal urine is **clear.** Amorphous materials (and mucoid material) cause the urine **Opalescent.**

2. **Chronic pyelonephritis.**
3. **Polycystic kidney.**
4. **Malignant hypertension.**

Normal sp. gr. 1010–1020; too much **sweating makes urine concentrated.** Urine is highly concentrated in **fever** and **after exercise. High sp. gr.** occurs in **diabetes mellitus** (presence of crystalloids), acute nephritis. **Low specific gravity** occurs in **chronic nephritis**, and after **drinking a large quantity of water. Low and Fixed Sp. gr.** occurs in late **chronic nephritis** (1010), the end stage kidney.

Reaction — usually acid (pH 6.8). **Alkaline urine** occurs after vomiting of meals (**alkaline tide**); or due to ammonia formation by **bacterial decomposition in cystitis.**

II. CHEMICAL (BIOCHEMICAL) EXAMINATION

Qualitative tests

Take a column of urine in a test tube; **boil the upper layer** by slight tilting, and holding the test tube at the bottom by left hand; and the opacity that forms may be:

(a) **Transient** — urates,

(b) **Turbid** on boiling , then add acetic acid; if turbidity disappears it is **phosphate** but in case of **carbonates** it **disappears** with **effervescence**.

Turbidity does not disappear in case of **albumen** or compound protein, and turbidity is increased by adding 10% acid.

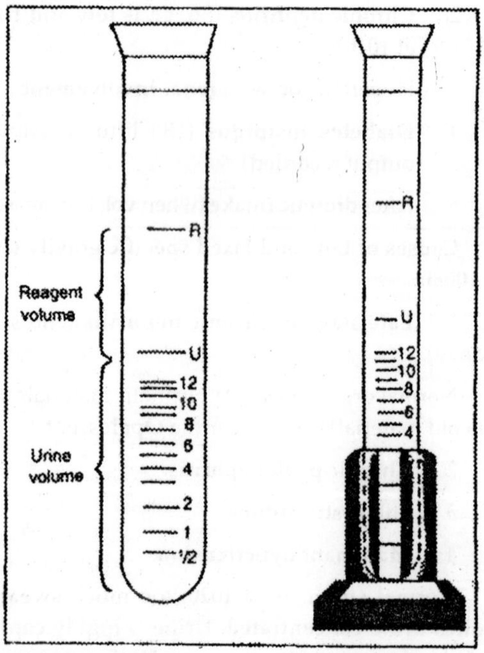

Fig. 10.2: Esbach's Albuminometer

TESTS FOR ALBUMEN (PROTEIN)

(a) **Heat** the upper part of urine in a test tube. **Haziness or turbidity appears. Add 10% acetic acid** when **haziness** becomes **marked and prominent** which indicates presence of albumen (protein coagulates around 62°C).

(b) **Heller's cold nitric acid test for albumen**

Take $\frac{1}{2}$ inch column of yellow nitric acid in a narrow test tube; slowly and carefully layer the surface by adding urine. A sharp white ring forms at the junction when albumen is present.

(c) **Sulpho-salicylic acid reagent for albumen**

Sulpho-salicylic acid — 20 g, magnesium sulphate — 50 g, Sodium sulphate — 10 g, water add 100 ml.

To 1 ml of urine in a test tube, add 1 ml of 20 per cent sulpho-salicylic acid reagent. A **white turbidity indicates the presence of albumen.**

N.B. Filter the urine if it is turbid. A ring test can be done in a similar manner.

(d) **Esbach's method**

Addition of Esbach's reagent in urine offers precipitation (render urine acid, if it is alkaline); filter and dilute if necessary. This test is done by Esbach's albuminometer (Fig. 10.2).

Preparation of Esbach's Solution

Picric Acid	......	1 G
Citric Acid	......	2 G
Distilled water	......	20 ml

Cool; make up the volume to 100 ml.

CAUSES OF ALBUMINURIA

I. **Functional Causes:**

1. Severe **muscular exertion**
2. Prolonged exposure to **cold**
3. Orthostatic (**postural**) albuminuria
4. Pregnancy — sometimes organic (cause) due to toxemia of pregnancy, i.e., **eclampsia**.

II. **Organic Causes:**

A. *PRERENAL*

1. Heart failure
2. Fever and toxemia
3. Ascites, or tumors, due to the rise in intra-abdominal tension that presses on renal veins.

4. After administration of drugs, like mercury, bismuth, etc.

B. *RENAL*

1. Carcinoma of the kidney
2. Infarction of kidney
3. Nephritis — acute glomerulonephritis, pyelonephritis
4. Nephrotic syndrome
5. Nephrosclerosis
6. Tuberculosis of the kidney.

C. *POST RENAL*

1. Cystitis
2. Prostatitis
3. Pyelitis
4. Urethritis
5. Admixture — when vaginal secretion is mixed up with urine.

Types of Proteins which may be found in the urine:

1. **Albumin**. 2. **Mucin**. 3. **Bence Jones' protein** (in multiple myeloma). 4. Lymph (**Chyle** in filariasis).

BENCE JONES' PROTEIN

(H. Bence Jones', 1847)

Osgood and Haskins' Test

For detection of Bence Jones' protein (**free light chain either kappa chain or lambda chain**).

Reagent (1):

Acetic acid, 50% aqueous solution (v/v).

Reagent (2):

Sodium chloride, saturated aqueous solution (approx. 36 g per 100 ml).

Procedure

If alkaline, **make urine slightly acidic** by a drop of **Glacial acetic acid**. To 5 volumes of urine, add **1 volume of reagent (1)**, and **3 volumes of reagent (2)**. The presence of Bence-Jones' protein is indicated by an immediate precipitate, that **forms in the cold**; it dissolves on boiling (or at **80°C**) and **reappears on cooling** (45°C to 55°C).

Other urinary proteins once precipitated, do not dissolve on boiling.

Bence Jones protein was first demonstrated by H. Bénce Jones in 1847. **These proteins are the circulating free light chains of both κ (kappa) and λ (lambda) types**, which are produced in excess (in **monoclonal gammopathies**, like **multiple myeloma**) to the **heavy chains** (**α, δ, ε, γ** and **μ**); and either of them appears in the urine. These free light chains (κ and λ) are electrophoretically homogeneous bearing the antigenic determinants κ and λ (For further information, see authors' "Medical Bacteriology", Chapter on Immunochemistry).

TESTS FOR CHYLE

(a) 10 ml of the (white, milky) urine is centrifuged. The supernatant fluid may be clear showing some **floating fat globules**.

(b) 5 or 10 ml of urine if shaken with equal volume of ether, the urine may be partially or completely clear.

(c) When a coverslip preparation of the chylous urine is examined microscopically it may show some fat globules.

(d) Tests for albumen should be positive.

EXCESS OF PHOSPHATES

Heat the upper portion of a sample of urine in a test tube. A turbidity appears, which **disappears on** addition of a **few drops of 10% acetic acid**.

Phosphaturia pathologically occurs in phosphatic calculi **in alkaline urine**. It may occur also physiologically in mental tension, worries, anxieties, etc.

TEST FOR CALCIUM

Sulkowitch Test

For detection of calcium in urine, as an arbitrary **indicator of the serum calcium level.**

Oxalic acid	...	2.5 g
Ammonium oxalate	...	2.5 g
Acetic acid, glacial	...	5 ml
Distilled water	...	to 150 ml

Mode of Preparation

Dissolve oxalic acid and ammonium oxalate in 100 ml of distilled water. Add acetic acid, mix and make up the volume to 150 ml with distilled water. Label and put date.

Procedure

To 5 ml of clear urine (if required, filter), add 5 ml of the reagent and mix. Allow to stand for 5 minutes and observe for turbidity.

Result

No turbidity — serum level **below 7.5 mg %** (Hypocalcemia).

Faint turbidity forming in a few seconds and not increasing (requires dark background for observation) — serum calcium level **8-9 mg % (Hypocalcemia)**.

Immediate faint **turbidity increasing on standing** (visible without the use of a dark background) — serum calcium level **9-11 mg % (normal range)**.

Immediate precipitate — serum calcium level above 11.5 mg % (**Hypercalcemia**).

TEST FOR SUGAR

To 5 ml of **Benedict's** reagent add **8 drops of urine**; boil vigorously for 2 minutes and then allow it to cool. **A red precipitation at the bottom indicates presence of sugar. Precipitation is more important than color change**, latter may occur in presence of oxalates, ascorbic acid, or some other **reducing agents** as well.

PREPARATION OF BENEDICT REAGENT

Tri-Sodium citrate	...	173 g
Sodium carbonate (Anhydrous)	...	100 g
Copper sulphate (Hydrated)	...	17.3 g
Distilled water, add up to	...	1 litre

Dissolve Trisodium citrate and sodium carbonate in 500 ml distilled water.

Dissolve copper sulphate in 500 ml distilled water **with gentle heat**. Mix the solutions. Label and put date.

Presence of glucose can be confirmed by **osazone reaction**. Quantitative estimation may be done, when glucose is present.

Osazone test method

Using **Phenylhydrazine Hydrochloride (PHH)**: Take about 10 ml of urine in a test-tube, and make it acidic with acetic acid. Then add as much **phenylhydrazine hydrochloride** as will lie on a piece of penny (**cent or sikka**), and **sodium acetate** (twice the bulk of PHH). Mix thoroughly; heat till the ingredients are dissolved; filter. Place the tube containing the filtrate in a boiling water bath for half to one hour. Then switch off the water bath and allow the filtrate to cool down slowly (in the water bath) to room temperature. **Examine the precipitate formed, by a cover-slip preparation under the microscope.**

Using Phenylhydrazine **(free base**; Neumann): To approximately 10 ml of urine, add 2 ml of saturated sodium acetate in 50 per cent acetic acid, and 5 or 6 drops of saturated solution of phenylhydrazine. Mix and place in a boiling water bath. There is no need to filter. Frequently osazone crystals will appear in ten or fifteen minutes. If not, leave for half an hour, and then switch off the water bath without removing the tube. Mount and examine crystals, if any, by a microscope (under **cover slip preparation**).

TESTS FOR ACETONE (ROTHERA'S TEST)

To 10 ml of urine saturated with **ammonium sulphate** (by adding an excess of the crystals), add 2 to 3 drops of strong freshly prepared solution of **sodium nitroprusside** in water; then layer in with 2 ml of strong ammonia (Liquor ammonia forte) carefully and gently along the wall of the test tube; a purple ring is formed at the junction, indicating presence of acetone (acetonuria).

Aceto-acetic acid & β-Hydroxybutyric acid constitute (DIACETIC ACID, and each of them is tested by GERHARDT'S TEST)

If Rothera's test is positive then only this may be positive. Take 10 ml of urine in a test tube; add 10 per cent **ferric chloride solution** drop by drop. A precipitate usually forms and disappears on adding more ferric chloride. Stop when no more ferric precipitate forms. Filter it and to the filtrate add an excess of ferric chloride solution. A clear **red color** indicates a positive test.

In Diabetic coma there is presence of these **3 ketone bodies:**

1. ACETONE, 2. ACETOACETIC ACID, 3. β-HYDROXY BUTYRIC ACID. Out of these **aceto-acetic acid is most important** which **acts on the brain cells to cause diabetic coma.**

> **N.B.** Whenever acetoacetic acid is present, β-hydroxy-butyric acid is always associated with it.

TESTS FOR BILE ACID (i.e., Bile salts)

Bile salts are sodium (Na-glyco-, Na-tauro-, and Na-desoxy-) CHOLATES.

HAY'S (sulphur granules floatation) TEST: Place fresh, clear and cool (room temperature) urine in a conical glass, and lightly sprinkle dry sulphur powder on its surface. The bile acid, in concentration of 0.01 per cent reduces the surface tension and sulphur powder sinks at the bottom. The test is positive when the liver is damaged or the duct is obstructed (with possible exclusion of nephritis).

TESTS FOR BILE PIGMENT (BILIRUBIN)

(a) **Gmelin's test** — put a drop of urine on the filter paper and also a drop of fuming nitric acid by the side of it; a play of colors develops when the test is positive.

(b) **Alcoholic Iodine test** — To about 1 ml column of urine **add a few drops of one per cent Alcoholic (tincture) Iodine — a green ring forms** at the junction.

(c) **Hunter's test** — To 5 ml of 10% barium chloride add 5 ml of urine. The precipitate of barium sulphate, on which the bile pigments are quantitatively present, is spun down and washed with water (centrifuged) several times. Add 0.5 ml of **van den Bergh's diazo reagent** and it shows a typical reaction of bile pigment; or add a drop of fuming nitric acid to the precipitate on the filter paper and this shows a display of color, e.g., green, red, yellow, etc.

(d) **Harrison's test (For Bile Pigment)** — This is the **best and most sensitive test** for bilirubin. 5 ml of Barium chloride (10%) solution, is mixed with 5 ml (equal part) of urine; it is centrifuged and the precipitate is spread on a filter paper and dried. Put a drop of **FOUCHET'S REAGENT** (Trichloroacetic acid — 25 g, Ferric chloride — 0.9 g, Distilled water — 150 ml) which turns the precipitate to **green color** in presence of bilirubin (pigment).

TEST FOR UROBILIN
(Schlesinger's method)

Add 3 drops of Lugol's iodine solution to 5 ml of urine. Add 5 ml of 10 per cent solution of alcoholic **zinc acetate**. Mix and filter. View the filtrate in sunlight against a dark background with **light** concentrated upon it by a lens. A **greenish fluorescence** indicates the presence of **urobilin**. **Bile pigment**, if present, **should be removed previously by adding $\frac{1}{5}$th volume of 10% solution of calcium chloride and filtering it.**

TEST FOR UROBILINOGEN

WALLACE-DIAMOND TEST (Reaction) (for urobilinogen):

Reagent — **Ehrlich's aldehyde reagent** (Paradimethyl aminobenzaldehyde — 2 g and 100 ml of 20% HCl).

Procedure

1 ml of Ehrlich's aldehyde reagent is added to 10 ml undiluted urine; allow to stand for 10 min. in the dark. An idea as to the quantity of urobilinogen is obtained by noting the **rapidity and the intensity of port wine color** seen best through the fluid from the top of the test tube.

When the reaction is marked, make a quantitative estimation by preparing a serial dilution of urine 1:10, 1:20, 1:30, etc., upto 1:200 or higher. Add 1 ml of the reagent to each of the dilutions and take the reading after 5 minutes. A faint pink color appears in diluted urine when the test is positive as assessed by looking down through the fluid against a white background.

Interpretation (Causes of excess urobilinogen):

Appearance of the color at **1:20 dilution** is regarded as **normal**, (constipation may also produce a temporary rise of urobilinogen). **Excess** of urobilinogen is present in **hepatic dysfunction, malaria, infectious diseases, alcoholic intoxication, hemolytic diseases** and after administration of **sulphones**.

Causes of absence of UROBILINOGEN in urine

1. Carcinoma of the head of the pancreas.
2. **Impaction of stone** in the ampulla of Vater, causing **Cholestasis** and **Cholangitis**.

Causes of excess of UROBILINOGEN in urine

1. **Constipation**
2. **Fever**
3. **Hemolytic Jaundice**
4. **Malignant tumors of the liver**
5. **Chronic venous congestion of the liver**

Table IV.1: Abnormal color of urine

Color	*Conditions/or due to the presence of*
Colourless:	Diabetes insipidus, chronic nephritis, increased water intake
High coloured:	Concentrated urine (Dehydration)
Brown to almost black:	Hemoglobinuria, acute nephritis, porphyrinuria, alkaptonuria, (due to the presence of homogentisic acid), melanuria (malignant melanoma), pyridium therapy
Red or pink:	Hematuria, hemoglobinuria, pyridium therapy
Brick red:	Urates
Yellowish green:	Bilirubinuria or jaundice (obstructive, early hepatocellular)
Milky: Chylous	Chyluria (filariasis)

6. **Pre-icteric phase of infective hepatitis**
7. **Cirrhosis of the liver**
8. **Pernicious anemia.**

TESTS FOR BLOOD

BENZIDINE TEST FOR BLOOD IN URINE

I. Saturated solution of benzidine in glacial acetic acid and hydrogen peroxide (or Barium peroxide) are mixed in equal volumes; a few ml of the reagent are added to an equal volume of urine. Appearance of a blue color indicates presence of blood or hemoglobin; most sensitive (**in 1 million dilution of urine**).

II. Ruttan and Hardisty's Ortho-Tolidine test for blood

Reagent (1):

Ortho-tolidine (4%)	...	4 g
Acetic acid (glacial)	...	100 ml

Reagent (2):

Hydrogen peroxide, 3% (10 volume O_2 content per 1 volume of H_2O_2).

Mode of Preparation

Reagent (1):

Dissolve **ortho-tolidine in acetic acid**. Label and put date. The solution keeps well for one month.

Procedure

To 1 ml of reagent: (1) In a test tube, take 1 ml of urine and then add 1 ml of **reagent (1)**.

(2) Appearance of a blue color indicates presence of blood in the sample. Any sample can be investigated for the presence of blood.

Merit of the test (Avoidance of carcinogen, i.e., Benzidine)

As benzidine is said to be carcinogenic, ortho-tolidine test can be safely done with similar sensitivity of the test.

III. Tincture Guiacum Test

This is just like Benzidine test; sensitivity is low (1 : 100,000 dilution).

CAUSES OF HEMATURIA

PRE-RENAL CAUSES:

Collagen disease

Filariasis (lymphatic obstruction)

Leukemia

Purpuric diseases

RENAL CAUSES:

Polycystic kidney

Acute glomerulonephritis (GN) and **PSGN**

Focal or embolic GN

Renal tuberculosis

Malignant hypertension

Nephrolithiasis

Renal tumors

POST-RENAL CAUSES:

Traumatic after catheterization
Stone in the bladder
Tumors of the bladder
Prostatitis and urethritis
Benign Prostatic Hypertrophy (BPH)
Cancer of the prostate

CAUSES OF PYURIA

Kidney abscess
Prostatitis
Pyelitis
Pyelonephritis
Tuberculosis of the kidney
Urethritis (gonorrhoeal)

CAUSES OF POLYURIA

A. Physiological

1. Excessive fluid intake
2. Nervousness, anxiety
3. Administration of Diuretics.

B. Pathological

1. Diabetes insipidus
2. Diabetes mellitus
3. Chronic nephritis (chronic GN)
4. Polycystic kidney
5. Hypertension with renal involvement
6. During disappearance of generalized edema or ascites

CAUSES OF OLIGURIA

A. Physiological

1. Low fluid intake.

B. Pathological

1. Dehydration, diarrhea, vomiting.
2. Fevers with low fluid intake.
3. Acute GN, terminal phases of Chronic Nephritis.
4. **Acute renal failure** due to: **hemolytic transfusion reaction, surgical shock, Massive hemorrhage**, and administration of **nephrotoxic agents**.

Test for real oliguria (differentiating) from anuria may be done **by careful insertion of a catheter**.

CAUSES OF ANURIA

Some type of **uremia**, **growth** in the bladder, big involvement of **ureteral openings**, **peripheral circulatory failure**.

Test for Oxyhemoglobin and **Methemoglobin** is done by **spectroscopic method**.

TEST FOR INDICAN

(Potassium Indoxyl Sulphate)

It is a derivative of indole and presence of it in urine signifies the presence of putrefactive substances from the bowel. **Normal urine may contain a trace of it.**

Indican can be demonstrated by Obermeyer's test as follows:

Obermeyer's Reagent

For detection of indican in urine

Reagent (1)

Ferric chloride ... 2 g
Hydrochloric acid (Conc. 11N)
(sp. gr. 1.19) ... 1000 ml

Mode of Preparation

Reagent (1)

Dissolve the ferric chloride in the acid and label.

Reagent (2): Chloroform.

1. OBERMEYER'S TEST FOR INDICAN (INDIGO-BLUE REACTION)

To 5 ml of urine add 5 ml of Obermeyer's reagent and 4 ml of chloroform; mix up inverting repeatedly and closing the mouth of the test tube with the left thumb. Now, do not shake any more. Chloroform becomes blue and settles at bottom. **Depth of the color** indicates the **quantity of indican present**. Acid liberates **indoxyl from potassium indoxyl sulphate** (indican). **Indoxyl is oxidized to indigo** by ferric chloride to give the **indigo-blue color**.

Caution:

(a) If **oxidation is slow**, a red color due to the formation of **indigo red** may develop.

(b) Thymol and iodides may interfere with the test, when present in urine. So addition of a crystal of sodium thiosulphate will discharge their color.

(c) **Bilirubin**, when present, must be **removed by** the addition of **one-fifth volume of a 10 per cent** solution of **calcium chloride** and then filtering it.

2. **JAFFE'S TEST FOR INDICAN**

For detection of indican in urine.

Solution (1): Hydrochloric acid conc. (11N; sp. gr. 1.19).

Solution (2): Chloroform.

Solution (3): Potassium chlorate, 1% aqueous solution.

Procedure:

To 5 ml of urine in a test tube, add 6 ml of **reagent (1)**, and 4 ml of **reagent (2)**. Mix thoroughly for 1 minute and allow the chloroform to settle. A blue color indicates the presence of indican. Add **reagent (3)**, drop at a time, to assess the approximate concentration of indican.

WATSON'S TEST FOR PORPHYRINS

For detection of **COPROPORPHYRIN** and **UROPORPHYRIN** in urine.

Reagent (1) : Acetic acid, glacial.

Reagent (2) : Ether.

Reagent (3) : Hydrochloric acid, 5% aqueous solution.

Procedure:

To 25 ml of urine in a separating funnel, add 10 ml of **reagent (1)**, to make urine acidified. Extract the acidified urine taking half with two 50 ml volumes of **reagent (2)**. Combine the two extracts and wash in a separating funnel with 10 ml of **reagent (3)**. Examine the (a) **washing** and the (b) **urine residue** after **extraction under ultraviolet light. A strong red fluorescence** of the former indicates the presence of a large amount of **coproporphyrin; red fluorescence** of the latter is indicative of the **presence of uroporphyrin.**

TEST FOR PORPHOBILINOGEN

For detection of porphobilinogen in urine.

Ehrlich's dimethylaminobenzaldehyde reagent

Reagent (1):

Hydrochloric acid Conc. 11N (sp. gr. 1.19)	...	150	ml
Distilled Water	...	100	ml
p-dimethylaminobenzaldehyde	...	0.7	g

Reagent (2):

Chloroform.

Reagent (3):

Sodium acetate, saturated aqueous solution.

Mode of Preparation

Solution 1

Add acid to water; dissolve **paradimethylaminobenzaldehyde** and label; put date.

Procedure

Adjust the reaction of 10 ml of urine to pH 3.5-5 with dilute hydrochloric acid. To 2.5 ml of the **acidified urine** in a large test tube, add 2.5 ml of **solution (1)** and mix. Quickly add 5 ml of **reagent (2)**. **If a red color develops, add 2 ml of reagent (3)** (solution); shake vigorously. The color due to urobilinogen or to indole is soluble in chloroform. If after repeated extraction with **reagent (3)** (solution); the aqueous fraction remains **red, and the test is said to be positive for porphobilinogen.**

TEST FOR MELANIN

von Jaksch-Pollak Test

For detection of melanin in urine.

Reagent

Ferric chloride, 10% aqueous solution.

Procedure

To 10 ml of urine in a test tube, add a few drops of the reagent. A grey color develops followed by a dark precipitate on addition of further reagent. The precipitate consists of phosphates and adhering melanin. **Excess reagent dissolves the precipitate.**

TEST FOR PPA

Phenylpyruvic Acid Test (PPA)

For detection of increased phenylpyruvic acid excretion **in phenylketonuria.**

Reagent (1):

Ferric chloride, 10% aqueous solution.

Regeant (2):

2, 4-dinitro phenylhydrazine (**DNPH**)		1.4	g
Hydrochloric acid, 1N, solution	...	500	ml

Mode of Preparation

Reagent (2):

Dissolve **2, 4 DNPH** in acid by gently heating, Allow the solution to cool. Label and store in a dark glass bottle.

Procedure (for PPA detection):

To 5 ml of urine (acidified with acetic acid or dilute sulphuric acid) add a few drops of **reagent (1).** An **intense green to green-blue color** which **gradually disappears indicates the test positive for PPA** or some other interfering substance. As a single test may be negative, while administering drugs, like chlorpromazine and aspirin that may give a positive reaction; the **following additional test** is recommended for routine use in parallel with that described above.

> **To 5 ml of clear urine, add 5 ml of reagent (2); mix and allow to stand; a yellow turbidity forming within a few minutes indicates a positive reaction for PPA.**

TEST OF ALKAPTON BODIES

For detection of alkapton bodies (homogentisic acid) in urine.

Reagent:

Sodium hydroxide, 10% aqueous solution.

Procedure

To 10 ml of urine in a test tube add the reagent drop by drop until the urine is alkaline. **Blackening** of urine indicates the **presence of homogentisic acid.**

> A **similar reaction** may be obtained, **if the test is applied to normal urine to which hydroquinone** has been **added.**

TEST FOR SULPHANILAMIDE

For detection of sulphanilamides in urine.

Reagent (1): Ehrlich's aldehyde reagent:

(a) *p*-dimethyl-amino-benzaldehyde

$(CH_3)_2NC_6H_4CHO$	...	4 g
Hydrochloric acid Conc. 11N (sp. gr. 1.19)	...	80 ml
Ethyl alcohol, absolute	...	380 ml

and

(b) Saturated solution of **potassium persulphate.**

Reagent (2): Chloroform.

Reagent (3):

Sodium acetate, (saturated aqueous solution).

Procedure

To 5 ml of urine in a test tube, add 1 ml of **reagent (1)**, 2 ml of **reagent (2)**, and 1 ml of **reagent (3)**. Mix carefully by inverting the tube several times and allow chloroform to settle. A **yellow color** in the chloroform layer indicates the presence of sulphanilamides.

Urobilinogen, if present, will interfere with the test. So urobilinogen must be converted to urobilin first, by adding 2 or **3 drops of Lugol's iodine solution** to about 5 ml of the urine and then warm. Allow to cool. Excess of iodine must be avoided as it will interfere with the test, but the pink color may be **removed by adding a few drops of a saturated solution of sodium thiosulphate.**

TEST FOR 5-HYDROXY-INDOLE-ACETIC ACID (HIAA)

For detection of abnormally large amounts of **5-HIAA** in urine (40 mg or more per 24 hours specimen). A positive test indicates the presence of **metastatic carcinoid tumor somewhere in the body.**

Sodium nitrite solution

(Half Strength DIAZO 'B' Reagent)

Sodium nitrite (Analar, i.e., A.R)	...	2.5 g
Distilled water	...	100 ml

Sulphuric acid solution

Sulphuric acid **Conc. (36N)** (sp. gr. 1.84) (Analar)	...	19.6 g
Distilled water	...	85 ml

Reagent (1):

1-nitroso-2-naphthol (Eastman)	...	100 mg
Ethyl alcohol, 95%	...	100 ml

Reagent (2):

Sodium nitrite solution (see below)	...	0.2 ml
Sulphuric acid solution (see below)	...	5 ml

Reagent (3):

Ethylene dichloride (purified)

Mode of Preparation

Sodium Nitrite Solution: Dissolve sodium nitrite in distilled water. Label and store in a refrigerator at 4°C, where the solution remains **stable for 3 weeks.**

Sulphuric Acid Solution: Weigh the sulphuric acid into a 50-ml beaker. Pour carefully into the distilled water in a pyrex flask by gentle shaking. Allow the solution to cool; transfer it to a suitable reagent bottle and label.

Reagent (1): Dissolve the 1-nitroso-2-naphthol in alcohol and label.

Reagent (2): Add the sodium nitrite solution to the acid and mix well. The reagent **must be used within 30 minutes**.

Procedure

Into two 5 inch test tubes labelled "T" **and** "C", measure 0.2 ml of test urine and 0.2 ml of known **negative urine** (control "C"), respectively. Add 0.8 ml of distilled water and 0.5 ml of **reagent (1)** to each tube, and mix well. To both tubes, add 0.5 ml of **reagent (2)** and again mix well. Allow the tubes to stand for 5 minutes and then add 5 ml of **reagent (3)** to each tube. Mix well to extract the excess of **1-nitroso-2-naphthol**. If turbid, the tubes should be centrifuged. A **purple to black color in the upper layer** denotes a **positive reaction** and indicates the presence of **5-HIAA** in excess of **8 mg per litre of urine**. A **yellow color** (which often appears) is of **no significance**.

QUANTITATIVE AND SEMI-QUANTITATIVE ESTIMATIONS

TEST FOR ALBUMIN

(**By Esbach's albuminometer**) (See Fig.10.2 – Pg.168)

ESBACH'S REAGENT IS PREPARED AS FOLLOWS:

By boiling **picric acid—1 g, citric acid—2 g**, in 20 ml of distilled water. Cool and make up the volume to 100 ml.

Method: If the urine is alkaline render it acid by acetic acid; filter it. Dilute the urine to make up the sp. gr. 1008. **Fill** the Esbach's albuminometer tube up to the **mark U with Urine**: pour in the **Reagent up to the mark R**. Put the rubber cork and invert several times to ensure thorough mixing. Set aside the tube (encased in wooden frame) carefully without moving for 24 hours and then read the level of the precipitate. Graduation represents dry albumin in grams per litre of urine.

TEST FOR SUGAR

Benedict's method: Take 25 ml of the Benedict's (quantitative) solution in an Ehrlenmeyer flask containing 5 g of sodium carbonate, and boil briskly. Dilute the urine 1:10 accurately and run from the burette, at first quickly and then slowly. When the blue color disappears, the end point of titration is reached. 50 mg of the glucose fully reduces 25 ml of **Benedict's reagent**. Therefore, the quantity of solution run from the burette contains 0.05 g of glucose.

Calculation:

$$\frac{0.05 \times 10}{\text{No. of ml of urine (undiluted)}} = \text{G \% of glucose}$$

TEST FOR CHLORIDES

(Volhard method)

Solutions required are —

A. **Standard silver nitrate solution**: 29.06 g silver nitrate is dissolved in 1000 ml of distilled water in a volumetric flask. 1 ml is equivalent to 0.01 g of NaCl.

B. **Standard ammonium thiocyanate solution**: Dissolve 13 g of ammonium thiocyanate in 80 ml of distilled water. Titrate this against **solution A**, using 1 ml solution C. Ferric alum indicator; calculate and dilute it so that 1 ml is just equivalent to 1 ml of silver nitrate solution C. 100 g ferric alum sulphate is dissolved in 100 ml of 25 per cent nitric acid.

Procedure

In a 50 ml flask, put 5 ml urine, 20 ml of distilled water, 10 ml of silver nitrate (**solution A**) and 2 ml of ferric alum indicator (**solution C**) (If the fluid is pink add a few drops of strong solution of pot. permanganate till the color is dispelled). Allow it to stand for 10 minutes. Run from a burette standard ammonium thiocyanate (**solution B**) until a yellow color appears. The **first trace of yellow color** indicates the point.

Calculation:

$$\frac{(A - B)}{5} \times 0.1 = \text{G of NaCl per ml}$$

Multiply by the volume in 24 hours = G of NaCl in 24 hours.

The normal excretion of chloride is 10 to 15 g a day. Excretion is diminished when the **blood chloride is reduced in pneumonia, pyloric obstruction, etc.**

ESTIMATION OF UREA IN URINE

(By Doremus Ureometer)

Reagent require: Fresh **sodium hypobromite solution**. For this, one **ampoule** of 2.55 ml of bromine is **crushed** in a stoppered bottle containing 25 ml of 50% **caustic soda solution**. Use the reagent freshly.

Estimation by Doremus ureometer:

In the closed limb of the ureometer, put a volume of sodium hypobromite solution. In the side tube (with stop cock), pour the urine up to the mark 0. Now turn the stop-cock and allow the urine to run slowly until 1 ml is used. When **nitrogen gas evolves,** it rises and collects at the top of the tube. Urea (nitrogen) percentage is read directly on the scale.

Calculation:

1 small division = 0.001 g of urea. Calculate the percentage from the number of ml of urine used. Normal excretion is 20 g (330 m. mole/*l*) to 35 g (500 m. mole/*l*) daily (approximately 2%).

Draw the diagram of Doremus ureometer.

ESTIMATION OF DIASTASE (AMYLASE)

(Window's method)

Adjust the reaction of urine slightly acidic. In a series of 10 small tubes put 1 ml quantities of 1 per cent **sodium chloride solution.** Put 1 ml of urine in the second tube, mix. Transfer 1 ml of the mixture to the 3rd tube and so on and discard extra 1 ml of the last tube. To each tube put 2 ml of 0.1 per cent **soluble starch solution in 0.5 per cent sodium chloride** and put in a water bath at 37°C for 30 mins. and then in cold water for 3 minutes. When cool, add 1 drop of Gram's iodine. **Determine the tube** which shows smallest amount of urine that shows **no blue color.** Units of diastase = 2 ÷ volume of undiluted urine in the tube. Diastatic index or "d" per ml of urine:

The unit is expressed as $d\ \frac{37°}{30'}$

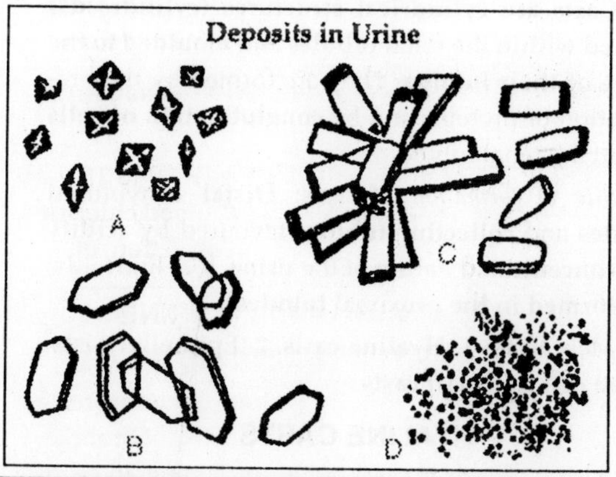

Fig. 10.3: Acid urine—A. Calcium oxalate, B. Cystine, C. Uric acid, D. Amorphous urates

The **normal figure is 8 to 32 units.** Excretion is **diminished in nephritis** but many times **increased in acute pancreatitis (100-200 units).**

MICROSCOPICAL EXAMINATION OF URINARY DEPOSITS

Centrifuge fresh urine for about 2-3 minutes at moderate speed (2000 R.P.M); reject almost all supernatant fluid and with a Pasteur pipette take a drop from centrifuge deposit; put it on a clean slide; make a coverslip preparation. Examine under low power and confirm it under high power.

UNORGANISED DEPOSITS

[See Figs. 10.3, 4, 5(a) and 5(b)]

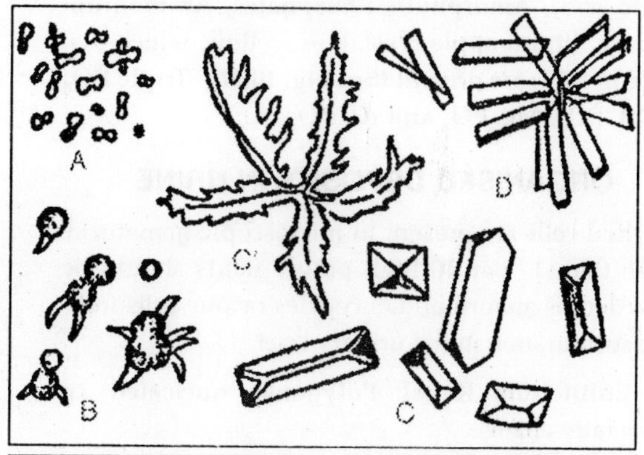

Fig. 10.4: Alkaline urine—A. "Dumbell" shaped crystals of calcium carbonate, B. Ammonium biurate, C. Triple phosphate (Prismatic), C'. Triple phosphate (Feathery), D. Calcium phosphate (weakly alkaline).

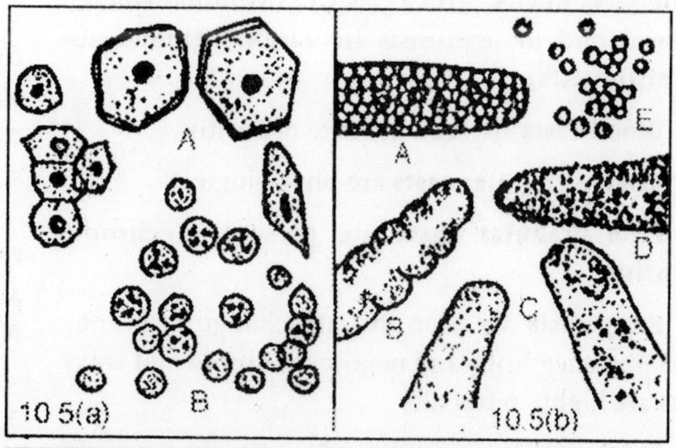

Fig. 10.5(a): A. Epithelial cells, B. Pus cells.

Fig. 10.5(b): A. Blood cast, B. Fatty cast, C. Hyaline cast, D. Granular cast, E. Red cells and Red cell (cellular) cast.

IN ACID URINE:

1. **Uric Acid (yellowish-red**, white-stone crystals);
2. Amorphous Acid Pot. or Sod. **Urates** (yellowish red); heating in alkali dissolves them;
3. Cholesterol, Cystine, Leucine (spheres), Tyrosine (needles) and Sulphonamides are found.

Calcium oxalate may be present (dumbell or biscuit or octahedral or envelop shaped crystals) in **both acid and alkaline urine**.

IN ALKALINE URINE:

Calcium Hydrogen Phosphate (Stellar), Triple Phosphate (Coffin lid or feathery crystals soluble in acetic acid), **Amorphous Phosphates, Ammonium Biurate** (thorn-apple crystals — yellow, which dissolve in HCl) are present **(See Fig. 10.4B). Triple PO_4 is Cal. PO_4, Mg. PO_4 and Al. PO_4.**

ORGANISED DEPOSITS IN URINE

Red cells are present in microscopic hematuria. More than 1 per 10 high power fields should be regarded as abnormal. Leucocytes or pus cells indicate suppuration in the urinary tract.

Epithelium Renal: **Polygonal**, nucleated; or show fatty change.

Bladder and Urinary passage — Transitional. Vaginal Epithelia are **Squamous** in character.

Tube Casts are narrow, homogeneous; found in **all forms of nephritis**. Epithelial casts are seen in Acute GN, RPGN, MPGN, MCD (Minimal change disease) and in nephrosis in various **glomerulonephritis**, (GN).

Blood casts are seen in acute nephritis.

Coarse granular casts are physiological.

Fine granular casts are present in **chronic nephritis.**

Fatty casts are seen in fatty change of kidney specially in nephritis and nephrosis; **Lipoid** and **waxy casts** are highly refractile.

Spermatozoa, parasites, *Microfilaria bancrofti* may be present in chylous urine; ova of **Schistosoma hematobium** may be present in the urine (see below).

EXAMINATION OF URINE FOR DETECTION OF OVA AND LARVA

Urine is primarily examined for:

(i) Ova of *S. **hematobium***.

(ii) Microfilaria of ***Wüchereria bancrofti***.

(iii) Larvae of ***S. stercoralis***.

(iv) Rarely ova of ***Dictophyma renale***, the dog kidney worm, a rare parasite of human. They are passed in the urine.

Sedimentation

A coverslip preparation is made from the sediment and examined for the detection of ova of *S. hematobium*.Look for microfilaria in **milky urine** (i.e., **chyluria**).

Centrifugation

Centrifugation is useful in the detection of ova of *S. hematobium, microfilaria* of *W. bancrofti* **(filariasis)**, and larvae of **S. stercoralis (Strongyloidosis)**.

URINE EXAMINATION FOR MALIGNANT CELL

Stain a smear with **H & E and Papanicolaou stain** and examine for malignant cells (**exfoliative cytology**).

A **histopathological** examination is done by preparation of a **cell block**. For this, the centrifuged deposits should be wet fixed in a mixture of equal parts of 70% Alcohol (50% vol. by vol.) and Ether (50% vol. by vol.).

Draw diagram to show — deposits in urine, [unorganised and organised (see Figure 10.5)].

CASTS [CYLINDROIDS]

Casts are cylindrical structures (cylindroids) formed within the renal tubules and moulded to the shape of their lumina. They are formed by the precipitation of proteins and by **conglutination of cells** within the renal tubule.

Site of formation of casts: **Distal** convoluted **tubules** and **collecting tubules** favoured **by acidity and concentrated** nature of the **urine**. [(Cylindroids) **Not formed in the proximal tubules**)].

Main types: **1. Hyaline casts. 2. Epithelial casts. 3. Red cell (cellular) casts.**

HYALINE CASTS

Appearance: In the unstained preparation, hyaline casts are homogeneous cylindrical structures. In

Table IV.2: Varieties of Telescoped sediment

Characteristics	*Diseases*
Red cell casts	Lupus nephritis
Red blood cells	Polyarteritis nodosa
Urinary lipids (oval fat bodies, etc.) Fatty casts (Waxy casts) (Waxy)	Acute exacerbation of nephritis during nephrotic phase
Cellular casts	Focal necrotizing GN
Colloid casts (Protein and hyaline casts)	See under hyaline casts
Granular casts (Fine)	Chronic nephritis and Renal sarcoidosis
Renal failure casts	Progressive systemic sclerosis

Sternheimer-Malbin preparations the hyaline matrix stains light pink in contrast to the dark staining inclusion elements.

Composition: **Mucoprotein** derived from the renal epithelium (major constituent) + small amounts of **plasma proteins**. There may be mucin threads.

Formation: Not completely understood. It may perhaps be due to precipitation of a mucoprotein by serum albumin in **salt free urine**.

Significance: A few **hyaline casts** may be present **in normal urine**. Temporary increase after **exercise, fever** and **congestive heart failure**. They are particularly important because of the messages carried by inclusions which they may contain. They may **contain cells, cellular debris, fat, bacteria and crystals.**

Red cells inclusion within hyaline casts **indicate intrarenal hemorrhage; pus cells or bacterial inclusions** are pathognomonic of **renal inflammation or infection** (pyelonephritis).

Tubular epithelial inclusions suggest **tubular degeneration**.

Fatty and waxy casts are commonly observed in **Nephrotic syndrome**.

Urate crystals in casts occur in gouty nephropathy.

EPITHELIAL CASTS

Epithelial casts are formed by the conglutination of tubular epithelial cells within the nephron. The **epithelial (cell) cast** and the **hyaline cellular cast degenerate to form granular** (coarse or fine) and waxy **casts**. The epithelial casts may contain fat droplets.

WAXY AND GRANULAR CASTS

Characteristics of **chronic renal disease**. Fat droplets in the cellular casts suggest fatty tubular (degenerative) change and are observed in **nephrotic syndrome**.

RED CELL CASTS

Red cell casts are formed by the conglutination of red cells within the tubular lumen. It is believed that **conversion of fibrinogen** (entering the tubular fluid from damaged glomeruli) **into fibrin within the tubular fluid** is important in the formation of red cell casts (immunological phenomenon in acute post streptococcal [(GN) (**PSGN**)].

Red cell casts are indicative of acute GN as in

1. **Acute glomerulonephritis** (GN).
2. **Polyarteritis nodosa**.
3. **Allergic vasculitis** e.g., **Schoenlein-Henoch** (purpura) disease.
4. **Malignant hypertension**.
5. **Embolic GN** (Subacute Bact. Endocarditis—SABE).

Broad Casts

This is 2-6 times bigger in diameter — sometimes referred to as **renal failure casts**. They are observed in chronic renal disease and during the **diuretic phase of acute renal failure**. **Stasis** of urine in the **kidney** and **dilation of nephron** appears to be necessary for its formation.

PIGMENTED CASTS

Myoglobin casts

Myoglobin casts are seen in **crushing injury, massive muscle necrosis** in gas gangrene and **idiopathic myoglobinuria**.

Hemoglobin casts (Hemosiderin granules containing casts): This occurs in **hemoglobinuric conditions** from any cause (hemolytic crises, transfusion reactions, etc).

> **Note: Hemoglobin and myoglobin cast** formations play significant role in the genesis of oliguria **in acute renal failure following crush injuries**, etc.

CYLINDROIDS

They are **similar to hyaline casts** and probably have the same significance. They are distinguished by having rather narrow and tapering to a slender tail often twisted or curled on itself. **They are associated with mild circulatory or inflammatory disorders of the urinary tract.**

PSEUDO CASTS

They are formed by masses of **amorphous urates, phosphates**, etc.

Mucus Threads

They appear as long strands or ribbon like structures with tapering ends which are often split or curled. They may be found normally or in **mild inflammatory conditions.**

Urinary Lipids

(Oval fat bodies): The oval fat bodies are epithelial cells containing fat droplets. They are usually found in **nephrotic syndrome**.

Bacteria

Normal urine is free of bacteria. Their presence may be demonstrated in **infections of the urinary tract (UTI)** and in **contaminated specimens.**

Spermatozoa

They are occasionally found in the urine of males and in females after coitus. It is of no significance.

***Trichomonads and Giardia lamblia:* Contaminants** in female urine, and urine after coitus in male.

Telescoped Sediment

It refers to the simultaneous appearance in the urinary sediment of elements characteristically found in the three classic stages of glomerulonephritis (GN).

Table IV.3: Examination of Feces: Color consideration

Color	Conditions
1. **Black**	(a) **Malena (Tarry)** (b) Iron, Bismuth, Manganese and Charcoal administration
2. **Green (greenish)**	(*E. coli*) Gastroenteritis in children
3. **Red**:	
(a) Blood on outer surface of formed stool	Hemorrhage, fissure in ano, and ano-rectal cancer
(b) Red current jelly	Intussusception
(c) Bright red intimately mixed with semisolid stool	Carcinoma colon and hemorrhage in Meckel's diverticulum
(d) Bright red: blood mixed with mucus and pus in liquid feces	Bacillary dysentery, ulcerative colitis and ulcerating cancer of the colon
4. **Clay colored** or **greyish white**	(a) Obstructive, or hepatic (regurgitation) jaundice
	(b) After barium meal
5. **Pale bulky (fatty) stool**	Steatorrhoea
6. Green	Green diarrhea in children (*Esch. coli* infection), after diet very rich in green vegetables, and **calomel administration**
7. Characteristic yellow	After administration of **senna, rhubarb, santonin**
8. Colourless (Rice-water)	Cholera

PROFORMA OF REPORT ON EXAMIANTION OF URINE

Name of Laboratory:
Address:
Telephone No.:

Patient's Name:
Referred by:
Date of Reference:
Date of Issuing Report:

Physical Examination:

Quantity (volume)	... ...	ml
Colour	... ...	
Odour	... ...	
Appearance	... ...	Turbid / Opalescent / Clear
Sp. Gravity	... ...	

Chemical Examination:

Reaction	... ...	Acid / Neutral / Alkaline
Albumin	... ...	Nil / Present (Trace +/++/+++; **Heat test** / Esbach's / Heller's method)
Excess of phosphate	... ...	Absent / Present
Sugar	... ...	Nil / Present (Trace +/++/+++/++++; **Benedict's** method)
Acetone	... ...	Nil / Present (**Rothera's test**)
Diacetic acid	... ...	Nil / Present (**Gerhardt's test in Acetoacetic and B-hydroxybutyric Acid**)
Bile pigment	... ...	Nil / Present (**Harrisons'** / Hunter's / Gmelin's method)
Bile salt	... ...	Nil / Present (Hay's sulfer test)
Blood	... ...	Absent / Present (Benzidine / Guaiacum / **Orthotolidine test**)
Urobilinogen	... ...	Nil / Present (dilution 1: ...... **Wallace-Diamond method**)
Urobilin	... ...	Nil / Present (Schleshinger's method)
Indican	... ...	Nil / Present (**Obermeyer's test**)
Others	... ...	

Microscopical Examiantion:

Cells	... ...	(a) **Pus cells** (inner **coarse granules**)	...	per H.P. Field
		(b) **Leukocytes (fine granules)**	...	per H.P. Field
		(c) Red cells	...	per H.P. Field
		(d) Epithelial cells:		
		(i) Squamous type	...	per H.P. Field
		(ii) Round (parabasal or basal) type	...	per H.P. Field
		(iii) Transitional type	...	per H.P. Field
		(e) Macrophages	...	per H.P. Field
Casts	... ...			

Crystals (see figures; sulphonamide crystal)
Amorphous (urates and phosphates)
Others (Mucin)

Quantitative Estimations:

Signature.................................

Pathologist

BACTERIOLOGICAL EXAMINATION OF URINE

Collect a midstream or whole urine **under aseptic precautions or preferably a catheter specimen of urine in a sterile container**. Centrifuge aseptically and inoculate in MacConkey's plate for coliform group, or in Blood agar plate for staphylococci, streptococci, etc. Inoculate after concentration in case of **M. tuberculosis**. Stain a smear prepared from the deposit by Ziehl-Neelsen (Z-N) **method** and examine under oil-immersion lens.

Culture in Loewenstein-Jensen (L-J) media, and finally inoculate a guinea-pig as usual.

EXAMINATION OF FECES

For detailed examination see section on authors' Parasitology and Practical Microbiology also.

CAUSES OF OCCULT BLOOD IN STOOL

1. **Peptic ulcer**.
2. Acute and chronic inflammatory bowel lesions, like amoebic dysentery, bacillary dysentery, ulcerative colitis, etc.
3. Esophageal varices.
4. Malignant tumors of the G.I. Tract, pancreas, ampulla of Vater, etc.
5. Ulcer in the Meckel's diverticulum.
6. **Diseases of bleeding diathesis**, e.g., hemophilia, purpura.
7. Hookworm disease.

CAUSES OF BLEEDING PER ANUM

1. Traumatic
2. Malena (peptic ulcer)
3. Hemorrrhage in enteric fever
4. **Bacillary dysentery**
5. **Colonic and rectal (colorectal) cancer**
6. Malignant tumor of the pancreas
7. Bleeding diathesis.

Diagrams/Notes

Diagrams/Notes

Diagrams/Notes

CHAPTER 11

MISCELLANEOUS INVESTIGATIONS

INVESTIGATION OF GASTRIC FUNCTION

FTM (FRACTIONAL TEST MEAL)

Preparation of the Patient

The patient is given a light supper at 8 P.M. in the previous night. (He is also stopped from chewing spices, betel nuts and paan). A charcoal biscuit is given with a glass of milk before retiring at 10 P.M. or four charcoal tablets are given instead of a biscuit.

Introduction of the Tube

In the morning at 8 A.M. the Ryle's tube is introduced; swab the throat of the patient, if necessary with 1 per cent xylocaine or any other local anesthetic. The patient should be comfortable either in the sitting or in lying position. The bulbous end of the tube is introduced on the posterior part of the dorsum of the tongue and allowed to drop slowly backwards and downwards. When it is in the pharynx, ask the patient to swallow and ask him to continue it slowly till the tube reaches the fundus of the stomach as is indicated by the 2nd mark in the tube.

Aspirate; content is acid reaction to the litmus (confirms correct insertion of the tube).

RYLE'S TUBE (Fig. 11.1)

This is a thin rubber or plastic tube of about 60 cm (24 inches) long. It has several markings to determine whether it is **inserted in the cardiac part** or the **pyloric part of the stomach**, or in the **duodenum**.

Fasting contents of the stomach is withdrawn when the tube is in the fundus. This is done by attaching a 50 ml syringe to the tube with the piston withdrawn; push the piston home; this will dislodge any mucus sticking to the tube. Now withdraw the piston and try to collect the fasting gastric juice as completely as possible by altering the position of the tube. This gives the total resting juice.

Preparation of the Test Meal

1. **Gruel test meal**: A tea-spoonful of quaker oats is put in two pints of water; add a pinch of salt; boil down to a pint and strain through a piece of fine muslin (cloth). Ask the patient to swallow. Sometimes it is difficult to swallow thick gruel; if so, then push through the tube in a 50 ml syringe.

2. **Alcohol meal**: 100 ml of **7 per cent alcohol** is taken in a beaker. The syringe is filled up with it and alcohol meal is introduced into the stomach. Alcohol is a more powerful stimulant for gastric juice secretion than the gruel meal.

N.B. The test and the interpretations are rather like those of the Rehfuss meal but the acidity is higher in gruel meal.

Collection of Samples

1. Resting juice. 2. Collection of 12 post-prandial samples (after test meal). **Total: 13 samples** are obtained.

Note the time of introduction of the meal and aspirate a little more than 10 ml of the gastric contents each time at an interval of every 15 minutes, up to $2\frac{1}{2}$ or better upto 3 hours (when the stomach is empty). The specimens are put in test tubes, labelled serially and sent to the laboratory for examination. Measure the quantity of resting juice. Normally it is about 20 to 25 ml. Over 50 ml indicates **hypomotility**, obstruction or hypersecretion; remnant of charcoal indicates **pyloric obstruction, gastric ptosis**, etc.

MACROSCOPIC EXAMINATION

Look for gross **mucus, starch, bile, blood**, etc., in all the specimens after arranging the tubes in order.

Interpretation: **Excess of mucus indicates gastritis.**

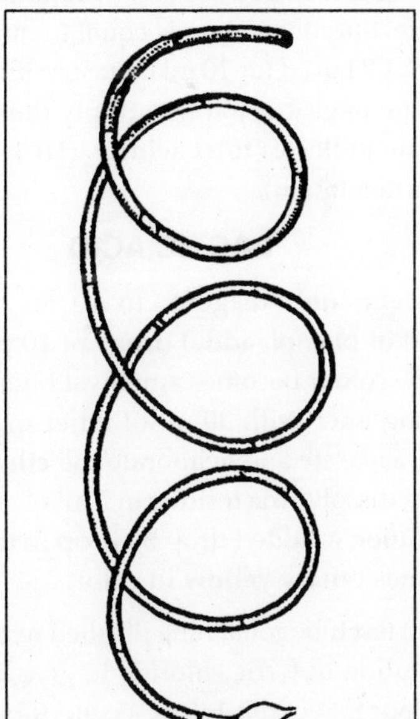

Fig. 11.1: Ryle's tube for Gastric juice collection

Bile when present in excess is pathological; it is **absent in pyloric stenosis**.

Presence of blood indicates varices, erosion, ulcerations including the **malignant conditions**.

CHEMICAL TEST

Acidimetry: To 10 ml of strained gastric juice in a porcelain dish add a drop of **Topfer's reagent** (0.5% dimethylaminoazobenzene in ethanol); note the color. A **cherry red or orange color** indicates the **presence of free HCl**. Titrate with N/10 NaOH from the burette; start from 0, stirring the contents all the time till **color changes to canary yellow**. Note the burette reading.

Now add a drop of **1 per cent phenolphthalein** in alcohol and titrate with N/10 NaOH (from the same burette) till a permanent pink colour develops. Stir the contents all the time while adding the solution. Note the final burette reading. Repeat the process in all the samples of gastric juice.

Calculation of free acid

The first burette reading minus the initial burette reading indicates the **number of ml of N/10 NaOH** used for 10 ml of gastric juice; for 100 ml multiply by 10. The figure thus obtained is expressed in terms of degree and percentage of **free-acidity** (i.e., HCl).

TOTAL ACIDITY: Final burette reading minus the initial burette reading is equal to number of ml of N/10 NaOH used for 10 ml of gastric juice. Therefore, for 100 ml of gastric juice, multiply the figures by 10; the figure indicates **total acidity**. **(HCl + Lactic Acid** from fermentation).

LACTIC ACID

Uffelmann's reagent: To 10 ml of 5 per cent solution of phenol, add 3 drops of 10 per cent ferric chloride, colour becomes amethyst blue. Extract 5 ml of resting juice with 30 ml of ether in a **separating funnel**; separate and evaporate the **etheral extract** to dryness; dissolve the residue in 2 ml of distilled water. The solution is added drop by drop to the reagent till it becomes **canary yellow in color**.

To a test tube containing distilled water, add 10 per cent solution of ferric chloride to give a faint yellow tinge. Pour half of this into a second tube to serve as a **control**. To the other half add a small amount of gastric juice. Then add **six drops of saturated solution of mercuric chloride** in both the tubes. **Lactic acid gives a distinct yellow colour** which is readily recognized by comparison with the control tube.

STARCH

To a few drops of unfiltered gastric juice, add dilute solution of **iodine drop by drop** and shake. **Blue colour** appears if **starch** is present.

BILE

When present in excess, it is easily recognised by its colour. **Bile pigment** can be recognized by **Fouchet's method in Harrison's test** (see previous chapter under urine).

To filtered juice add a couple of drops of 1 per cent alcoholic iodine. A **green ring** formed at the junction indicates the presence of **bile pigment**.

Hay's (sulphur) test

Sprinkle dry flour of sulphur on the surface of the gastric juice. Presence of **bile (salt) acid** is indicated by **sinking of the sulphur powder (granules)**.

BLOOD

Benzidine test is the best of all (for test see under urine examination, previous chapter). The test detects blood in dilution of in 1 : 1,000,000. But benzidine being carcinogenic, ortho-tolidine test is done.

Ortho-tolidine Test: Take 2 per cent of ortho-tolidine (in acetic acid) and add several drops on the sample to be tested. Add equal proportion of 1 : 10 dilution of hydrogen peroxide.

MICROSCOPIC EXAMINATION OF THE RESTING JUICE

Examine the residue after centrifuging by a wet preparation under **high power for red cells, pus cells, malignant cells**. Make a thin film of the contents. Heat to fix and stain with Lugol's iodine. Look for **Boas-Oppler-bacillus, Helicobacters**, etc. under oil-immersion lens. They are stained yellow to brown.

GASTRIC ANALYSIS REPORT (Make a graphic representation):

Name, age, sex, ward, diagnosis ...... Date of Examination. Free acid (Red line); Total acid (Blue line); Resting juice — quantity, lactic acid, starch, bile, mucus, blood and other special points.

N.B. In case of gastric carcinoma, appearance of resting juice is coffee ground due to interaction of acid with blood forming acid hematin.

Make a Graphic Representation of Curves Interpretations:

(1) Normal, (2) Peptic ulcer, (3) Peptic ulcer with pyloric stenosis, (4) Gastric carcinoma, (5) Pernicious anemia, etc.

HISTAMINE TEST

0.6 to **1 mg of histamine** is injected subcutaneously. This is effective in stimulating gastric secretion at the end of 1st hour and may help to detect true **achylia gastrica (histamine-fast achlorhydria)**.

LIVER FUNCTION TESTS

The tests usually employed may be classified as to differentiate the hepato-cellular or **medical jaundice** from the **surgical (extrahepatic or obstructive surgical) jaundice** and to detect the activity of the liver damage for prognosis.

LIVER FUNCTION TESTS USED ARE

(a) To assist in differential diagnosis of jaundice, namely; **urobilinogen in urine** (bile pigment metabolism), **van den Bergh test** (excretory function) and **thymol turbidity test** (if increased indicates **Globulin quantitatively is more than Albumin**).

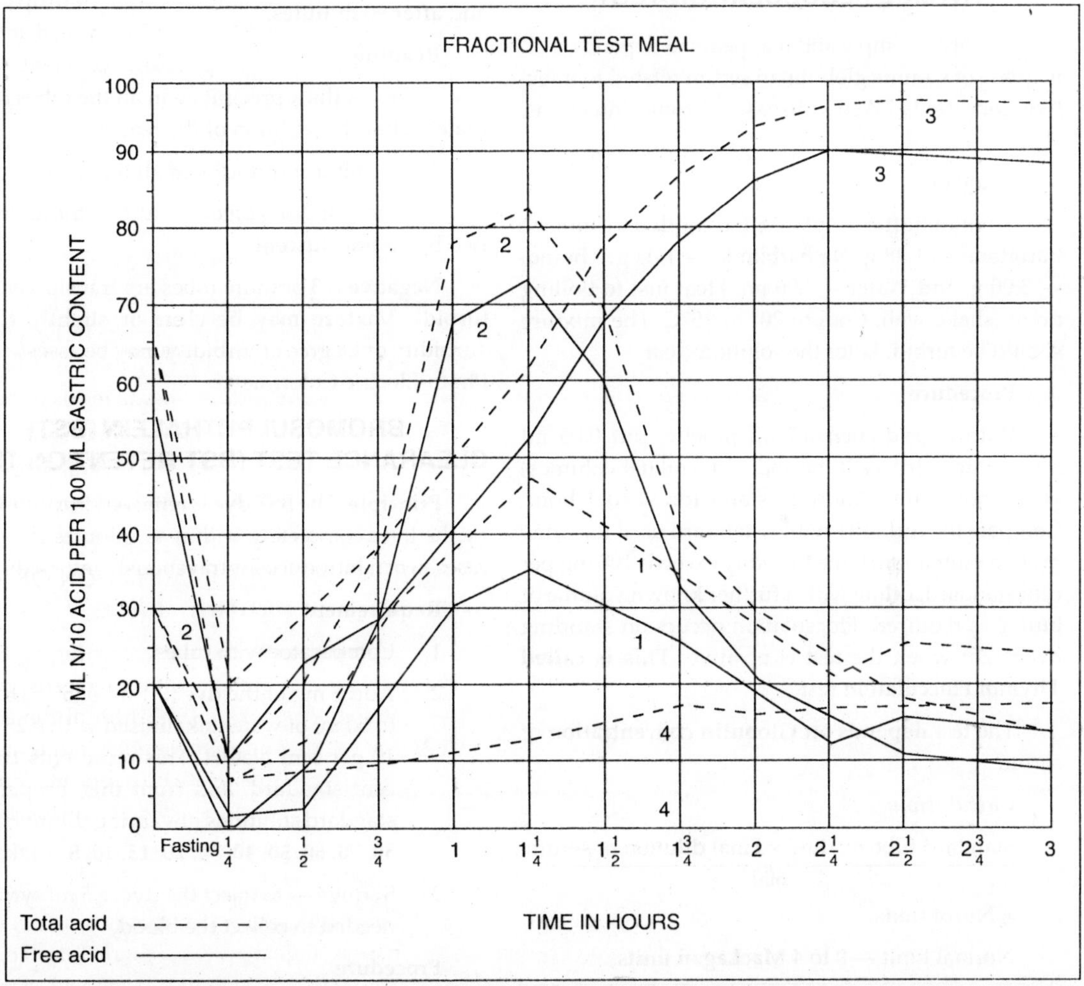

Fig. 11.2: 1. Normal Result—**Resting juice** 15–20 ml

2. Hyperacidity curve in case of hypermotility of stomach with rapid emptying time (**Duodenal ulcer**: **Resting juice—30 ml)**
3. Hyperacidity curve in case of **pylorospasm** with delayed emptying time (**Gastric ulcer; Resting juice**—110 ml)
4. **Achlorhydria** in case of carcinoma of the stomach **with pyloric obstruction (Resting juice**—300 ml or more)

(b) To estimate the extent of the hepatic insufficiency (extent of liver damage and degree of surgical risk). Tests are **hippuric acid** test (detoxicating function), **bromosulphalein test** (excretory function), serum protein estimation (power to form protein), laevulose or **galactose tolerance test** (Carbohydrate metabolism), plasma prothrombin synthesis and its response to vitamin K administration.

To detect and follow the activity of liver damage for prognosis in hepatic disease, **thymol turbidity test** and **Takata-Ara test** are used.

THYMOL TURBIDITY TEST AND THYMOL FLOCCULATION TEST

The test is simple and it appears to depend on an increase of gamma globulin in serum related to infective conditions (Weil's disease, chronic infections, etc.).

Reagents

Thymol buffer — pH 7.8 (strength 0.01 molar), Barbitone — 1.38 g, Na-barbitone — 1.03 g, Thymol — 3.00 g, and Water — 500 ml. Heat just to boiling point; shake well. Cool to 20° to 25°C. The mixture should be turbid. Filter the solution clear.

Procedure

With a graduated 0.2 ml pipette, put 0.05 ml serum into a dry test tube and add 3 ml (60 volumes) of thymol buffer. Allow to stand for $\frac{1}{2}$ to 1 hour. Compare the turbidity with a standard used for urine protein estimation. If the turbidity exceeds 100 mg per cent standard, dilute with a further known volume of buffer as required. Flocculation occurs on standing overnight when the test is positive. **This is called Thymol Flocculation test.**

The test **depends on Globulin concentration** of serum.

Calculation:

$$\frac{\text{Standard tube reading} \times \text{Final dilution of serum}}{600}$$

= No. of units.

Normal limit — 0 to 4 **MacLagan units**.

N.B. Inactivated serum should not be used. Check standard every two months against diluted serum of known protein content (1 ml of serum in varying dilutions and 3 ml of 3 per cent sulphosalicylic acid).

TAKATA-ARA TEST (UCKO'S MODIFICATION)

Reagents

0.3 per cent solution of **anhydrous sodium carbonate**, 0.5 per cent solution of **mercuric chloride**.

Procedure

Into 5 clean test tubes, each containing **0.2 ml of serum** where 0.1, 0.15, 0.20, 0.25 and 0.3 ml of **sodium carbonate** is added **(Saturated Solution)**. Shake the tubes, and same quantities of mercuric chloride are added to each tube like sodium carbonate solution. Shake and allow to settle. Reading is taken **at once** and **after 90 minutes**.

Reading

+ + + = A thick precipitate in all the tubes immediately after the addition of the reagents.

+ + = Uniform turbidity in all the tubes.

+ = The first 2 or 3 tubes are turbid; the remaining two being transluscent.

Negative = 3 or more tubes are transluscent (not turbid). Mixture may be clear or slightly turbid. Turbidity or Degree of turbidity may be assessed by a Photo-Electric Colorimeter.

BROMOSULPHTHALEIN (BST) CLEARANCE TEST (BST RETENTION TEST)

Principle: The BST dye is removed from the blood by the liver completely within 45 minutes in normal cases, when introduced intravenously into body.

Requirement

1. Comparator with tubes.
2. Add 5 mg of the dye (0.1 ml of 5% solution) to 50 ml of water alkalinised with 0.25 ml of 10 per cent NaOH. This represents 100 per cent standard, and from this, prepare the standard solutions of varying dilutions, e.g., **80, 70, 60, 50, 40, 30, 20, 15, 10, 5**.
3. Syringe — to inject the dye, a 5 ml syringe is needed to collect the blood.

Procedure

Inject 5 mg of the dye per kg of body weight intravenously in 1 minute without any leakage. **Blood samples (5 ml) are withdrawn at intervals of 5 and 45 minutes**. From these samples, put about 1 ml of clear serum in each of the two comparator tubes; to one add 1 to 2 drops of 10 per cent NaOH to secure the maximum depth of color, and to the other **add 1 drop of 5% HCl (acidified serum)**.

Read at once in the comparator matching with the standard. Match the standard tube with the acidified serum, and the alkalinised tube with a tube of distilled water. Reading can also be taken in a colorimeter at **540 nm (green-yellow filter)**.

Interpretation

Normally 5 minutes after the injection of the BST 20-50 per cent (average 35 per cent), and **30-45 minutes after the injection whole of the dye disappears from blood**.

Remarks

Retention of dye in blood **indicates liver insufficiency**. The test is sensitive and reliable for detecting **liver insufficiency in absence of jaundice**. It is of great prognostic value in surgical cases.

GALACTOSE TOLERANCE TEST

Theory

Liver is solely concerned with metabolism of galactose (converted into glycogen without any insulin) and galactose is not utilised by the muscle. Any galactose that escapes through the liver is excreted by the kidney; the **renal threshold for galactose being nil**.

Procedure

No food is allowed at night or at breakfast time. The patient empties the bladder completely before the test. Give a drink of **40 g of pure galactose in 250 ml** or more of **water. Collect urine** hourly for 5 hours. Make sure that the initial sample does not show any glycosuria before the administration of galactose. **Examine** qualitatively all the samples **by Benedict's method**. Pool all the positive samples; determine quantitatively from the **volume of urine** (0.053 g reduces 25 ml of Benedict's quantitative reagent).

Interpretation

Normal excretion — 0 to 2 g. Decreased tolerance is indicated by total excretion of more than 3 g. The test is positive in 70 per cent cases of parenchymatous **medical (hepatic) jaundice**, but negative in 80 per cent **obstructive jaundice**.

N.B. In case of glycosuria, the mixed urine is treated with a 10 per cent suspension of yeast (1 part of urine and 7.7 parts of yeast). Keep for 45 minutes at room temperature; centrifuge or filter. Then determine the remaining quantity of **sugar (galactose)** by **Benedict's method** (Shey et al., 1931).

Intravenous Method

Inject intravenously 1 ml of 50 per cent galactose solution per kg body weight. Estimate blood 75 minutes after the injection, when the blood is free from galactose in normal case.

HIPPURIC ACID TEST (H.A. TEST)

Principle

The test depends upon the **synthesis of hippuric acid from benzoic acid administered as sodium benzoate. Benzoic acid is conjugated with glycine** in the liver **to form hippuric acid** and water.

Method

1. QUICK'S PRECIPITATION METHOD

Quick's precipitation method by weighing of the precipitate gives only partial recovery of hippuric acid from urine. **Addition of 30 per cent NaCl is better** than one by addition of 50 per cent ammonium sulphate.

2. ORAL TEST METHOD

After a light breakfast, ask the patient to empty the bladder, and give a dose of 4 or 6 g of sodium benzoate in 30 ml of water, flavoured with Oil menth. pip. This is followed by drinking a glass of water. Samples of urine passed during the next 4 hours are collected for examination and the volume is measured. Reduce the volume in a water bath, if the total volume is above 600 ml. Add 30 g of sodium chloride per 100 ml of urine; heat until the salt is dissolved completely. Put the flask in iced water and cool the solution to 15°C to 20°C. Add 2 ml of concentrated HCl and scratch inside the flask vigorously until there is a complete precipitation of hippuric acid. Allow the flask to stand for 15 minutes in the cold water. Filter through a filter paper rinsing and including the precipitate in the flask with cold 30 per cent NaCl from the wash bottle, till the precipitate is free from HCl. **Transfer all the precipitate in the flask and heat till whole of hippuric acid dissolves in water**. Titrate while hot with 0.5N. NaOH with **phenolphthalein as indicator**.

Calculation

No. of ml of NaOH used for neutralization × 0.072 g = **Hippuric acid is precipitated** in terms of

Na-benzoate. Add 0.1 g of Na-benzoate per 100 ml as correction for solubility of **HA** in solution.

Intravenous Method

After a light breakfast, give a glass a water (200 ml) to drink and ask the patient to evacuate the bladder. Inject intravenously **1.77 g of Na benzoate (= 1.5 g of benzoic acid)** in 20 ml of distilled water, taking 5 minutes or more for the injection. Just at the **end of one hour** after completion of the injection, collect the entire amount of urine (if necessary by catheter). Measure the volume of urine and if it is **over 100 ml, add a few drops of glacial acetic acid**, concentrate the urine to 50 ml to 100 ml (if high coloured or contains bile, add one teaspoonful of charcoal). Filter while hot through a coarse filter paper and then through a fine filter paper. **Add 53 g of NaCl per 100 ml of filtrate** and dissolve completely. Other steps are same as in the oral method.

Interpretation

Normal excretion by oral route in 4 hours after a 4 g dose on average is 3.2 g (80 per cent). Recovery less than 40 per cent means a definitely low excretion.

N.B. (1) **Renal disease** invalidates the test. (2) **Bile and protein** in urine **interferes** with estimation. In that case **remove them by adding 5 ml of 30 per cent zinc sulphate** and 2.5 ml of 2.5 N.NaOH per 100 ml of urine . Shake and filter. Large quantities of protein are precipitated by boiling the urine.

After intravenous injection of 1.77 g of Na-benzoate, excretion at the end of 1 hour should be 1 g.

RENAL FUNCTION TEST

Renal function tests can be divided into three:

1. *Changes in the blood*: Retention of urea and NPN in blood (due to failure in excretion of urine)—urea may rise up to 280 mg or higher in acute and chronic nephritis.

2. *Presence of abnormal constituents in urine are*: albumin, casts, etc.

3. *Eliminating power of excretion of the kidney*: It is judged by excretion of water, urea, phenolsulphenolphthalein.

I. FOR TUBULAR FUNCTIONS

UREA CONCENTRATION TEST

(MacLean and De Wesselow, 1920)

Procedure

Light food is given to the patient in the previous night. He should not take any fluid some hours previous to the test. In the morning at 7 A.M. he empties the bladder and a drink of 15 g of urea in 100 ml of water, flavoured with little tincture of orange is given. Urine passed after 1, 2 and 3 hours are collected in separate bottles. Estimate urea percentage in all the specimens of urine. If the amount of urine **after one hour exceeds 120 ml discard** it; as it is the result of **diruetic effect of urea**.

Interpretation

Normally a healthy person excretes about 2 g per cent of urea in urine but under this observation, urea will be 4 g per cent or more. **Less than 3 g per cent urea in urine indicates renal insufficiency**.

WATER TEST

(Volhard's test modified by Rosenberg)

A. Dilution test

On the first day the patient takes 1,500 ml of water in 30 minutes after micturition. He can then take his breakfast but **should not take any drink till** the test is completed. **Samples** of urine are collected. **Every half an hour** for next four hours, separately. The volume and specific gravity of each sample is measured. A normal individual excretes the whole amount of water within 4 hours and the **specific gravity falls to 1002 or below that.**

B. Concentration test

On the second day ordinary meals are given to the patient and the amount of the **fluid is restricted to 500 ml during the whole 24 hours** taken in **four** roughly **equal intervals**. Fruits are avoided. Urine is passed as the patient desires. Samples are collected separately and **tested for volume and specific gravity. Total urine should not exceed 750 ml** and the **specific gravity should rise to 1027**. In a case of chronic nephritis with impaired renal functions, the patient is unable to pass the full amount of urine on the first day and total volume exceeds 750 ml on the second day.

FIXATION OF SPECIFIC GRAVITY TEST

In this the patient does not take fluid, drink, liquid foods or fruits from his breakfast time (no fluid) till the breakfast time next day. The urine passed in first 12 hours is not collected but urine passed in second 12 hours is collected and pooled. In case the renal function is satisfactory, the specific gravity should be **at least 1024 and concentration of urea**

should be more than 2 per cent. In case of fixation, the specific gravity is 1010.

II. FOR GLOMERULAR FUNCTIONS

1. BLOOD UREA CLEARANCE TEST (Moeller, McIntosh and Van Slyke)

Procedure

The patient is given his usual breakfast at 8 A.M. without tea or coffee **but water as desired**. At 9 A.M. he empties the bladder completely just before the test. He is then given 100 ml of water. At 10 A.M. he empties the bladder completely and the sample of urine is **collected (sample 1)**.

Then 100 ml of water is again given to him as drink and **immediately collect blood** from the vein and **urea estimated**. The patient empties his bladder completely at 11 A.M. and the sample is collected (**sample II**).

Measure the volume of urine in each specimen separately and calculate the output per minute in ml (by dividing the number of ml by number of minutes lapsed between voiding). Determine:

(a) **Concentration of urine urea in each sample of urine**,

(b) **Concentration of blood urea**. If the volume of urine excreted is more than 2 ml per minute, calculate the **standard clearance (Cs)**:

Cm = Clearance maximum.

Cs = Clearance standard (normal).

$$Cm = \frac{U \times V \times 1.33}{B}; \quad Cs = \frac{U \times \sqrt{V} \times 1.85}{B}$$

(Percentage of normal clearance is $^{100}/_{75} = 1.33$ in case of Cm. The percentage of normal clearance is $^{100}/_{54} = 1.85$ in case of Cs).

U = Urea concentration in urine, **V** = Volume of urine excreted per min. **B** = Urea concentration of blood

2. INULIN CLEARANCE TEST

This is a more specific **test of glomerular filtration** than the urea clearance test as inulin is completely filterable through the glomerulus. Inulin is neither reabsorbed nor synthesized by the tubules.

Procedure

25 g of **inulin** is injected by intravenous route, and clearance is measured by determination of inulin in blood and urine. The process is similar to that employed for Urea Clearance Test.

Interpretation

Average adult clearance = **120 ml of plasma per minute** as GFR. The range varies from 100–150 ml per minute.

Percentage of average of normal renal function clearance.

Over 70%	...	Normal
70 to 40%	...	Mild deficit
40 to 20%	...	Moderate deficit
Below 20%	...	Severe deficit
Below 5%	...	**Uraemic coma** present or imminent

2. DIODRAST CLEARANCE TEST

Diodrast is removed by the kidney through glomerular filtration and tubular excretion. It serves as a basis for **clearance determination**. The material used is the same as intravenous pyelography (I.V.P.). In adults the average diodrast clearance is 700 ml of blood per minute; but the **normal range is 520 to 1,560 ml per minute**.

PREGNANCY TESTS

Various methods are used for pregnancy tests but the following tests gave a very satisfactory result in the past.

1. FROG TEST

Select male frog (Rana tigrina) — 150 g in weight. Be sure that it is a male one, by the presence of pads on the thumbs (thenar eminence). Inject 5 ml of fresh urine (**when delayed**, use **urine treated with ether**) in the region near the dorsal lymph sac. For this take a long needle and introduce it in the skin to reach the dorsal lymph sac. Wait for 1 to 2 hours; then take a sample of cloacal fluid and examine it under the microscope. Presence of motile, rod-shaped spermatozoa indicates a positive test which means the presence of A.P.L. (anterior pituitary-like) hormone in urine of a pregnant woman.

Concentration of the hormone rises in the earlier months of pregnancy. A well-marked concentration is **noticed in hydatidiform mole, chorionepithelioma and seminoma**.

It is a nonspecific type of test.

2. FRIEDMAN'S TEST

Rabbits ovulate only when their ovary is specially stimulated as after their mating. A mature female rabbit is isolated in a cage three weeks before the test; inject 10 ml of urine to be tested into the marginal ear vein. Ovaries are examined 24 hours later. A positive reaction is marked by reddish protrusion of recent **hemorrhage in the follicles of the ovaries**. The abdomen is opened under anaesthesia; ovaries are inspected and abdomen is stitched again. The same rabbit can be used some weeks later, when the corpora lutea (formed) disappear.

IMMUNOLOGICAL TESTS

(Immunological tests for pregnancy)

A number of immunological tests have been worked out for the determination of **human chorionic gonadotropin** (HCG) in pregnancy (McKean, 1960). These are **precipitin** (Coombs et al., 1951), **inhibition of latex agglutination** (Henry and Little, 1962), **hemagglutination inhibition** (Wide and Gamzell; 1960) and **complement-fixation test** (Brody and Carl-strom, 1960). Inhibition of latex agglutination with GRAVINDEX (Ethnor) and hemagglutination inhibition with **Pregnosticon (Organon)** are popular, the latter being most reliable.

Another test is there indicating positivity of the test by **color Reaction is given by β-component of hCG**.

The latest in the field are **SPECIFIC β-GRAVINDEX**, and ELISA.

This is a test with a specificity of HCG hormone 0.3 I. U/ml.

SEMINAL FLUID ANALYSIS

(SEMINOGRAM)

The investigation is done to assess the possibility of fertilization of ovum.

The patient (husband) should be advised to maintain strictly a period of abstinence for 3 to 5 days.

The sample may be collected by:

(a) Prostatic massage.

(b) By masturbation in a Petri dish or wide mouthed bottle. The latter method is easier.

Quantity: 3.5 to 5 ml.

Viscosity: Should be fairly viscous.

Appearance: Opalescent.

Reaction: Alkaline.

Motility: 90% to 100% should be motile.

Movement should be scorpioid in all directions.

Stages of Maturation

Mature spermatozoa — 95%.

IMMATURE FORMS MAY INCLUDE:

(a) Spermatogonia.

(b) Primary Spermatocyte.

(c) Secondary Spermatocyte.

(d) Spermatid.

(e) Mature sperm.

Morphological Defects

Defect in the head: It may be double head, spherical head, etc., instead of normal pointed one (**triangular head**).

Defect in the tail: Rudimentary tail, short tail, excessively long tail, etc., are the defects.

Report of semen analysis (Normal sample)

Time of ejaculation: 5 minutes

Time of complete liquefication: 3 Hours/more

Volume: 4-10 ml.

Viscosity: **Average**/Less/More

Reaction: **Alkali**/Neutral/Acid

Total Cell Count of the Series: 60 million/More/Less per ml.

Motility

	1st hr.	2nd hr.	3rd hr.	24 hrs.
Motile	90%	75%	60%	Nil
Sluggishly motile	5%	10%	15%	Nil
Non motile	5%	15%	25%	100%

Mature form: 95% **Immature form**:

Primary Spermatocytes

1%

Secondary Spermatocytes

1%

Spermatids

Teratological Forms: **Absent**/Present % (Giant headed)

Slender Form: **Nil**/Present %

Other Cellular Elements

Pus Cells: **Nil**/Present per HPF

Red cells: **Nil**/Present per HPF

Squamous Epithelial Cells: **Nil**/Present per HPF.

Others

Trichomonad not Detected/Detected.

THYROID FUNCTION TESTS

SEVERAL TESTS ARE THERE:

1. **Determination of basal metabolic rate (BMR)**. This is not in much use today as it has been found that there is a wide range of variation for the normal values of BMR, and **alterations of the BMR may occur due to nonthyroidal factors** also. However, the BMR is increased in hyperthyroidism and minimized in hypothyroidism (infant type, cretinism; adult type, myxedema).

2. **Protein-bound Iodine** (PBI). Serum protein bound iodine is **increased in hypothyroidism**. Normal value: 4-8 mg.

3. **T_3 resin uptake**. Tri-iodothyronine resin uptake is **increased in hyperthyroidism**.

4. **Estimation of serum thyroxine level**. It is **increased in hyperthyroidism**.

5. **Radioactive (RA) iodine (RAL) uptake**. It is directly dependant upon the iodide uptake by the thyroid gland. **RA iodine is trapped in the hyperactive thyroid gland**, so **R A I will be low**.

6. **Estimation of Cholesterol**. Cholesterol **level** goes **high in hypothyroidism** and is **depressed in hyperthyroidism**.

7. **Urinary hydroxyproline excretion**. It is **depressed in hypothyroidism**.

8. **Creatine phosphokinase (CPK)**. It is **elevated in hypothyroidism**.

9. **S.G.O.T.** The level is increased in hypothyroidism.

10. **Lactic dehydrogenase (LDH)**. The level is elevated in hypothyroidism.

11. **Tanned red cell (TRC) agglutination test**. This is **positive in hypothyroidism in Hashimoto's disease**.

Choice of thyroid function tests

Initially it is wise to estimate PBI or serum thyroxine level, the free thyroxine index if available, and the radioactive iodine uptake test. In the initial evaluation of many patients TRC agglutination test to be performed. If a good laboratory is available, the BMR is to be estimated. The serial record of patient's weight is also a good prognostic index. **In hypothyroidism** the weight is increased.

SPECIFIC TESTS

Estimation of Serum T3, T4 and TSH is the best index. The test is done by 2 methods:

1. **Radio-Immuno Assay (RIA).**
2. **Chemical Assay by ELISA method (see Practical Microbiology in Serology Chapter).**

Diagrams/Notes

Diagrams/Notes

CHAPTER 12

HEMATOLOGY

COLLECTION OF BLOOD
(Wintrobe's technique)

ANTICOAGULANT

A. DOUBLE OXALATE

For each ml of blood, use 2 mg of oxalate as an anticoagulant. Pot. oxalate causes shrinkage of cells and therefore a combination of **ammon, pot. oxalate in proportion of 3:2 respectively should be used.**

Prepare a solution of **ammonium oxalate 0.6 g, pot. oxalate 0.4** g and distilled water 100 ml. Distribute 1 ml in some and in others 0.4 ml of the above solution into clean rubber-capped penicillin vials. Put them without the rubber cap in a hot air oven and allow to evaporate to dryness. Remove them as soon as they dry to avoid charring. Put the cap back on vials. They contain 10 mg and 4 mg of oxalate for 5 ml and 2 ml samples of blood respectively. For full hematological investigation collect 10 ml and in other cases 2 or 5 ml of blood. A few blood smears are first of all prepared on the slides from the blood drawn. Remove the needle and put blood into the vial and mix.

Various other anticoagulants may be used. **Double oxalate**, as described above **is unsuitable for collection of blood for estimation of urea**. So blood may be collected in **Potassium oxalate for urea** estimation.

B. SODIUM FLUORIDE

Sugar in blood is constantly metabolized by red cells mainly. If the blood in anticoagulant is left out for sometime, sugar level falls down. So a *toxic anticoagulant sodium fluoride* is added to stop the metabolism of cells and bacteria, and the sugar level remains constant on preservation of the blood sample.

Blood group and Hemoglobin are not to be determined by Fluoride Blood

Sodium fluoride used is 0.25 mg/2ml. or 0.5 mg/4 ml of blood in a vial for blood collection.

C. UNIVERSAL ANTICOAGULANTS

They are: (1) Ethylene Diamine Tetra-Acetic acid (EDTA), and (2) Lithium oxalate. They are used as 1-2 mg of EDTA/ml of blood.

D. SODIUM CITRATE

3.8% g aqueous solution is used for E.S.R. estimation by **Westergren method only. 1 part of citrate solution and 4 parts of blood** is mixed for E.S.R. estimation by Westergren method only.

3% sodium citrate solution is used for collection of blood for estimation of **prothrombin time by old method.**

For cross matching in blood transfusion one sample is essential to take in Sod. citrate.

Finger Prick Method is used for estimation of hemoglobin, total leukocyte and red cell count, films for differential leukocyte count, malaria parasites, etc. This method is also used for modern technique of Blood Glucose Estimation by a glucometer.

GENERAL STEPS FOR BLOOD COLLECTION

STEPS:

1. Patient (Pt.) is **asked to take his seat** on a chair with arm rest.
2. Patient is asked to **stretch his arm.**
3. **Select** the most prominent **vein (ante-cubital** vein)
4. **Bind the tourniquet** "1 to 2" above the venous prominence (i.e., at the site of possible prick).
5. **Sterilize the skin** at the site of prick.
6. **Fix the vein** by stretching of the skin downward on the forearm by the left thumb of the blood collector (botamist).
7. Prick the vein by a sterile **needle** (No. 22 or No. 23) fitted to a sterile disposable syringe.
8. A feel of **sudden loss of resistance** indicates that the needle is in the lumen of the vein.
9. **Draw** the required amount (volume) of blood.
10. **Loosen** (and take out) **the tourniquet**; first Dab the pricked area with sterile dry unabsorbable cotton, and then **withdraw the syringe.**
11. **Fold the forearm** on the dry sterile non-absorbable cotton and ask the patient to wait in that posture.
12. **Put blood in** respective vials and shake the vial that contains anticoagulant.
13. **After 3 minutes stretch the hand** and the forearm and put steripad or band-aid if required.

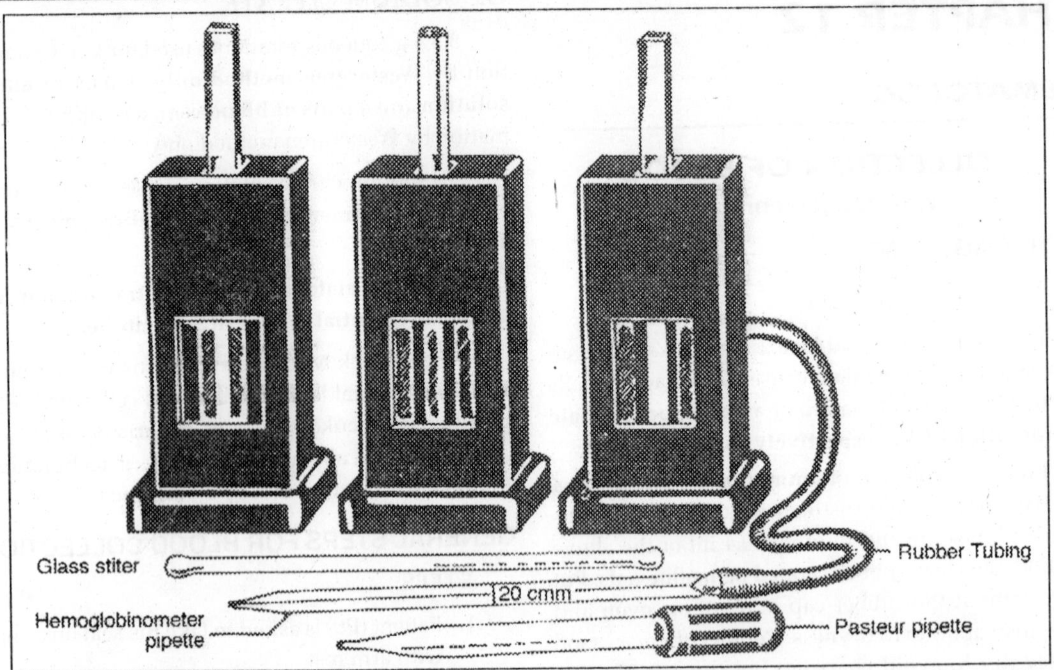

Fig. 12.1: Sahli hemoglobinometers. Acid-hematin mixture is formed by addition of Hydrochloric acid; and Hemoglobinometer pipette with glass rod (Stirrer) and a dropper (Pasteur pipette)

ESTIMATION OF HEMOGLOBIN

(by Hellige's Hemoglobinometer or Hemometer and Hemoglobinometer pipette, See Fig. 12.1)

By Acid Hematin Method: Put 5 drops of $^N/_{10}$ HCl in the graduated hemoglobinometer tube. Fill up the pipette with well shaken oxalated blood or directly from freely flowing drop of blood (by pricking the finger tip), exactly up to the mark 20 cmm (μl) carefully avoiding air bubble.

Wipe off surplus blood from outside the pipette with a gauge and transfer the blood into the hemoglobinometer tube by immersing the tip of the pipette in HCl solution. Wash off the blood in the capillary portion by repeatedly filling and emptying the pipette. Finally wash off the blank pipette. Stir until the blood is well mixed, wait for 5 minutes when the color appears uniformly brown (i.e. **acid hematin formation**). Then add distilled water, one drop at a time from the dropper and stir it every time, comparing, till it matches the standard glass prism of the hemometer. Read the result from the scale in the graduated tube by noting the graduation at the lower meniscus of the liquid column.

100% in Hellige tube is equal to 13.75 g (or 14 g) of Hb. per 100 ml of blood but 100% of Wintrobe's scale is equal to 14.5 g, and 100% Sahli's scale is equal to 17.3 g of Hb. So **absolute percentage is more expressive**, when there is no mention of the method. But the international standard is 14.5G per 100 ml of blood, which corresponds to Wintrobe's scale. The most modern method today is the colorimetric one by conversion of Hb. into cyanomethemoglobin.

TOTAL BLOOD COUNT

(See Figs. 12.2–12.6)

Use Thoma or (Neubauer) counting chamber and RBC pipette for total red cell count and improved Neubauer counting chamber (See Figs. 12.3–12.6), and WBC pipette (see Fig. 12.2) for total WBC count.

A. **TOTAL RED CELL COUNT (Red cell pipette and Red cell count; See Figs. 12.2 to 12.6)**

Diluting Fluids:

(a) **Hayem's fluid** — Mercuric chloride — 0.5 g Sodium chloride — 1 g Sodium sulphate — 5.0 g and distilled water — 200 ml. Or,

(b) **Toisson's fluid** — It is satisfactory. Sodium chloride — 1 g, Sodium sulphate — 8 g, glycerine — 30 ml, water — 160 ml.

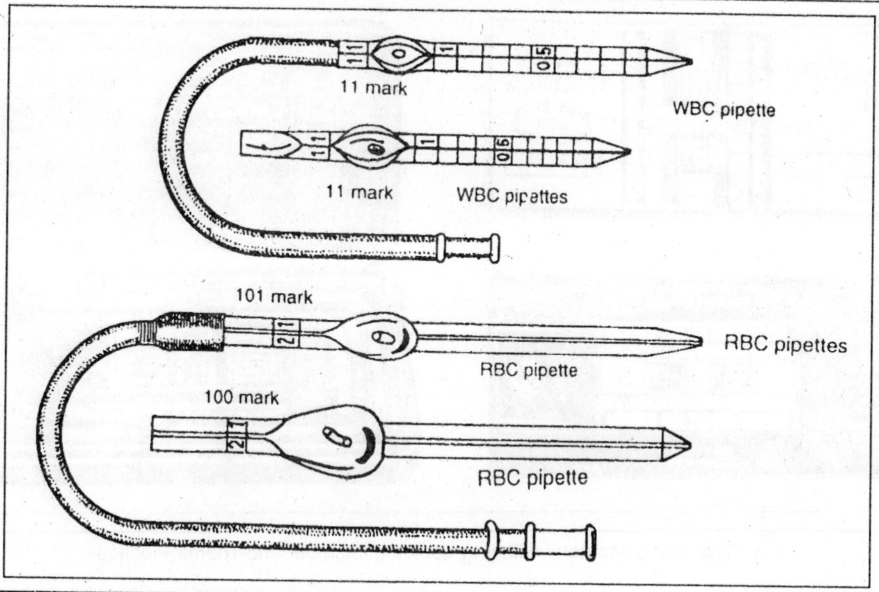

Fig. 12.2: Various diluting pipettes for counting blood cells. Above are the Thoma pipettes, left, Trenner automatic pipettes and right, cross sections of the Thoma and Trenner pipettes

Technique

Take the dry RBC pipette and draw blood by gentle suction into that pipette either from a finger prick or from oxalated blood exactly up to the mark 0.5 (or **1 in case of severe anemia**) without any air bubble.

Wipe off the surplus blood from outside the pipette and draw diluting fluid from a watch glass to fill up the bulb exactly up to the mark 101, during which the pipette is rotated in the vertical axis. Do not include air bubble. The fluid in the bulb is mixed uniformly by closing the tip by pressure and rolling the pipette for about 3 minutes. **Reject the fluid in the capillary portion of the pipette.**

Put the cover-slip on the counting chamber placed in a level surface and allow the thoroughly mixed diluted blood to pass under the cover-slip. Put the counting chamber on the stage of the microscope; allow the cells to settle for a few minutes, focus under $\frac{2}{3}$" objective to locate the field, examine with $\frac{1}{6}$" objective and × 6 eye-piece, with draw tube at 160 mm. **Count** RBCs included in *5 big squares bounded by double ruling, each containing 16 small squares*. To avoid counting a cell twice, cells which touch the right hand and lower line, are not counted but **those touching the upper and left hand line are counted in the square** (while moving the chamber down and to the right).

Calculation:

The depth of the chamber, when cover-slip is in position is $\frac{1}{10}$ mm and each side of a small square is $\frac{1}{20}$ mm. Therefore, the volume of a small square is $\frac{1}{20} \times \frac{1}{20} \times \frac{1}{10} = \frac{1}{4000}$ cmm.

Let the **number of cells in 80 small squares** be x.

Then $x \times \frac{1}{80} \times 4000 \times$ dilution = Number of red cells per cmm. Or, the number of cells counted in 80 small squares and then put 4 siphers i.e. (0000) (× 10,000) on the right of it. That is the red cell count; (or No. of million × 10^{12}).

TOTAL LEUCOCYTE WBC (COUNT)

(WBC pipette, See Fig. 12.2 –12.6)

Turk's Fluid is the Diluting Fluid that consists of: (a) **Glacial acetic acid — 2 ml, Mercuric chloride — 0.1 g, Water — 100 ml,** or (b) **Acetic acid alone can lyse red cells.**

Preparation:

One per cent solution of acetic acid in distilled water. Add a drop of methyl violet solution to give a color to the solution.

Technique

Follow the technique as in the case of red cell count but use WBC pipette (with **mark 11**). Suck

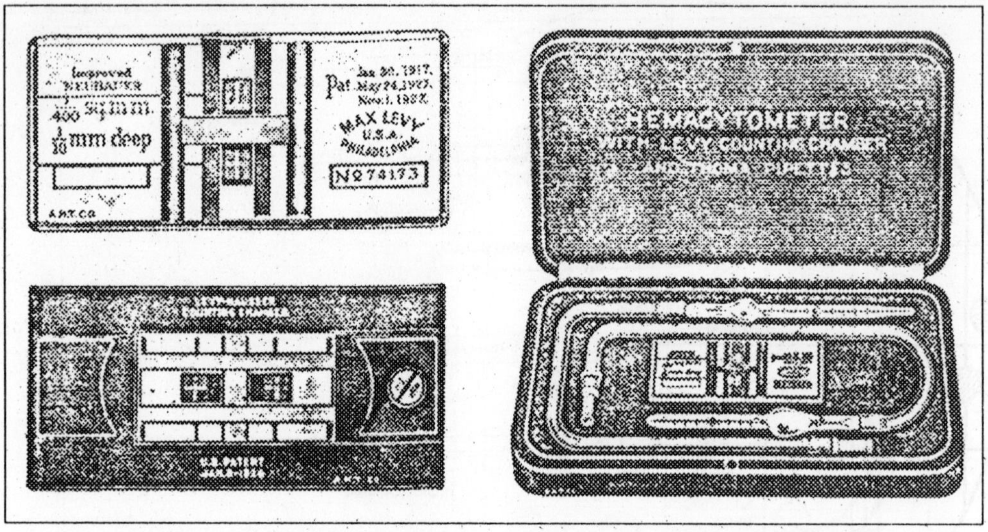

Fig. 12.3: Hemocytometer with levy counting chamber and Thoma Pipettes

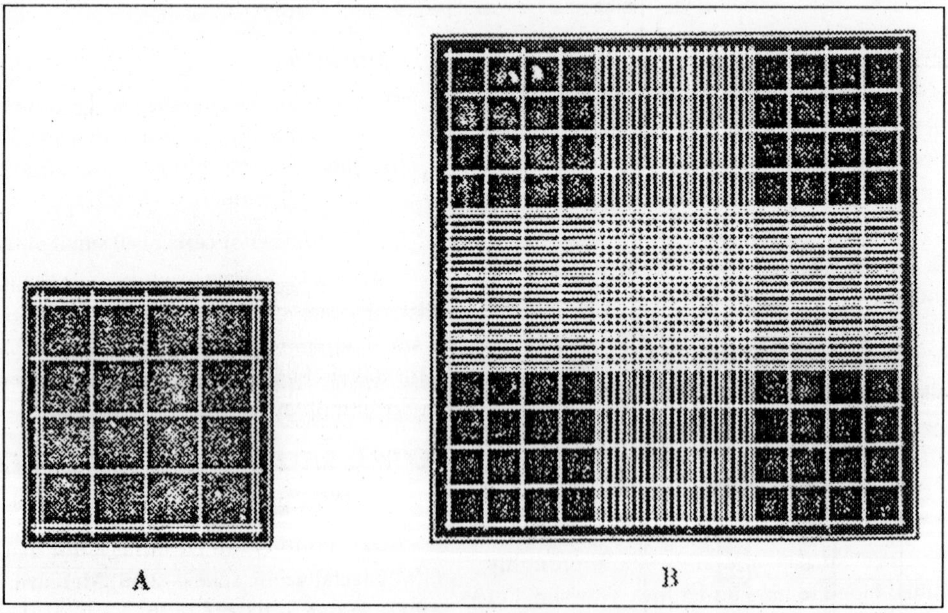

Fig. 12.4: A. A group of sixteen smallest squares of Improved Neubauer Ruling, showing transparent boundary enclosed between two engraved furrows. B. Entire area of Improved Neubauer Ruling; A total of 9 big squares, the 4 block corners are for WBC count and the central big square containing 400 smallest squares and 25 intermediate squares are meant for red cell count

Volume of primary or "large squares" are $1 \times 1 \times {}^{1}/_{10}$ cu mm (μl)

Volume of secondary or "intermediate squares" are ${}^{1}/_{4} \times {}^{1}/_{4} \times {}^{1}/_{10}$ mm $= {}^{1}/_{160}$ cu mm (μl)

Volume of tertiary or "small squares" are ${}^{1}/_{20} \times {}^{1}/_{20} \times {}^{1}/_{10}$ mm $= {}^{1}/_{4000}$ cu mm (μl)

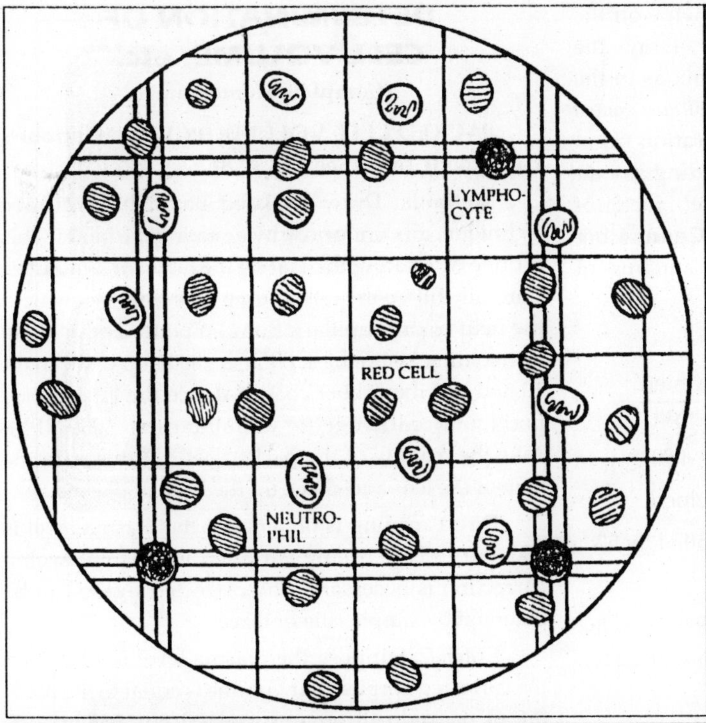

Fig. 12.5: Neubauer or Improved Neubauer. Showing high power view of one big (16 small) squares for counting of leukocytes

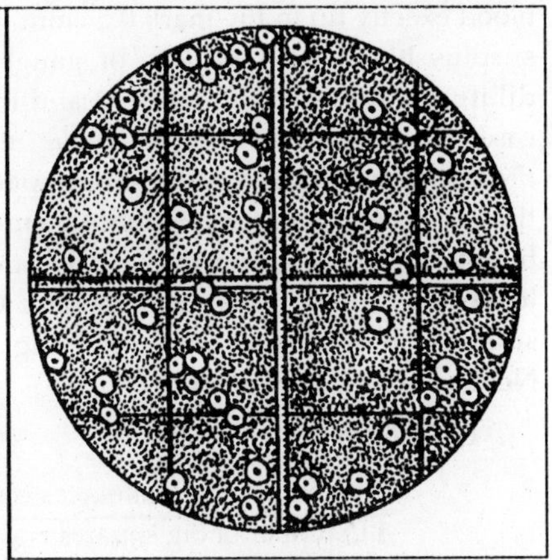

Fig. 12.6: Neubauer Ruling Chamber

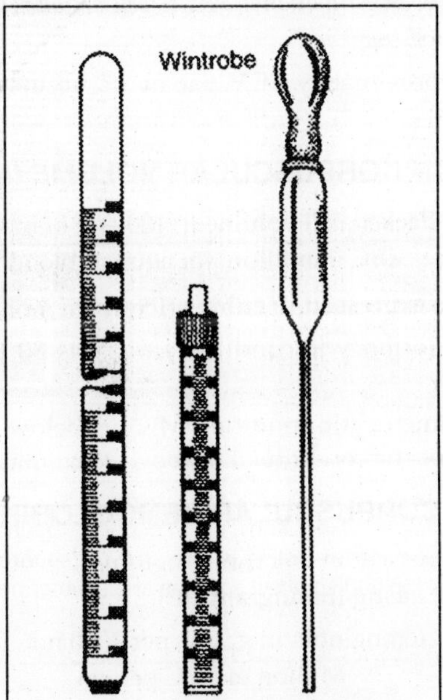

Fig. 12.7: Wintrobe sedimentation tube

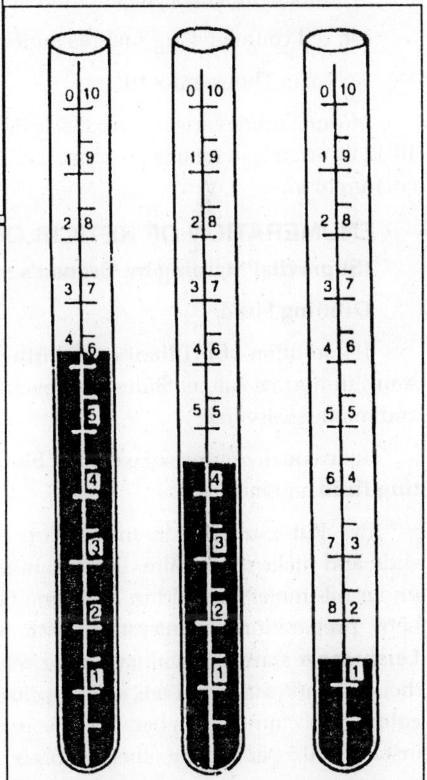

Fig. 12.8: Wintrobes' Hematocrit Tube showing PCV and ESR by Wintrobe's method. A. Greater than normal (Erythrocytosis, or Polycythemia, 62%), B. Normal (45%), C. Less than normal e.g., Anemia. Figures on left side of Tubes indicate for ESR and those on right side indicate PCV% (determination)

blood exactly up to the mark 0.5 cmm, wipe off the surplus blood with a piece of gauge. Draw the diluting fluid up to the **mark 11** and mix as in the case of red cell. *Discard the fluid in the capillary part of the pipette* and make a cover-slip preparation (as in the case of red cell count) without including any air bubble. Examine under the microscope. Nuclei of leukocytes appear as refractile bodies. **Count 4 big squares in 4 corners** out of 9 big squares of Neubauer ruling chamber.

Calculation

$$\frac{\text{Total number of leukocytes counted}}{\text{4 (Number of big squares counted)}}$$

× 20 (dilution) × 10 (depth for cover slip).

= Number of leucocyte per cmm of blood.

Or, cell count of 4 big squares multiplied by 50;

∴ No. in Thousand × 10^9.

Normal count varies from 6,000 to 8,000 in adults; 10-12 thousands in infants per cmm. i.e., 6 × 10^9 cells/ cu. mm or *μl*.

ENUMERATION OF RETICULOCYTES

(Supravital Staining by Osgood's method)

Diluting Fluid

1% solution of **brilliant cresyl blue** (supravital stain) in normal saline. Slides are specially polished and made grease free.

Take equal volumes of oxalated **blood and diluting fluid** and mix.

(a) Put a drop of the mixture on a grease free slide and make a thin film. Dry in air and examine under oil-immersion within 24 hours. For a permanent preparation, counterstain with **Wright's** or **Leishman's stain**. Reticulocytes are recognized by their network within red cell, staining **chromatin blue color**. The count is higher by this method (1.5% instead of 0.5 per cent by other methods).

(b) Make a ringed vaseline cover-slip preparation and examine through a small window in the eye-piece; count at least one thousand red cells in a normal case but, if the reticulocyte count is high, **500 red cells may be counted** preferably by using **Veeder counter**. Reticulocyte count is expressed as percentage of red cell count (**Red cell + Reticulocytes = 100**).

DETERMINATION OF CELL VOLUME, etc.

(Complete Hemogram)

PACKED CELL VOLUME (PCV) by **Wintrobe's Hematocrit Tube (See Fig. 12.8).**

Methods: Draw oxalated blood by Wintrobe technique, mix uniformly by agitating the blood. This is done by rotating the vial on the table for 3 minutes. Carefully fill up the cell volume tube from below with the help of dry capillary (long) pipette. This is done by avoiding air bubbles. Fill up exactly up to the mark 10 and put the rubber cork. **Balance** the bucket properly and **centrifuge** for 30 minutes at 3,000 RPM. Take the reading of the packed-cell volume with the help of the lens and check up the level of plasma also.

Direct reading is obtained if the plasma level is 100, but in case of any variation in plasma level, a correction is necessary. The corrected figure can be obtained by simple rule of three.

Example: Suppose the plasma level is 103. Then the corrected corpuscular volume is equal to the reading of packed cell volume i.e. 100 divided by 103. When **pot.** (single) **oxalate** is used instead of ammonium and pot. (**double**) **oxalate** as an anticoagulant, the factor for correction is 1.09.

Make an estimation of packed cell volume of the sample of blood supplied.

Approximately **PCV rise of 3% occurs per g of Hb**.

MEAN CORPUSCULAR VOLUME (MCV)

$$\text{MCV} = \frac{\text{Packed cell volume in 1000 ml of blood}}{\text{RBC in million per cmm of blood}} \left(\frac{450}{5}\right)$$

It is expressed in cubic micron (cu *μ* or, μ^3).

In normocytic conditions MCV is 80 to 96 cu microns.

In microcytic condition MCV is below normal. In macrocytic condition it is above 96 cu microns.

MEAN CORPUSCULAR HEMOGLOBIN (MCH)

Expressed in micromicrograms (γγ or gamma gamma), i.e. **ng (nanogram 10^9)**

$$\text{MCH} = \frac{\text{Hemoglobin in grams per 1000 ml of blood}}{\text{Million of RBC per cm}}$$

= micro-microgram (10^{-10}) or $^1/_{10}$ mg or (γγ)/cell

Therefore, MCH $= \frac{145}{5}$ = 29 (**ng**) γγ

Table IV.4: Average normal blood cell values at different age levels in infants and children

	At Birth	At 2 days	At 15 days	At 3 months	At 6 months	At 1 year	At 2 years	At 4 years	At 8-12 years
Red cells/cmm (in millions)	5.1	5.3	5.0	4.3	4.6	4.7	4.8	4.8	5.1
Hemoglobin: Grams %*	16.9	17.0	16.0	10.7	10.7	11.5	12.2	12.3	13.3
(Absolute percentage)	113	115	109	73	74	78	83	84	90
White cells/cmm (in thousands)	15.0	21.0	11.0	9.5	9.2	9.0	8.5	8.0	8.0
Platelets/cmm (in thousands)	350.0	400.0	300.0	260.0	250.0	250.0	250.0	250.0	250.0
Differential Count									
Percentages / Absolute count:									
Polymorphonuclear neutrophils	47/7,500	55/11,500	35/3,850	35/3,325	40/3,680	40/3,600	40/3,400	50/4,000	52/4,160
Eosinophils and basophils together	3/450	5/1,050	3/330	3/285	3/276	2/180	2/170	2/160	3/240
Lymphocytes	30/4,500	22/4,620	55/6,050	56/5,320	53/4,876	54/4,860	53/4,505	48/3,440	40/3,200
Monocytes	10/1,500	13/2,730	7/770	6/570	4/368	4/360	5/425	5/400	5/400
Immature white cells	10/1,500	5/1,050	—	—	—	—	—	—	—
Percentage of nucleated red cells in total nucleated (red & white) cells of blood	1–5	2	...	...	...	...	...	...	...
Percentage of reticulocytes in total red cells	2	3	1	0.5	0.8	1	1	1	1

* Value of Hemoglobin 14.6 g corresponds to absolute value of 100 per cent (Hellige)

Determine the MCH of a blood with Hb 14.5 g per 100 ml and red cell 5 million per cmm.

Normal MCH is 29.5 γγ or ng. This indicates the average color (Hb content) of a single RBC. Variations are expressed in terms of hypo-, hyper- or orthochromic (normal) conditions. In **orthochromia** MCH is **25 to 33, in hypochromia MCH is below 25,** in **hyperchromia** MCH is **above 33 γγ** (ng).

MEAN CORPUSCULAR HEMOGLOBIN CONCENTRATION (MCHC)

This is expressed as percentage of hemoglobin in each cell:

$$MCHC = \frac{\text{Hb. in g per 100 ml of blood}}{\text{Vol. of packed cells per 100 ml}} \times 100 \left(\begin{matrix}\text{For}\\ \text{per cent}\end{matrix}\right)$$

Determine the MCHC of a sample of blood with Hb. 14 g per 100 ml and cell volume 42%

The **MCHC** = $^{14}/_{42} \times 100 = 33.3G\%$.

COLOR INDEX (CI) =

$$\frac{\text{Hb. per cent (14.5 g as 100\%)}}{\text{Red cell per cent (5 million as 100\%)}}, \text{ i.e.,} \frac{100}{100} = 1$$

The other method is:

$$\frac{\text{MCH of a particular case}}{\text{Normal MCH of population to}}$$

which the patient belongs.

Normal color index is 1 but figures between 0.9 to 1.1 are not abnormal.

VOLUME INDEX =

$$\frac{\begin{matrix}\text{Packed cell volume per cent}\\ \text{(calculated 47 ml for man per 100 ml)}\end{matrix}}{\text{RBC per cent (5 million as 100\%)}}$$

Normal volume index is 0.95 to 1.05.

It is high in pernicious anemia (1.2) and low in microcytic anemia (< 0.9).

ENUMERATION OF BLOOD PLATELETS

Direct Method: The diluting fluid is **Rees and Ecker's solution**. Formula for other solutions are also given below:

PROCEDURE NO. 1

Rees-Ecker Solution for Thrombocyte Count.

Sodium citrate, $Na_3C_6H_5O_7 \cdot 2H_2O$	3.8	g
Brilliant cresyl blue	0.05	g
Distilled water	100	ml
Concentrated formaldehyde neutral solution (40%)	0.2	ml

Mode of Preparation

Dissolve sodium citrate and the dye (brilliant cresyl blue) in distilled water. Add concentrated formaldehyde solution. Mix well, label, and put date. **Store at 4°C** and filter before use. This may be used for years.

PROCEDURE NO. 2

Kristensen's Diluting Fluid for Platelet Count.

Stock Solution (A):

Sodium citrate, $Na_3C_6H_5O_7 \cdot 2H_2O$	1	g
Mercuric chloride	0.002	g
Brilliant cresyl blue	0.2	g
Distilled water	100	ml

Stock Solution (B):

Urea	20	g
Distilled water	100	ml

Working Solution:

Stock Solution (A)	1	vol.
Stock Solution (B)	1	vol.

Mode of Preparation

Stock Solution (A)

Heat distilled water to 45°C. Dissolve the ingredients and label. Put date.

Stock Solution (B)

Dissolve urea in distilled water. Label, put date, and store at 4°C. This can be used up to 3 to 6 months.

Working Solution

Mix equal volumes of the stock solutions as required. The mixture remains stable for several days but should be centrifuged or filtered before use.

PROCEDURE NO. 3

AMMONIUM OXALATE SOLUTION FOR PLATELET COUNT

Quite satisfactory and simple.

The most satisfactory fluid for platelet count is 1 per cent **ammonium oxalate** crystals in distilled water to get a clear view of platelets.

Oxalated Blood

Draw oxalated blood in red cell pipette up to 0.5 and diluting fluid up to 101. Mix thoroughly; make a preparation in the counting chamber as in red cell count. Wait for 20 minutes to settle and count as in the case of red cell but count 25 groups of 16 small squares. The total count is multiplied by 2000 to give the number per cm of blood. Normal count is 250,000 per cmm by this method.

Venipuncture Method (Tocanti's Procedure): Draw **0.4 ml of Rees and Ecker fluid** in the tuberculin (1 ml) syringe and expel the fluid into a 2 ml sterile vial. Draw exactly **0.1 ml of blood** from a vein. Empty the contents of the syringe under the level of fluid. Wash the syringe 3 or 4 times with fluid and count as above. Average normal count is 310,000 per cmm or per μl by this method.

Direct approximate counting may be done from stained peripheral blood smear by an expert. If at least 3 to 4 platelets are genuinely observed, the count may be taken as normal about 1,50,000 or little more. But this should not be practised regularly.

Normal count varies from 150,000 to 350,000 per cmm. i.e. per μl.

INCREASE OF PLATELETS occurs in acute infections, hemorrhage, chronic myelogenous leukemia, polycythemia, Hodgkin's disease.

DECREASE OF PLATELETS occurs in idiopathic (primary) thrombocytopenic purpura (ITP); pernicious anemia, acute leukemia or acute and chronic poisoning of benzol, arsphenamine and gold, excessive radiation (radium), secondary thrombocytopenia, viral infections, like Dengue with **NS1 antigen** in serum.

ERYTHROCYTE SEDIMENTATION RATE (ESR)

I. **WINTROBE'S METHOD (1933)**: Estimated in Wintrobe's cell volume (PCV) tube (see **Fig. 12.7**).

Procedure

Shake the oxalated blood vial for 3 minutes and then fill up the PCV tube accurately up to the mark O with a long capillary pipette starting from the bottom of the PCV tube. Note the time and allow the tubes to stand perfectly upright in a vertical position in Wintrobe tube stand. Take the reading after 1 hour at room temperature of 20° to 25°C. The length of the column of clear plasma shows the sedimentation from mark zero at the bottom up to the top of the red cell column. Give the report as sedimentation rate in millimeter for one hour by Wintrobe method (at the top of red cell level).

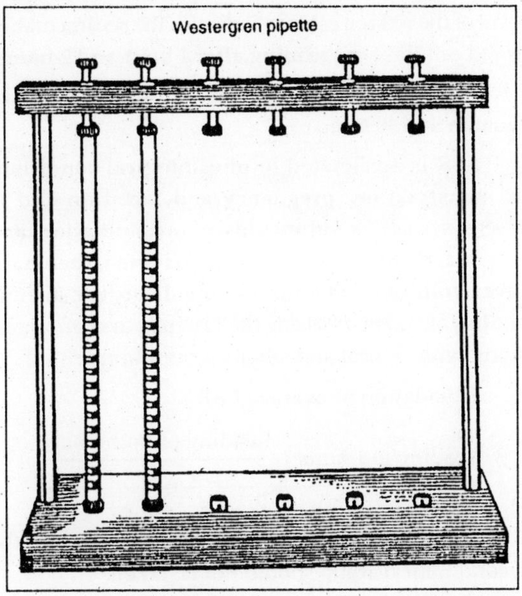

Fig. 12.9: Sedimentation tube stand for Westergren tubes (provision of 6 pipettes)

Also find out the packed cell volume in the same tube. Correction for anemia (when there is reduction in number of red cells, the sedimentation rate increases); and compensated rate for male and female subjects are also considered according to the **chart of Hynes and Whitby**.

Normal limit in Indians (Das Gupta and Napier) — In man 2–10 mm and in woman 4–20 mm per hour. In aged and old people it is 25–35 mm (Dey, 2013).

II. **WESTERGREN METHOD**: (See **Fig. 12.9**, ESR Tubes and stand)

Procedure

Take 0.6 ml of 3.8% citrated solution in a dry vial. Collect exactly 2.4 ml of blood from the vein without any air bubble and put the whole into the vial containing citrate solution; mix thoroughly. Draw well-mixed citrated blood into the Westergren pipette up to the mark 0. The pipette is set upright in the stand with a rubber cork (bung) below and spring clip above, the pipette being between these two fixtures without leakage. The length of the plasma form 0 to the upper level of the red cell column indicates the sedimentation of red cell. Take the **reading after 1 hour and 2 hours.**

Normal Limits in Indians: In man 3 to 20 mm; **woman 5 to 30 mm.**

ESR is accelerated in physiological conditions as **menstruation, pregnancy** and **lactation** and in diseases such as **tuberculosis, inflammation and toxemia, rheumatoid arthritis, carcinoma, rheumatic fever, collagen and autoimmune disorders, anemia** etc. It is an aid in assessing the progress and prognosis along with clinical and laboratory findings.

Calculation of average ESR

$$\frac{\text{Reading of 1 hour} + \dfrac{\text{Reading of both hours}}{2}}{2}$$

when ESR level descends to 100 mm or more, the second hour reading should not be taken.

If the reading of the 1st hour crosses 100 mm, usually it reminds the following 3 diagnosis sequentially: **(a) Tuberculosis, (b) Cancer, and (c) Rheumatoid arthritis and rheumatic fever, or some types of Polyarthritis in children.**

COAGULATION TIME

Wright's Capillary Tube Method (Dale & Laidlaw, 1911-12): Clean the tip of the finger with ether alcohol mixture or propanol. Apply tourniquet or holding and make sharp puncture with a blood gun to get a free flow of **capillary blood**. Discard the first two drops and then fill up $\frac{3}{4}$th of the capillary tubes; note the time of prick on a stop watch and seal one end of the capillary tube. **Place the tube in a water bath at 37°C**. After one minute, take out the first tube and gently **break off a small piece of the capillary tube** from the distal end and draw them apart. Repeat it every 15 seconds *till a slender thread of unbroken fibrin has formed*, stretching between the two broken ends. Note the time of commencement of clotting. Repeat the process with other tubes and take the mean. Normal coagulation time by this method is 3 minutes (Range 3-5 minutes, and even up to 11 minutes).

Method of Lee and White (1913, **Venous Blood** Method): Collect 5 ml of blood from the vein in an all glass syringe washed in normal saline. Set on the stop watch when blood enters the syringe.

1. **Tube Method**: Put exactly 1 ml of blood into each of **3 tubes**; insert the rubber cork and allow them to stand in a **water bath for 3 minutes at 37°C**. Then *take out* ***one of the two tubes every 15 seconds*** *in rotation*. Tilt the tube to see whether the blood has set completely. There is no spilling of blood when clot has formed. The **3rd tube serves as a control** and a check of the two tubes. As **agitation hastens coagulation**. Note the time and take the reading.

Normal time of coagulation by this method is 3 to **6 minutes**. The time is **increased in hemophilia**.

2. **Slide Method**: Take a big drop of blood on a clean polished slide. Scratch with a needle every 30 seconds. Record the time of appearance of fibrin with a stop watch.

Normal C.T. i.e., **coagulation time is 6 minutes.**

BLEEDING TIME (B.T.)

Technique

Clean the ear lobule with ether alcohol mixture or propyl alcohol (propanol) and prick the most dependent part of the lobule just enough to get a free flow of blood without squeezing. Set the stop watch to action. Touch the blood every 30 seconds with a filter paper without touching the skin. Observe the last appearance of blood on the filter paper. Note the time. **It may be done on a finger also.**

Normal bleeding time by this method is **3 minutes. Purpura** shows a **prolonged bleeding time**, but hemophilia does not.

FRAGILITY TEST OF RED CELLS

Principle

When blood cells are suspended in **0.6 per cent saline (isotonic)** they remain unaltered. They become **crenated and laked when concentration** of the solution is **lowered to 0.45 per cent or less.**

Procedure

Make an accurate solution of sodium chloride (AR), standardized against 0.5% and 1% silver nitrate solution. Small test tubes (30 in number) are arranged in two rows (or 2 series). Put drops of solution with a standard pipette by Dreyer's technique as shown in **Table IV.5**.

Control series with similar arrangement is set (See Table IV.5).

Shake each tube individually and get a uniform mixture of water and saline. In series (a), add one

Table IV.5							
Drops of 0.5% saline	0...	12	13	14	15....	24	25
Drops of distilled water	25...	13	12	11	10....	1	0
Final conc. of sodium chloride	0%...	0.24%	0.26%	0.28%	0.30	0.48	0.5%

drop of blood either directly from the patient's vein with a syringe, or oxalated blood, or red cells washed with normal saline; mix properly. In series (b), add normal blood under similar conditions. This provides a check upon the accuracy of saline. Place both the racks on the table at room temperature for 2 hours. Centrifuge the tubes for 10 minutes and take the reading. A colored supernatant fluid (SNF) indicates hemolysis. Drops of saline in the tube **multiplied by 0.02 give the percentage of sodium chloride in solution**.

Example: Normally hemolysis begins in the tube containing 22 drops and is complete in the tube containing 15 drops of 0.5 per cent saline; i.e., the tube containing 22, drops (22 × 0.02) or 0.44 per cent sodium chloride shows commencement of hemolysis; the tube containing 15 drops (15 × 0.02) or 0.3% sodium chloride shows complete hemolysis. In the report, mention the concentration at which hemolysis begins and also the concentration at which it is complete.

Fragility is **increased in pernicious anemia and acholuric jaundice** (beginning at about 0.7 per cent and completing at 0.44 per cent saline); it is **decreased in hypochromic microcytic anemia** (beginning at 0.35% and completing at 0.24% saline).

DETERMINATION OF PROTHROMBIN TIME

(Modified Quick's method)

Requirements

(a) Prepare a uniform suspension of thrombokinase (Geigy 10 mg in a tablet) in 25 ml of 0.25 per cent solution of calcium chloride; warm at 37°C for 15 mins., in a water bath.

(b) Blood is withdrawn from a vein (4 ml) and mixed with 1 ml of 3.8 per cent sodium citrate. Centrifuge; supernatant fluid (SNF) is separated and collected in a dry test tube with a capillary pipette. The blood should be used within 2 to 4 hours.

Procedure

I. Transfer 0.1 ml of plasma in a test tube and put in the water bath at 37°C. To this add 0.2 ml of the suspension of thrombokinase at 37°C, while the tube is in the water bath; at the same time set the **chronometer** in motion.

The time which elapses before the plasma clots is determined. The process is repeated 2 or 3 times and average is taken. The normal result varies from 15-25 seconds. The mean value gives the final result. Express the result in terms of the percentage of normal clotting activity by this process, i.e., =

$$\frac{\text{Clotting time of } \textbf{normal plasma}}{\text{Clotting time of } \textbf{patient's plasma}}$$

II. The test can be performed with Geigy's readymade tablet as follows:

1. Carefully crush 1 Thrombokinase 'Geigy' tablet to a very fine powder by a glass rod.
2. Add 2 drops of distilled water.
3. Triturate with the glass rod to a homogeneous paste (1 minute).
4. Add 2.5 ml of distilled water. Stir with the rod for 30 seconds. Leave the rod in the test-tube.
5. Warm in the water bath to 37°C (99°F) for 15 minutes.
6. After 10 minutes, replace the glass rod by a 0.2 ml graduated pipette.
7. The citrate solution used consists of 3.0 g of trisodium citrate [dihydrate] (sodium citrate B.P.: $C_6H_5O_7Na_3 \cdot 2H_2O$) dissolved in distilled water to 100 ml. For all practical purposes, **3% sodium citrate** will do. **1 ml of this solution is mixed with 4 ml of freshly drawn blood**; alternatively half the volume of citrate and blood will also do. Mix thoroughly.
8. Centrifuge the sample in a normal laboratory centrifuge at the maximum speed of **2,000-3,000 rev/min for 10 minutes**. Separate off the citrated plasma.
9. Place 0.1 ml of citrated plasma into a test-tube 9-11 mm in diameter and 10-11 cm in length.

10. Warm in the waterbath to **37°C (99°F)** for 2 minutes.
11. Re-mix the warm thrombokinase suspension (as in step 6) with the aid of the pipette.
12. Rapidly add 0.2 ml of this warm homogeneous suspension to the warm sample of citrated plasma.
13. At the same moment, set the **stopwatch** in motion.
14. **Agitate the test-tube sharply and briefly** in the waterbath in order to mix the thrombokinase with the plasma. Then once per second swing the tube briefly out of the waterbath to a nearly horizontal position and back.
15. As soon as the **sample coagulates, stop the watch**. The reading of the watch in seconds is converted into a percentage.
16. Repeat the measurement with 2 further 0.1 ml portions of the plasma. **Use the mean of the 3 readings**. This gives the Prothrombin Time.

The Prothrombin index is calculated as follows:

PROTHROMBIN INDEX (Clotting activity) =

$$\frac{\text{Clotting time of normal plasma (control)}}{\text{Clotting time of patient's plasma}} \times 100$$

If the prothrombin index is more than hundred per cent, prothrombin time will be less than the control and vice versa. So **lesser the prothrombin index, the worse it is and the prothrombin time will be more**.

DIFFERENTIAL LEUKOCYTE COUNT

(See Figs. 12.3–12.5)

Make thin blood film and stain with Leishman's stain: make a differential leukocyte count.

N.B. In a report, the total number of each type of cell may be mentioned per cmm from the figure obtained by total count (absolute figures).

Abnormal variation in differential leukocyte count:

EOSINOPHILS CAUSE OF EOSINOPHILIA

Eosinophils are **increased in allergic state,** e.g., **asthma, urticaria, skin diseases, infection with intestinal worms** (i.e., **helminthic infestation**), **filariasis, tropical eosinophilia; blood diseases,** e.g., **myeloid leukemia, Hodgkin's disease.**

1. RANDOLPH'S DILUTING FLUID FOR EOSINOPHIL COUNT

After Randolph, T. G. (1949). *J. lab. clin. med.* 34,

***Stock Solution* (A):**

Methylene blue	...	0.1 g
Propylene glycol	...	50 ml
Distilled water	...	50 ml

***Stock Solution* (B):**

Phloxine	...	0.1 g
Propylene glycol	...	50 ml
Distilled water	...	50 ml

***Working Solution*:**

Stock solution (A)	...	1 vol.
Stock solution (B)	...	1 vol.

Mode of Preparation

Solution (A) and (B):

Mix propylene glycol and distilled water. Dissolve the dyes. Label and put date.

Working Solution

Combine the stock solutions, filter and label. The solution is not stable and should only be used within 3 hours of preparation.

Procedure

The staining solution may be used for both leukocytes as well as eosinophil count. The eosinophil granules stain bright red.

2. DILUTING FLUID FOR EOSINOPHIL COUNT (PILOT'S STAIN)

Pilot, M. L. (1950). *Amer. J. clin. Path.* 20, 870

Propylene glycol	...	50 ml
Distilled water	...	40 ml
Phloxine, 0.1% aqueous solution	...	10 ml
Sodium carbonate, 1% aqueous sol.	...	1 ml

Mode of Preparation

Combine the ingredients, filter, label and record date. The solution should be stored at room temperature.

Procedure

Dilute the sample of blood in a WBC pipette 1 : 20 with the staining solution and mix it for ½ minute.

Charge the hemocytometer. Allow 10 minutes to settle the cells. Count with a 10 × ocular and 16 mm (low power objective).

CAUSES OF EOSINOPENIA: TYPHOID FEVER, TUBERCULOSIS (PULMONARY), NEUTROPENIA WITH RELATIVE LYMPHOCYTOSIS, PERNICIOUS ANEMIA, ENTERIC FEVER

NEUTROPHILS: CAUSES OF NEUTROPHILOSIS

Polymorphonuclear neutrophils are increased in **acute infection** specially **pyogenic ones**. They are **decreased** specially in agranulocytosis.

In Macrocytic anemia, emergence of **Macropoly (hypersegmented poly or macropoly) occurs**.

MONONUCLEAR CELLS

Monocytes are increased in chronic protozoal infections, e.g., **malaria, kala-azar: monocytic leukemia, Hodgkin's disease, viral infections, infectious mononucleosis and malaria.**

Lymphocytes are **increased in chronic infections**, e.g., **tuberculosis, syphilis, glandular fever, infectious mononucleosis, whooping cough**. They are **RELATIVELY Increased in typhoid fever and kala-azar. They are ENORMOUSLY increased in chronic lymphatic leukemia**.

CAUSES OF LEUKOCYTOSIS

1. Various kinds of inflammatory conditions specially associated with acute pyogenic infections, and **leukemoid reaction** as in acute lobar pneumonia (**Neutrophilia**).
2. Various intoxications, e.g., uremia, diabetic coma, eclampsia, gout, etc.
3. Rapidly progressing malignant growth especially of the **liver, alimentary canal and bone marrow**.

CAUSES OF LEUKOPENIA

1. **Bacterial Causes: Typhoid fever**, brucellosis, bacillary dysentery (**Neutroperia**).
2. **Viral and Rickettsial Causes**: Influenza, small pox, **dengue**, measles, relapsing fever, etc.
3. **Protozoal Causes**: Chronic kala-azar.
4. **In disorders of blood: Nutritional macrocytic anemia**, pernicious anemia, splenic anemia (**Banti's syndrome**) and also in **agranulocytosis** and **aleukemic-leukemia**.
5. **In chronic intoxications**: By lead, mercury and arsenic.
6. **Iatrogenic (Drug induced)**: Sulphonamides, amidopyrine, thiouracil, chloramphenicol and (in leprosy) sulphones.
7. **Physical Conditions**: Exposure to radium and X-rays.

CAUSES OF LYMPHOCYTOSIS

1. **Bacterial Causes**: Enteric fever, brucellosis, tuberculosis, secondary syphilis, **pertussis (whooping cough)**, and in convalescent stage of acute infections.
2. **Viral Causes**: Influenza, infectious hepatitis, in various exanthemata, like rubella, chicken pox, measles, mumps especially after the initial phase **infectious lymphocytosis** and **infectious mononucleosis.**
3. **Protozoal Cause**: **Toxoplasmosis**
4. **Neoplastic Conditions**: Chronic lymphatic leukemia, lymphosarcoma, (giant) **follicular lymphoma**.
5. **Miscellaneous**: Thyrotoxicosis, hypopituitarism, myasthenia gravis, carcinoma and multiple myeloma.

ABSOLUTE LYMPHOCYTOSIS

It occurs in conditions, like **pertussis, infectious lymphocytosis, infectious mononucleosis, chronic lymphatic leukemia**, etc.

RELATIVE LYMPHOCYTOSIS

It occurs commonly in conditions like **enteric fever, lymphosarcomas, viral infections** (exanthemata), etc.

LEUKOPENIA WITH RELATIVE LYMPHOCYTOSIS

It occurs in **enteric fever**.

NUCLEAR INDICES

Neutrophils show wide variations in the **number of segmentation** and **degree of lobulation of the nuclei** depending **on the age and maturation of the cell**. The number of segmentations is in proportion to the age of the cell. In the normal mature cells, there are 2 to 4 nuclear lobes and occasionally 5 with better resisting power than the immature cells having one or two nuclear lobes. **Hypersegmented neutrophils** are seen in megaloblastic anemia (**Macropoly**). For interpretation of the age of Neutrophils the indices used are **Arneth's index** and **Cooke's weighted mean**.

ARNETH'S INDEX

Neutrophils are divided into 5 classes according to the number of lobes of the nuclei.

Class I: One lobe 10 to 12 per cent including M cell: Myelocyte,

W cells: Cells with slightly indented nuclei;

T cells: with bent horse shoe nuclei.

Class II: Two lobes pointed by thin filament of chromatin — 25 per cent.

Class III: Three lobes are completely separated and connected by 2 slender filaments of chromatin — 46 to 48 per cent.

Class IV: Four lobes — 15 to 16 per cent.

Class V: Five lobes (**hypersegmented or macropoly**) — 2 to 3 per cent.

Procedure

Make a differential count of 100 successive neutrophils in a film according to lobes of nuclei and determine the percentage of cells of each class (as above). In case of doubt regarding lobes of a nucleus, **always place it to the lower class.**

NORMAL INDEX

Class I, Class II, and ½ of Class III added together is 60%. In case of increase in percentage of less complex forms, i.e., **Class I** and **Class II** (at the expense of those with 3 or more lobes), **a shift to the left occurs in infections**; and increase of more complex *lobed-forms gives a shift to the right*, as found *in pernicious anemia.*

COOKE'S WEIGHTED MEAN

The weighted mean of the nuclear lobes of 100 neutrophils counted is calculated by multiplying the number of cells of Class I by 1, cells in Class II by 2, cells in Class III by 3, cells in Class IV by 4 and cells in Class V by 5.

Example:

Table IV.6: Cooke's Weighted Mean

Normal		Shift to left		Shift to right	
1 × 10 =	10	1 × 40 =	40	1 × 3 =	3
2 × 25 =	50	2 × 45 =	90	2 × 27 =	54
3 × 47 =	141	3 × 14 =	42	3 × 35 =	105
4 × 16 =	64	4 × 1 =	4	4 × 25 =	100
5 × 2 =	10	5 × 0 =	0	5 × 10 =	50
Total	275		176		312

Therefore, Cooke's weighted means are 2.75 (Normal), 1.76 (Shift to the left) and 3.12 (Shift to the right)

DETERMINATION OF BILIRUBIN* IN BLOOD

[van den Bergh (VB) Reaction]

1. *Ehrlich's diazo reagent*:
   (a) Sulphanilic acid 1 mg, Conc. (11N) HCl 15 ml and distilled water — 1,000 ml.
   (b) Sodium nitrite 0.5 g, distilled water — 100 ml.
2. Saturated solution of Ammon. sulphate.
3. Absolute or 96% alcohol.
4. ½" × 4" test tube used to centrifuge.
5. 1 ml and 5 ml graduated pipette, etc.

Tests are either from serum or plasma. Supernatant plasma above cell volume may be used. When this test is done alone, 4 ml of blood is drawn and placed in a dry oxalated or EDTA vial. Hemolysis is avoided and specimens are examined within two hours; otherwise the result may be paradoxical.

Technique

Diazo reagent (for preparation see Bilirubin in Chemical Pathology) — **10 ml of (a)**, and **0.3 ml of (b)** are mixed in a small flask just before use, the mixture should not be used later than 1 hour after it is prepared. Take 1 ml of plasma or serum in a centrifuge tube. Run down the wall of the slanting tube exactly 0.5 ml of **Diazo reagent** to be overlaid **on the plasma or serum.**

IMMEDIATE DIRECT REACTION

Reddish-violet color which is maximum in 30 seconds appear immediately.

* See also Chemical Pathology section.

GRANULOCYTIC SERIES

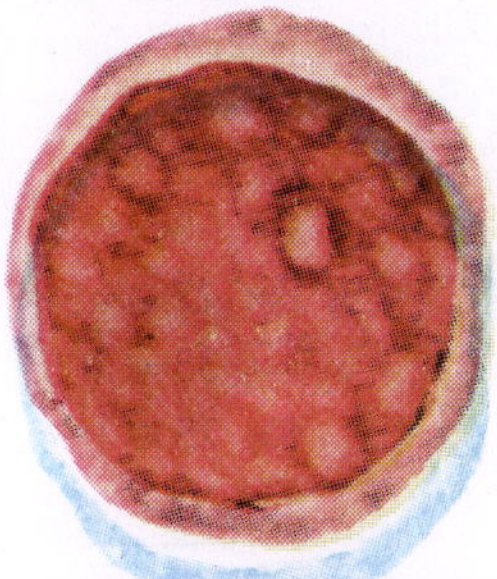

MYELOBLAST

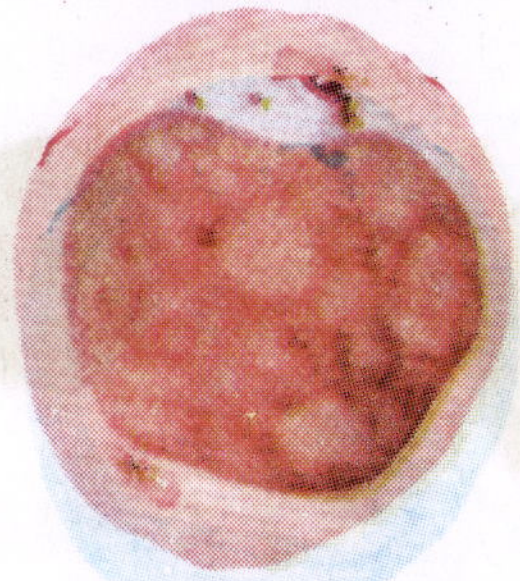

PROMYELOCYTE

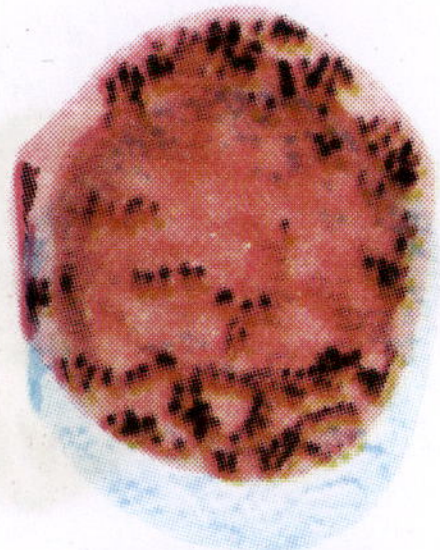

MYEIOCYTE

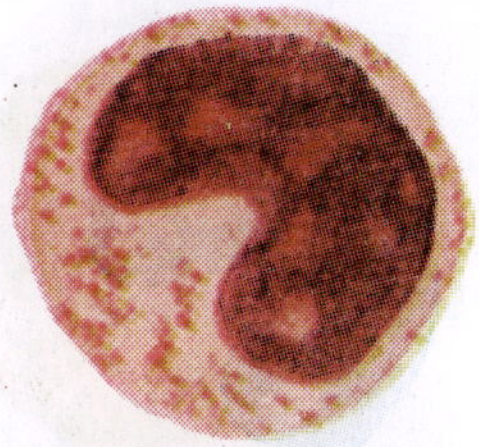

BAND OR STAB FORM (after METAMYELOCYTE FORM)

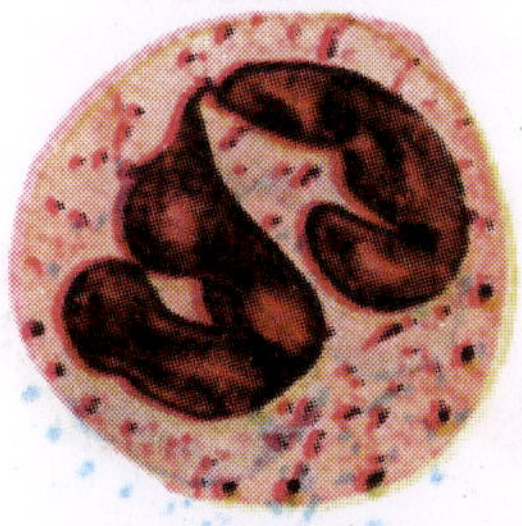

NEUTROPHIL

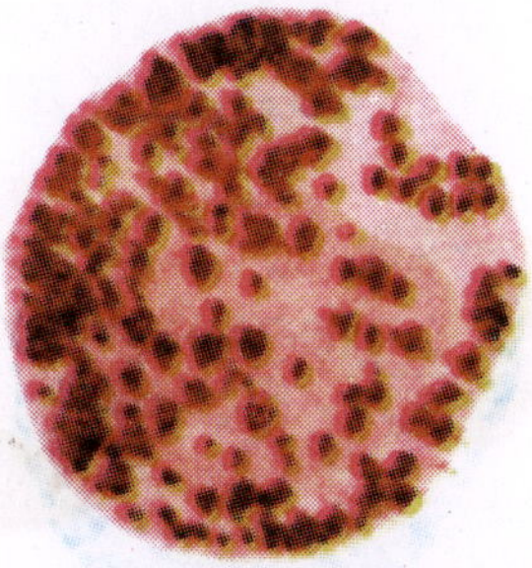

EOSINOPHIL

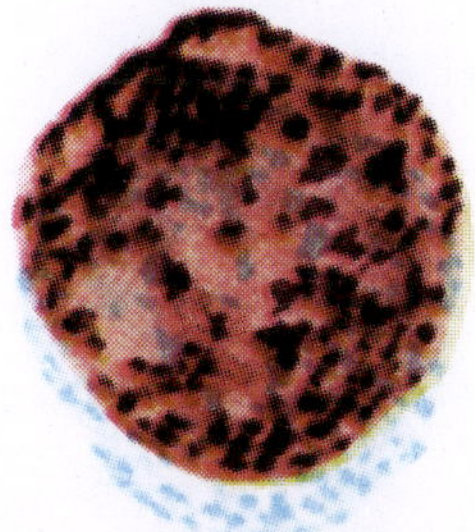

BASOPHIL

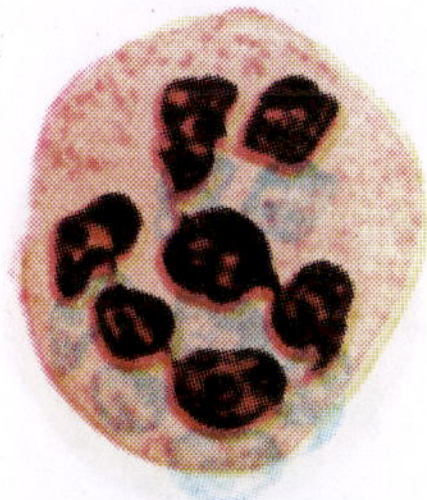

MACROPOLY

LYMPHO-MONOCYTIC SERIES

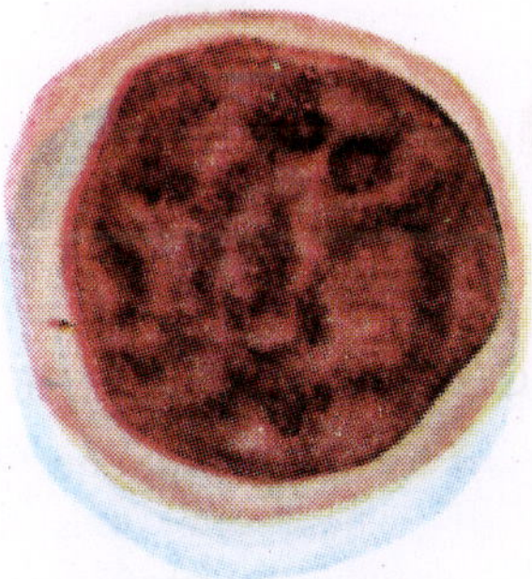

LYMPHOBLAST

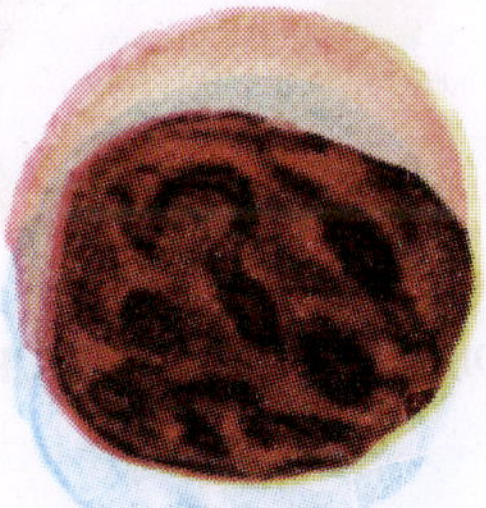

LARGE LYMPHOCYTE

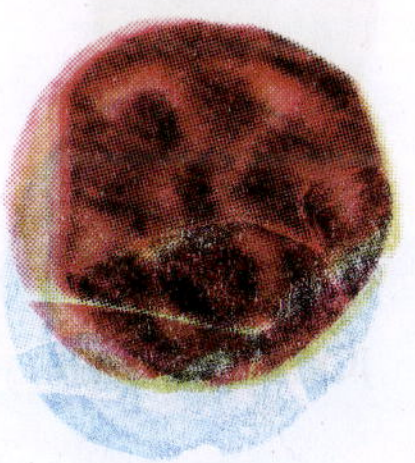

SMALL LYMPHOCYTE

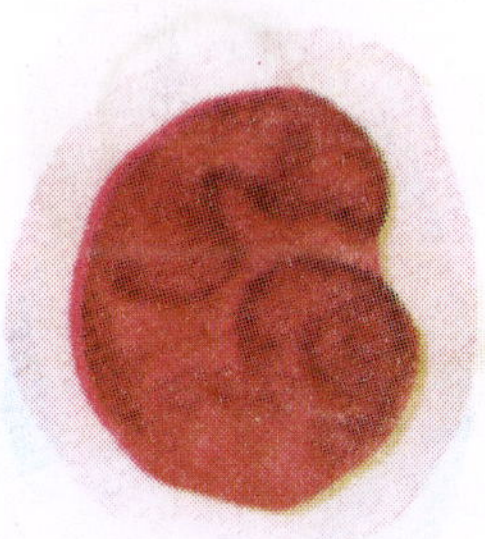

MONOCYTE

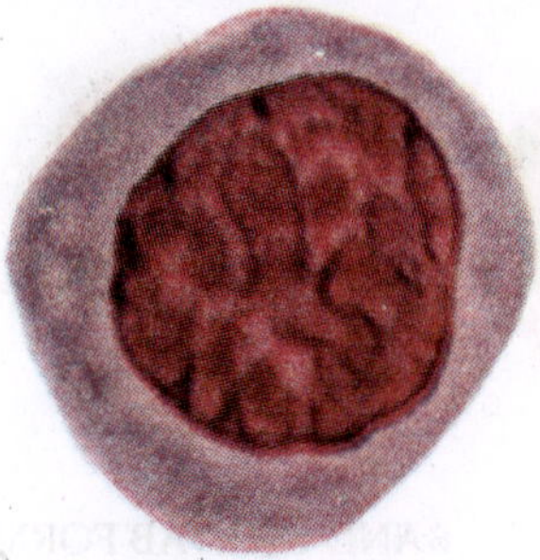

MEYELOBLAST

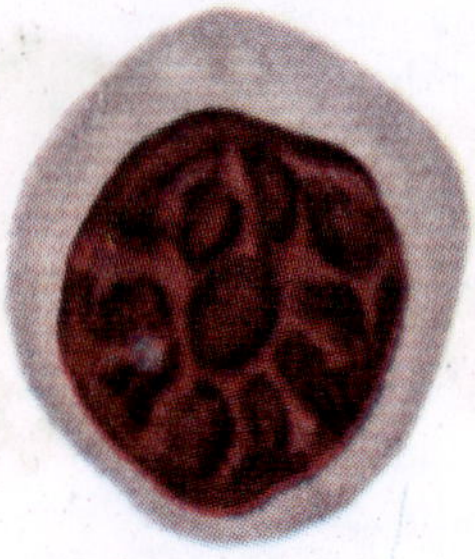

MACROBLAST
(MEGALOBLAST)

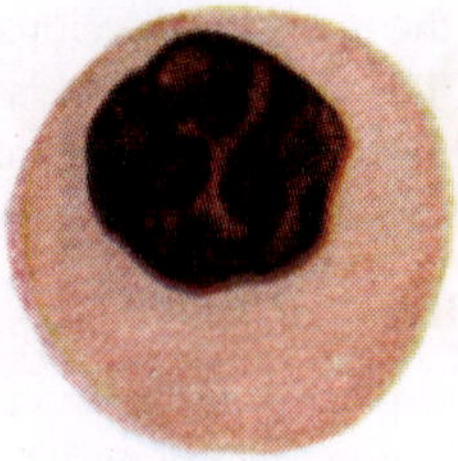

NORMOBLAST

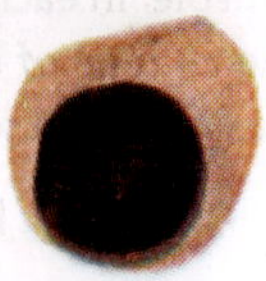

MICROBLAST

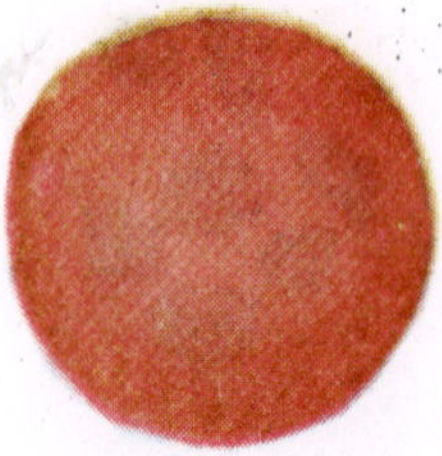

MACROCYTE
(MEGALOCYTE)

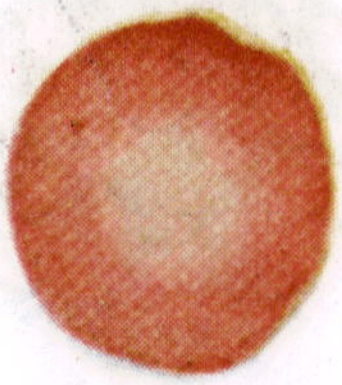

NORMOCYTE

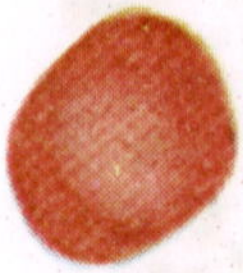

MICROCYTE

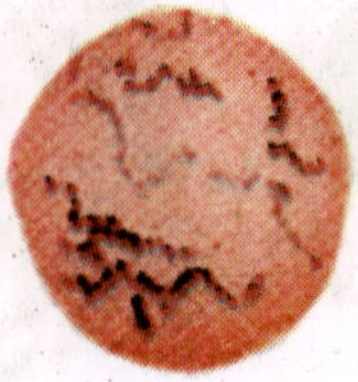

RETICULOCYTE

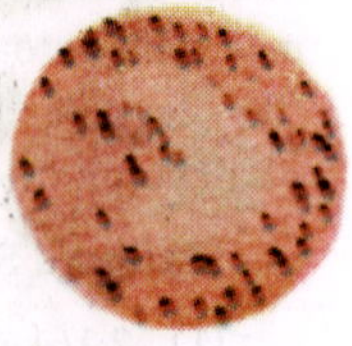

BASOPHILIC
STIPPLING
(IN RED CELL)

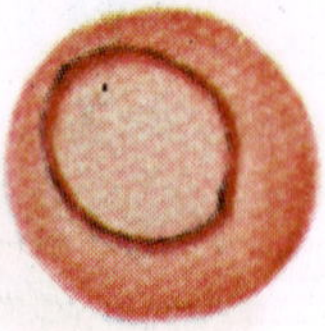

CABOT RING

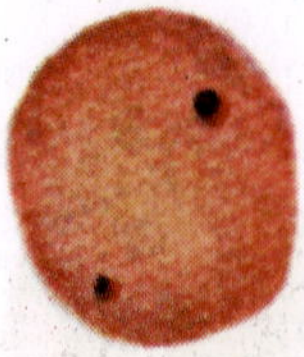

HOWELL
JOLLY BODIES

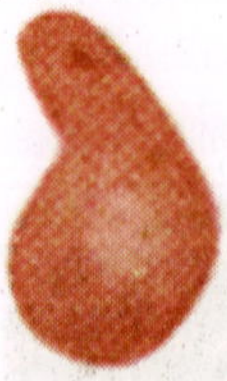

POIKILOCYTE

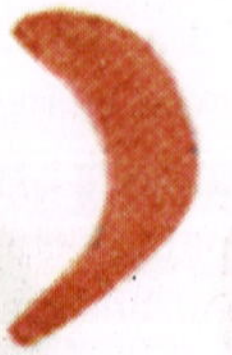

SICKLE CELL

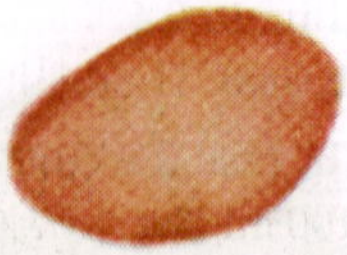

OVALOCYTE

BIPHASIC REACTION

It is indicated by the appearance of color either in 30 seconds (**Prompt biphasic**) or in 60 seconds (**delayed biphasic**), the red color develops to reddish purple in each case. **The direct reaction is negative if no change of color takes place in 10 minutes**; in that case proceed to the next stage for indirect reaction.

INDIRECT REACTION

To the mixture of plasma and diazo reagent add 2.5 ml of 96% or absolute alcohol and 1 ml of saturated solution of ammonium sulphate. Mix well by inverting the tube and allow it to stand for 2 minutes and centrifuge for 10 minutes.

INDIRECT (QUANTITATIVE)

Compare the color of the supernatant fluid with the bilirubin disc in Lovibond comparator or in a colorimeter and autoanalyzer too. Range of disc varies from 0.2 to 2 mg per 100 ml of blood. A standard solution of **cobalt sulphate or pot. permanganate** may also be used.

Standard Solution

(1) 2.161 g of anhydrous or 3.92 g of recrystallized salt of **cobalt sulphate** in 100 ml of distilled water containing 0.4 ml of **conc. H_2SO_4** (36N). This solution may be sealed in uniform-bore test tubes for matching, and this keeps well. The **color corresponds to 0.5 mg bilirubin (one unit) in 100 ml.** (2) 0.7 ml of $N/_{10}$ **Pot. permanganate** in 50 ml of distilled water. Different dilutions are made from the standard corresponding to 0.4, 0.3, 0.2, 0.1 and 0.05 mg of bilirubin per 100 ml. The solution must be fresh.

In case the concentration is higher than 0.5 mg per 100 ml, the supernatant fluid may be diluted with normal saline or 65% alcohol and the color is matched with a suitable standard.

Calculation:

$$\frac{\text{Reading of standard}}{\text{Reading of unknown}} \times 4 \times 0.5 \times \text{dilution}$$

= mg bilirubin per 100 ml.

(Take 0.5 mg as van den Bergh unit).

The test is positive when the supernatant fluid gives a distinct **bluish violet color**; the intensity of color depends on the amount of bilirubin present. Bilirubin is present in normal blood and faint violet color appears. Normal — 0.2 to 0.8 mg of bilirubin per 100 ml of blood. In latent jaundice it is 0.5 to 2 mg. Clinical jaundice does not appear until the concentration of bilirubin rises to about 2 mg per 100 ml.

Interpretation

The serum showing immediate direct reaction may give positive indirect reaction. The former indicates obstructive jaundice.

Biphasic reaction is positive in toxic and infective jaundice.

A **delayed biphasic reaction** is indicative of toxic jaundice.

Indirect reaction when positive indicates bilirubinemia due to hemolysis (hemobilirubin).

For biochemical test, see chapter on chemical pathology.

ICTERUS INDEX

It is a ratio which indicates a measure of the amount of bilirubin in the blood. The index is obtained by comparing the color of 1:10 dilutions of plasma/serum in a **colorimeter** with that of **1 : 100,000 sol. of pot. bichromate** (to which sulphuric acid has been added a "drop to" **a litre** as a preservative) which is considered **as one unit.**

Table IV.7: Relation of bilirubin concentration to vB reaction

	Total bilirubin per 100 ml of plasma	van den Bergh reaction
Normal	0.2 to 0.5 mg	**Indirect**
Pernicious anemia	0.7 to 3 mg	Indirect or delayed
Hemolytic jaundice	Up to 50 mg	Indirect (hemobilirubin-unconjugated)
Obstructive jaundice	2 to 6 mg	Direct (cholebilirubin–conjugated; formation of bilirubin glucuronides)
Hepatitis	1 to 20 mg	Direct or delayed
Cirrhosis of liver	0.4 to 6 mg	Delayed direct

Stock standard solution

Potassium dichromate ... 1 g

Sulphuric acid (sp. gr. 1.84)(36N) ... 0.1 ml

Distilled water ... upto 100 ml

Mix pot. dichromate in distilled water. Add sulphuric acid.

Working standard solution:

Stock standard solution ... 10 ml

Distilled water upto ... 1000 ml

Add stock standard solution to distilled water. Mix thoroughly.

Procedure

Take **Pot. bichromate** solution in a tube and in the other put 2 ml of clear plasma or serum without hemolysis.

Dilute plasma with normal saline to match the solution approximately. In the left hand cup of a *Duboscq colorimeter* put the standard sol. bichromate and in the right hand cup put the unknown (dilute plasma). Fix the standard at 20 mm. Match the unknown by moving the plunger down.

Or,

Dilute *1 ml patient's serum with 9 ml sodium citrate (5 per cent)*. Read in a colorimeter, using a **blue filter (420 nm) using the citrate solution as reagent blank** to set the galvanometer needle at zero.

Icterus Index Unit =

$$\frac{\text{Reading of the standard solution}}{\text{Reading of diluted plasma}} \times \text{dilution factor}$$

This calculation is for the Duboscq colorimeter.

Example: standard = 20 mm; plasma reading = 10 mm; dilution = 5.

Normal range is 4 to 6.

Therefore, Icterus index is $^{20}/_{10} \times 5 = 10$, or, $^{U}/_{S} \times 10$

DEVELOPMENT OF BLOOD CELLS

Draw diagram showing the stages of development of cells of **Erythroid series (Normoblastic).**

The cells in the order of their development are:

NORMOCYTE:

Hemocytoblast (Hemohistioblast) → **Proerythroblast** → **Normoblast A** (early erythroblast) → **Normoblast B** (late erythroblast) → **Normoblast C** (normoblast) → **Reticulocyte** → **Erythrocyte** (Normocyte).

Draw diagram comparing the normoblastic with megaloblastic series of red cell.

MEGALOBLAST:

Stages: Promegaloblast → Basophilic, **Polychromatic and Orthochromatic Megaloblast** (macroblast) → Megalocyte (macrocyte).

Megaloblastic Series

The **mature cells (macrocytes)** of this series are large (**10–20μ or more**) in diameter, nucleus larger, central with no pale perinuclear zone.

Promegaloblasts are large (about 30μ) with intensely blue cytoplasm and 3–5 nucleoli. The chromatin network in the nucleus is intensely blue, nuclear pale zone is absent in this series of cells. In later cells no clumping of chromatin is seen as occurs in the normoblastic series.

Draw diagram to show stages of development of leukocytes of **MYELOID ORDER:**

Myeloblast → **Premyelocyte** → **Myelocyte** → **Metamyelocyte** (these cells may be **neutrophilic, eosinophilic** or **basophilic**) → **Band** cells (**stab** form) → **Mature granulocyte** (Neutrophil, Eosinophil, Basophil).

Draw diagram showing stages of development of **LYMPHOCYTES:**

Stem cell → Lymphoblast → large lymphocyte (12 to 18μ) → small lymphocyte (7 to 12μ).

LEUKEMIA, ETC.

Draw diagrams showing cells in the peripheral blood of **(a) Acute Lymphatic** Leukemia, **(b) Chronic Lymphatic** Leukemia, **(c) Acute Myeloid** Leukemia, **(d) Chronic Myeloid** Leukemia, and **(e) Tropical Eosinophilia.**

STUDY OF PERIPHERAL BLOOD SMEARS

(See Figs. 12.13–12.14)

CASE HISTORY AND SPOT IDENTIFICATION OF HEMATOLOGY CASES

1. Acute Osteomyelitis

History

Boy aged 9 years, history of trauma, following boils has chills with high fever development, and severe pain and tenderness in the upper third of the

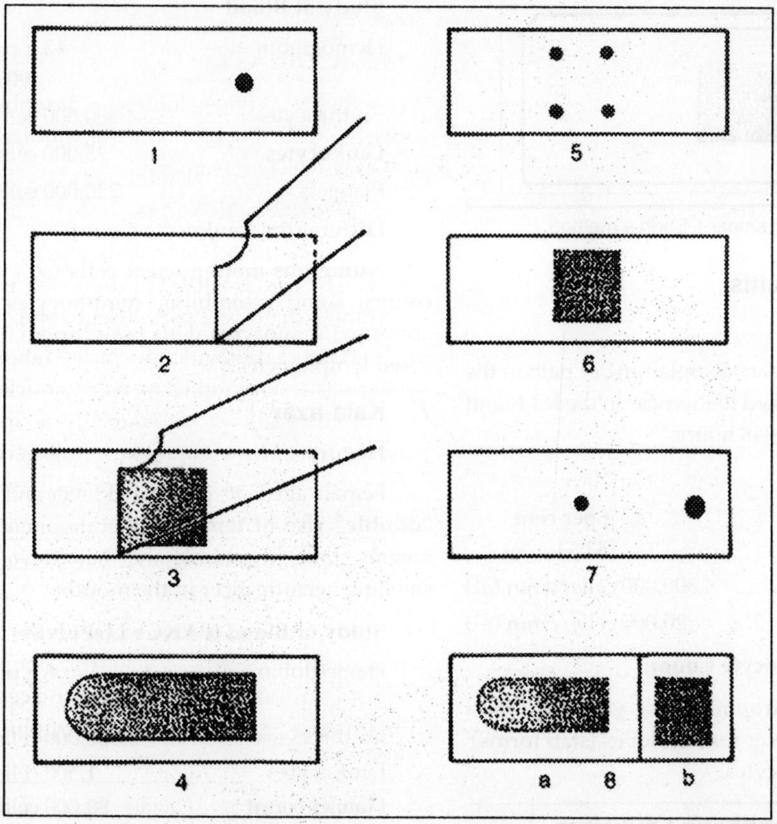

Fig. 12.12: Thin film (1 to 4), thick film (5 and 6). Sinton's method of thin and thick film (7, 8a and 8b)

leg which is somewhat red and swollen. Duration — 5 days.

Study of Blood

Hemoglobin	...	11 g per cent (76%)
Erythrocytes	...	4,500,000 cells/cmm (μl)
Leukocytes	...	18,000 cells/cmm (μl)

Differential Leukocyte Count shows:

85% neutrophils and a few stab forms.

2. Aplastic Anemia

History

Female aged 30 has a history of recurrent enteric fever treated with antibiotics 6 months ago. Presenting with lassitude, shortness of breath and palpitation.

Study of Blood

Hemoglobin	...	11 g per cent (76%)
Erythrocytes	...	1,00,000 cells/cmm (μl)
Leukocytes	...	18,000 cells/cmm (μl)
Platelets	...	80,000 cells/cmm (μl)

Abnormal Cells: None whatsoever.

3. Acute Lobar Pneumonia

History

A patient aged 30 with cough, stitching pain in the chest and high fever of 4 days duration. Breathing is somewhat laboured (**dyspnea**).

Study of Blood (Leukemoid Reaction)

Hemoglobin	...	14.5 g per cent (100%)
Erythrocytes	...	5,600,000 cells/cmm (μl)
Leukocytes	...	30,000 cells/cmm (μl)

Differential Leukocyte Count shows:

85% neutrophils with a few stab forms and metamyelocytes.

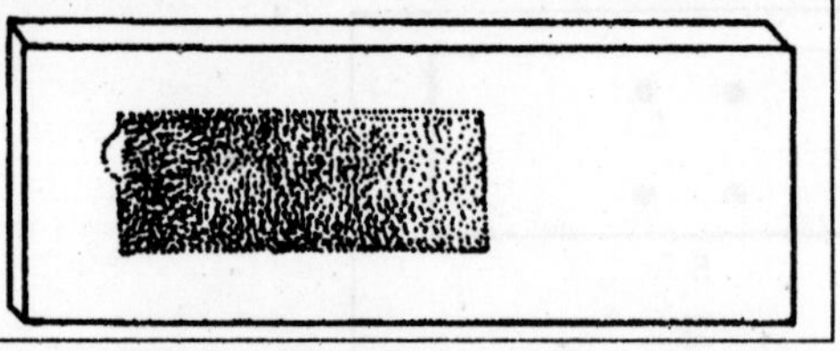

Fig. 12.13: Blood smear—Short's method

4. Acute Appendicitis

History

A patient aged 8 years complaining of pain in the abdomen, nausea; marked tenderness in the R.I.F. and Tachycardia for the last 48 hours.

Study of Blood

Hemoglobin	...	12 g per cent (82%)
Erythrocytes	...	4,800,000 cells/cmm (μl)
Leukocytes	...	20,000 cells/cmm (μl)

Differential Leukocyte Count:

5% of many neutrophil being young in Band (or Stab) form with fewer nuclear lobes (stab forms); Occasional metamyelocytes.

5. (Aleukemic) Lymphatic Leukemia

History

Male aged 50 with anemia and enlargement of neck glands: not responding to treatment.

Study of Blood

Hemoglobin	...	7 g per cent (48%)
Erythrocytes	...	4,500,000 cells/cmm (μl)
Leukocytes	...	18,000 cells/cmm (μl)
Lymphocytes	...	70%
Platelet count	...	80,000 cells/cmm (μl)

Abnormal Cells

A few lymphoblasts, anisocytes and Poikilocytes and Polychromasia.

6. Infectious Mononucleosis

History

A male aged 13 years has fever, enlargement of neck glands and sore throat following a similar illness occurring in his sister, who got cured.

Study of Blood

Hemoglobin	...	13 g per cent (90%)
Erythrocytes	...	4,900,000 cells/cmm (μl)
Leukocytes	...	25,000 cells/cmm (μl)
Platelets	...	220,000 cells/cmm (μl)

Differential Leukocyte Count:

Numerous mononuclear cells (60% of the total count); some resembling lymphocytes others as abnormal monocytes with pseudopodial outline or lobed lymphocytes.

7. Kala-azar

History

Female aged 30; prolonged fever and sometimes **"double" rise of temp.**; moderate anemia; splenomegaly and hepatomegaly; has developed foul smelling necrotic ulcer in the mouth.

Study of Blood (PANCYTOPENIA)

Hemoglobin	...	8 g per cent (54%)
Erythrocytes	...	2,560,000 cells/cmm (μl)
Leukocytes	...	1,500 cells/cmm (μl)
Platelet count	...	80,000 cells/cmm (μl)

Differential Leukocyte Count

Marked **reduction in neutrophils** and relative **increase in number of lymphocytes and monocytes** (above 10%).

8. Thalassemia (Hemolytic anemia)

History

Boy aged eleven: **Mongoloid appearance: muddy yellow skin, mild splenomegaly and hepatomegaly: chronic ulcer in a leg.**

Study of Blood

Hemoglobin	...	6 g per cent (40%)
Erythrocytes	...	25,000,000 cells/cmm (μl)
Leukocytes	...	14,000 cells/cmm (μl)
Lymphocytes	...	70%
Platelet count	...	80,000 cells/cmm (μl)

Abnormal Cells:

1. Target cells ... 15%
2. Numerous microcytes, anisocytes, poikilocytes, **leptocytes** (thin cells), schistocytes (residual left

after lysis of red cells) and **target cells — a few normoblasts, polychromatic cells and marked hypochromia.**

2. **Appearance of giant metamyelocytes.**

9. Tuberculosis

History

Male of 28 years has sudden attack of fever with **profound prostration and dry hacking cough, cyanosis and dyspnea**; period of **illness 24 hrs**. only.

Study of Blood

Hemoglobin	...	14 g per cent (98%)
Erythrocytes	...	6,000,000 cells/cmm (μl)
Leukocytes	...	3,800 cells/cmm (μl)

Differential Leukocyte Count:

Marked **reduction of neutrophils — relative lymphocytosis and absence of eosinophils (Eosinopenia before treatment starts).**

10. Eruptive Fever (? Viral origin)

History

A patient aged 20 has continued fever ranging between 103° to 104° Fht. for the past 2 weeks, he is constipated, toxic: with coated tongue and a few **rashes on the chest and abdomen.**

Study of Blood
(Leukopenia with relative lymphocytosis)

Hemoglobin	...	12 g per cent (82%)
Erythrocytes	...	4,350,000 cells/cmm (μl)
Leukocytes	...	3,800 cells/cmm (μl)
Platelet count	...	100,000 cells/cmm (μl)

Differential Leukocyte Count shows

Monocytes — 10%
Eosinophils — Absent
Lymphocytes — 50%.

11. Polycythemia

History

Plethoric, cyanotic female aged 50; Persistent **headache and sense of fullness in the head: abdominal pain left upper quadrant; pain over the shin bones.**

Study of Blood

Hemoglobin	...	19.5 g per cent (......%)
Erythrocytes	...	8.5 million cells/cmm (μl)
Leukocytes	...	13,000 cells/cmm (μl)
Platelet count	...	10,000,000 cells/cmm (μl)

Differential Leukocyte Count

80% granulocytes with a few myelocytes, normoblasts and polychromatic cells-plenty.

12. Aleukemic Myelocytic Leukemia

History

Male aged 30 complaining of chronic loss of strength and breathlessness, anemia and petechie, refractory to treatment and moderate enlargement of spleen.

Study of Blood

Hemoglobin	...	8 g per cent (54%)
Erythrocytes	...	2,000,000 cells/cmm (μl)
Leukocytes	...	4,800 cells/cmm (μl)
Platelet count	...	40,000 cells/cmm (μl)

Differential Leukocyte count shows:

70% neutrophils.

Abnormal cells:

A few myelocytes, metamyelocytes, occasional macrocytes and nucleated red cells.

13. Anemia in Malaria

History

Male aged 35; anemic; history of recurrent fever **on alternate days, preceded by shivering; moderate** enlargement of spleen.

Study of Blood

Hemoglobin	...	7 g per cent (48%)
Erythrocytes	...	3,000,000 cells/cmm (μl)
Leukocytes	...	4,600 cells/cmm (μl)

Differential Leukocyte count shows:

9-12% large mononuclear cells (monocytes) occasionally containing brown pigments, **anisocytosis, poikilocytosis, polychromasia** of red cells.

14. Congenital (Spherocytic) Hemolytic Anemia

History

Male aged 35 presenting with slight fever, ulcer (chronic) of the leg and mild splenomegaly of some duration.

Study of Blood

Hemoglobin	...	10 g per cent (68%)
Erythrocytes	...	3,000,000 cells/cmm (μl)
Leukocytes	...	12,000 cells/cmm (μl)
Color Index	...	**1.2**

Smear Shows

Many spherocytes, normoblasts, Reticulocytes polychromasia and a few stippled red cells.

15. Macrocytic (Nutritional) or Pernicious Anemia

History

Male aged 40, with chronic history of pallor, tiredness, sore tongue, palpitations, digestive disturbances and paresthesia (numbness and tingling).

Study of Blood

Hemoglobin	...	7 g per cent (48%)
Erythrocytes	...	2,000,000 cells/cmm (μl)
Leukocytes	...	4,8000 cells/cmm (μl)
Platelet count	...	45,000 cells/cmm (μl)
Color Index	...	**1.25**

Smear Shows

Neutropenia with relative Lymphocytosis.

Abnormal cells

Numerous macrocytes, occasional nucleated megaloblasts, anisocytosis, poikilocytosis, polychromasia and **hypersegmented neutrophils (macropoly).**

16. Chronic Lymphatic Leukemia

History

A male aged 60 years with enlarged lymph nodes and spleen, and general weakness with loss of weight.

Study of Blood

Hemoglobin	...	8 g per cent (54%)
Erythrocytes	...	3,800,000 cells/cmm (μl)
Leukocytes	...	100,000 cells/cmm (μl)
Platelet count	...	200,000 cells/cmm (μl)

Differential Leukocyte Count shows

About 90% of cells are small lymphocytes with occasional myelocytes. There are numerous smudged (smear) cells.

17. Agranulocytosis (Agranulocytic Angina): Absence of Granulocytes (Leukopenia with relative lymphocytosis)

History

An adult female aged 40 years with fever and painful throat showing necrotic ulcerations in the throat.

Study of Blood

Hemoglobin	...	8 g per cent (54%)
Erythrocytes	...	3,200,000 cells/cmm (μl)
Leukocytes	...	2,300 cells/cmm (μl)
Platelet count	...	3,500,000 cells/cmm (μl)

Differential Leukocyte Count Shows:

Marked **Neutropenia** with **relative Lymphocytosis.**

Abnormal cells

A few anisocytes only. The polymorphonuclear neutrophils are hardly 5-6 per cmm (absolute count).

18. Tropical Eosinophilia

[As the spleen is palpable, it may be a case of **visceral bilharziasis (Schistosomiasis).**]

History (Loeffler's acute pneumonia):

A patient aged 30 years suffering from repeated bouts of cough and breathlessness accompanied with fever and palpable spleen for some weeks with no loss of weight or deterioration in general health.

Study of Blood

Hemoglobin	...	13 g per cent (90%)
Erythrocytes	...	4,500,000 cells/cmm (μl)
Leukocytes	...	34,000 cells/cmm (μl)

Differential Count Shows

63% of Eosinophils and no other abnormality.

19. Acute Myeloid Leukemia

History

Male child aged 10 years with fever, sore throat, bleeding gums and purpuric rashes.

Study of Blood

Hemoglobin	...	6 g per cent (40%)

Erythrocytes	...	2,250,000 cells/cmm (μl)
Leukocytes	...	40,000 cells/cmm (μl)
Platelet count	...	60,000 cells/cmm (μl)

Abnormal Cells

Numerous **Blast cells**; a few myelocytes, many polychromatic cells, anisocytes and poikilocytes, and occasional normoblasts.

20. Thrombocytopenic Purpura

History

A girl aged 10 years had mild sore throat with fever a week before; has epistaxis; shows fine purpuric and larger **ecchymotic patches** over the lower legs. The gums bleed on mildest injury and continue bleeding for sometime.

Study of Blood

Hemoglobin	...	8 g per cent (54%)
Erythrocytes	...	3,200,000 cells/cmm (μl)
Leukocytes	...	5,300 cells/cmm (μl)
Platelet count	...	5,000 cells/cmm (μl)

Abnormal cells

None seen, except occasional monocytes with phagocytosed platelets.

21. Chronic Myeloid Leukemia (with Anemia)

History

Male aged 38 years complaining of fatigue, loss of strength, pallor, swelling of abdomen for 18 months.

Study of Blood

Hemoglobin	...	7 g per cent (48%)
Erythrocytes	...	2,300,000 cells/cmm (μl)
Leukocytes	...	250,000 cells/cmm (μl)
Platelet count	...	3,500,000 cells/cmm (μl)

Abnormal cells

Large number of Neutrophilic myelocytes, a few myeloblasts, *metamyelocytes*, stab cells, nucleated red cells (normoblasts), polychromatic and stippled cells.

22. Monocytic Leukemia (Acute)

History

An adult male aged 42 years with marked anemia, breathlessness on exertion, and soreness, swelling and bleeding ulcerations of the gums, tonsils and soft palate.

Study of Blood

Hemoglobin	...	6 g per cent (40%)
Erythrocytes	...	2,300,000 cells/cmm (μl)
Leukocytes	...	21,000 cells/cmm (μl)
Platelet count	...	230,000 cells/cmm (μl)

Differential Leukocyte Count Shows

54 per cent monocytes.

Abnormal Cells

Many large cells — a few pseudopodial outline with **fine azure granules (monoblasts)**; occasional cells **show vacuoles and even nucleoli.**

23. Microcytic Anemia

History

A lady multipara aged 38 years with chronic history of weakness, palpitation and headache and fullness after meals in the left hypochondrial and epigastric region plus findings of Plummer Vinson syndrome.

Study of Blood

Hemoglobin	...	6 g per cent (40%)
Erythrocytes	...	3,500,000 cells/cmm (μl)
Leukocytes	...	4,800 cells/cmm (μl)
Color Index	...	0.6

Abnormal Cells

Many **microcytes, anisocytosis, poikilocytosis and marked hypochromia.**

THE PEROXIDASE REACTION

(Myeloperoxidase)

[After Dacie, J. V. (1956). Practical Hematology, 3rd Edn., P. 77 London; Churchill]

For the demonstration of oxidase granules in myelocytes and myeloblasts.

Solution (1):

Concentrated formaldehyde solution (40%)	...	10 ml
Ethyl alcohol, absolute	...	90 ml

Stock Solution (A)

Benzidine, saturated aqueous soln.	...	99 vol.

Sodium nitroprusside, saturated aqueous solution ... 1 vol.

Stock Solution (B)

Hydrogen peroxide, 10 volume (freshly prepared) (0.04 ml added to 10 ml of distilled water)

Solution (2):

Stock solution (A) ... 2 vol.

Stock solution (B) ... 1 vol.

Solution (3):

Safranin, 0.1% aqueous solution

Mode of Preparation

Solution (1):

Add the concentrated formaldehyde solution to the alcohol, mix and label.

Solution (2):

Combine the two stock solutions just before use.

Procedure for staining

(1) Prepare thin films of peripheral blood or marrow; dry at room temperature and fix in **solution (1)** for 1 minute.

(2) Wash in distilled water and dry at room temperature.

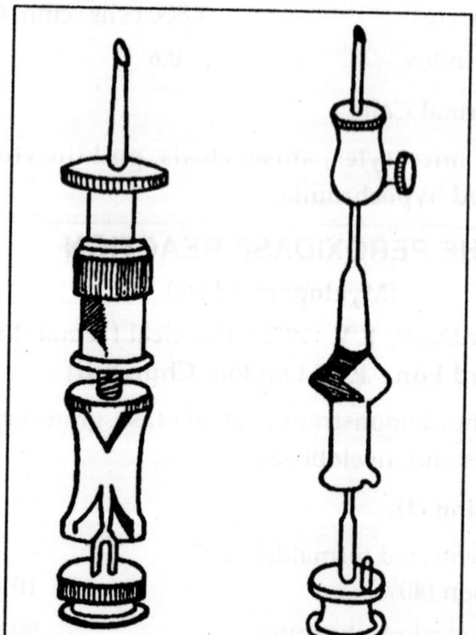

Fig. 12.14: Marrow (Sternal) Puncture Needle

(3) Flood the slide with **solution (2)** for one minute.

(4) Wash in distilled water.

(5) **Counterstain** in **solution (3)** for one minute.

(6) Rinse with distilled water and dry at room temperature.

Result

Oxidase granules — Deep blue-black.

Bone Marrow (Sternal) Puncture (Biopsy) Needle; see Sternal (Marrow) Puncture Needle Fig. 12.14.

LEISHMAN STAIN FOR STAINING PERIPHERAL BLOOD SMEAR (FILM)

(A differential stain)

Smear Examination or (PBSE)

Peripheral Blood Smear Examination (PBSE)

Original Romanowsky Stain. It is a **compound stain**, made by mixing two aniline dyes — (1) Medicinal **methylene blue** (polychrome) and (2) Eosin; the former contains an **OXIDATION PRODUCT CALLED Azure**. When both the stains are mixed, there is a range of loose chemical compounds like **Azure I Methylene Blue**, and **Azure II Eosin**, etc. It has different affinities for different elements in nucleoplasm and hence, gives **differential staining**. It therefore, consists of 2 solutions:

Leishman's Stain is universally used, as it has the advantage of both fixing and staining. **METHYL ALCOHOL FIXES THE BLOOD SMEAR**. Prepare an approximate amount of stain for 2 to 3 month's use. The stain **deteriorates on keeping for a long time**.

1 G of **Leishman powder** (*E. Merck*) is dissolved in Original 500 ml pack of **acetone free methyl alcohol** (2%) and **allowed to mature for some (15) days in the incubator.**

Method of Leishman's stain (Procedure)

Put name or a number by a permanent marker on the slide. Dry the glass rods on an **accurately levelled staining rack** by rubbing with a filter paper and place the slide with the **film side upwards** on the rack.

Cover the film with 9 drops of Leishman's stain from a drop bottle—wait for ½ min. **(methyl alcohol in the stain fixes the film).**

From another similar drop bottle add double the number of drops of distilled water (pH—7.0). The best result is obtained by using a **buffer solution.***

Mix the stain with distilled water quickly by rocking the slide gently or with the help of a capillary pipette, or blowing through a pipette, drawing in and blowing out the solution, or simply by blowing on the stain by mouth. A **golden scum** forms on the surface; this indicates good staining. Allow to act for 10 minutes.

Wash (by a flush) the slide with distilled water from a wash bottle without disturbing the slide.

Differentiate in distilled water or tap water if weakly alkaline for a minute.

Place the slide in a vertical position to dry with film-side backwards [(a) To avoid smear to erase, (b) To prevent dust falling on the smear].

Observe under low power. Leukocytes (neutrophils) should be well stained and stand out prominently. Then examine under oil immersion lens.

For quick counting High Power view helps an expert.

Result

In a properly stained slide, the film appears pinkish grey to the naked eye.

Erythrocytes — pink or orange buff.

Nuclei of Leukocytes—purple to dark blue (lymphocytes); *Cytoplasm* of lymphocytes—sky-blue.

Monocytes—have a kidney shaped nucleus of a lighter color with finely granular **(Azure granules)** cytoplasm.

Neutrophil (*Azure*) **granules are pinkish violet** (purple).

***Eosinophil* granules—vermilion red** (coarse granules).

Basophil granules—**deep purple or blue** (coarse granules).

Areas between the cells should be clear and without any precipitate. **When water is alkaline, the film is stained deep and appears bluish grey. Eosinophil granules** also take up deep greyish or blue color.

Variations

The slide may be: **(i) pink and understained and leukocytes not properly stained due to acid water, (ii) blue due to alkaline water**. Blue color does not interfere with the finding of parasites, and leukocytes; **parasites stand out prominently** on such a slide. **(iii)** When the slide is pink and leukocytes have been stained light, the **stain can be improved** (within limitation) **by putting in 1: 1,000 pot. carbonate solution, till the film is slightly bluish.**

Causes of deposits in Leishman's stain

(1) **Old stain** with sediment or old and scratched slide. (2) **Evaporation of stain on the slide** at the time of fixing. (3) **Delay in mixing** after putting distilled water. (4) **Draining of the stain** from the slide at any time before washing off finally, (5) **Overstaining** or staining for the **2nd time,** the same slide invariably gives a deposit.

Caution

For proper staining the following should be carefully observed. **Slides** should be scrupulously **cleaned,** grease-free and films nicely prepared. (1) **Films** should be properly **fixed.** (2) **Never allow the stain** (alcoholic) to evaporate on the film. (3) **Use** carbon-dioxide-free, **neutral distilled water (pH 7.0),** or a buffer solution for diluting the stain in all the stages if possible. (4) **Never allow the stain to drain** in any stage of staining until final washing is done. A deposit will surely form if the stain drains.

THE PROFORMA OF (ROUTINE) BLOOD EXAMINATION REPORT

Hemoglobin (Hellige 14.5G) ... g per cent

Total leukocyte count ... cells per cmm

Differential leukocyte count

Normal figures are within brackets.

Neutrophils (50-70) ... per cent

Lymphocytes (25-45) ... per cent

Monocytes (2-8) ... per cent

Eosinophils (up to 5) ... per cent

Basophils (0.5-1) ... per cent

---

* Buffer solution. Disodium hydrogen phosphate (anhydrous)—5.447 g.

Potassium dihydrogen phosphate—4.752 g.

Mix together in a mortar. Add 1 g of the mixture to 2000 ml (2 L) of distilled water that gives a pH of 7 to the solution.

Abnormal Cells: Red cell/White cell

Platelet Count
(150,000-350,000)/cum (μl)

Bleeding time
(1-3 minutes) mins. ... secs.

Coagulation time
(3-11 minutes) mins. ... secs.

Prothrombin time
(11-23 seconds or according to control) mins. ... secs.

Erythrocyte sedimentation rate (ESR):
(Westergren — up to 20 mm) 1st Hour ... mm
2nd Hour ... mm
Mean ... mm

Parasites:
Malaria parasite
Microfilaria

BLOOD CHEMISTRY (BIOCHEMICAL PARAMETERS)

*Blood (Plasma) Sugar
(Fasting: 60–100 mg %) ... mg per cent

*Blood Sugar (Post Prandial: up to 125–130 mg %) ... mg per cent

Blood Urea (15–45 mg %) ... mg per cent

Serum Cholesterol
(125–250 mg %) ... mg per cent

Blood NPN (25–35 mg %) ... mg per cent

Serum Bilirubin
(0.2–0.8 mg %) ... mg per cent

van den Bergh Reaction

Serum Sodium (135–140 MEq/Lt.)

Serum Potassium
(15–22 mg %; 3.9–5.6 MEq/Lt.)

Serum Calcium (9–11 mg %) ... mg per cent

Blood Chloride as NaCl
(450–510 mg %) ... mg per cent

Plasma Chloride
(560–620 mg %) ... mg per cent

Plasma Bicarbonate
(55–71 mg %) ... mg per cent

(26–32 MEq/Lt.) ... MEq/Lt.

Total Protein (6–8 G %) ... G per cent

Albumin (3.5–5.5 G %) ... G per cent

Globulin (1.5–3.5 G %) ... G per cent

Albumin: Globulin Ratio (1 : 7 : 1):

Serum Uric acid
(2.0–7.0 mg % Cyanide method) ... mg per cent
(2.7–7.2 mg % Phosphotungstic Acid Method)

Blood Creatine (2–7 mg %) ... mg per cent

Serum Creatinine (0.8–1.2) ... mg per cent

Serum Alkaline Phosphatase
(3–13 K–A units) ... units

Serum Acid Phosphatase
(1–3 K–A units) ... units

SGOT (Colorimetric method and Analyser 10–40 I.U. or 8-40 Karmen Units)

SGPT (Colorimetric method and Analyser method; 10–45 I.U. or 5–35 Karmen Units)

Thymol Turbidity Test
(0–4.7 MacLagan units) ... units

Zinc sulphate Turbidity Test
(0–4.7 MacLagan units) ... units

Serum Amylase
(80–180 Somogyi units) ... units

Inorganic Phosphate
(Child 4-6 mg %
Adult 2.5-4.5 mg %) ... mg per cent

Figures in bracket indicate normal range.

PERIPHERAL BLOOD PICTURE IN HEMOLYTIC ANEMIA (THALASSEMIA)

1. Anisocytosis
2. Poikilocytosis
3. Microcytosis
4. Hypochromia
5. Presence of Target cells (10–15%)
6. (a) Basophilic stippling, and
   (b) Howell-Jolly bodies, also in sickle cell anemia
7. Presence of **SCHISTOCYTES** (remnants of lyzed red cells)

* Requested to restrict administration of pyridoxin HCl and ascorbic acid 16 hrs. before the test.

IRON DEFICIENCY ANEMIA

A. **Parameters in Peripheral blood:**

1. Hemoglobin and hematocrit (PCV, MCH, MCHC and ESR) values are low (below 25); ESR above 25 mm
2. Presence of microcytes (6 μ in diameter)
3. Hypochromia—It is a constant feature
4. Serum transferrin level is low
5. Serum iron level is low.

B. **Bone Marrow Findings**

1. **Increase in erythroid progenitors.**
2. Absence of stainable iron in macrophages (**Prussian blue reaction is of low intensity**).

Microcytes are small cells of 6 μ diameter with a central **pallor which occupies $^1/_3$rd of the red cells**. Sometimes the whole cell looks vacuolated where hemoglobin occupies only a thin peripheral rim.

MEGALOBLASTIC ANEMIAS

Fundamentally, megaloblastic anemia occurs from impairment of DNA synthesis that leads to distinctive morphologic changes in the Erythroid series of cells, e.g., abnormally large erythroid precursors as well as the red cells.

PERIPHERAL BLOOD PICTURE

1. The red cells are macrocytes; they may be oval and called ovalocytes; hence there is presence of **macro-ovalocytes**.
2. The red cells lack central pallor (of normal red cells) and look **hyperchromic** and **normochromic but MCHC is not elevated**.
3. There is marked **variation** in red cell **sizes**. This is called **ANISOCYTOSIS**.
4. There is **variation in shape**, so it is called **POIKILOCYTOSIS**.
5. Presence of characteristic oval macrocytes called **MACRO-OVALOCYTES**.
6. **Presence of macropolys. Macro Polys** are larger neutrophils (polymorphonuclear leukocytes; macropolymorphonuclears) with **hypersegmentation (more than 4 lobes)** of neutrophils.
7. Presence of **giant metamyelocytes**.
8. There is mild-degree of hemolysis which remains unexplained.
9. Presence of **Reticulocytes above 5 to 10% red cells** called **Reticulocyte crisis**.

BONE MARROW FINDINGS IN MEGALOBLASTIC (MACROCYTIC) ANEMIA

1. **Hypercellular bone marrow** (due to increased hemopoietic precursor cells.
2. **Megaloblastic changes** in all stages of red cell development.
3. **Hyperplasia** of the most primitive **precursor cells**, i.e., **PROMEGALOBLASTS** which have (a) **nuclei with (i) fine nuclear pattern** and (ii) prominent nucleoli, and (b) **deep basophilic cytoplasm**.
4. **Nuclear maturation is delayed** as opposed to (a) cytoplasmic maturation and (b) acquisition of hemoglobin.
5. Presence of **GIANT METAMYELOCYTES** and **band forms**, i.e., **stab cells** due to **impaired DNA synthesis** in all types of proliferating cells including the myeloid series. This may also cause **PANCYTOPENIA (Robbins, Ed. VIII)**.

Diagrams/Notes

Diagrams/Notes

Diagrams/Notes

Diagrams/Notes

PART FIVE

Chemical Pathology

CHAPTER 13

CHEMICAL PATHOLOGY

USE OF A COLORIMETER

Biochemical estimations are often made colorimetrically by matching the color of the unknown with a standard. The exact quantity of the chemical present in the unknown may thus be easily determined, compared with that of the standard by color reaction.

In a photo-electric colorimeter, error arising from personal factor are excluded owing to the fact that the reading is automatically recorded by the photosensitive cell. In this a calibration chart is always obtained for the standard solutions and the unknown is matched and compared with the graph to obtain the percentage of the chemical. Thus, preparation of a standard solution every time, as is required in an ordinary Duboscq (old design) or Klett's (old) colorimeter can be avoided. In the latter instances, there are cups to contain the standard and unknown solution and plungers are dipped into them. The standard is usually fixed at a particular distance (say 20 mm); the unknown is matched with it, and the distance at which it matches is recorded. Formula for calculating the result is as follows:

X = concentration of the unknown substance mg per ml; U = reading in mm of the unknown; Y = concentration of the standard in mg per ml; S = reading of the standard in mm.

Then $X \times U = S \times Y$, or $X = \dfrac{S \times Y}{U}$

The result is expressed in mg per 100 ml (or per dl) considering the dilutions of the original blood used in the test.

OLDER METHOD WITH OPTICAL (DUBOSCQ) COLORIMETER

Estimation of Fasting Blood Sugar

Principle

The protein-free blood filtrate is treated with alkaline cupric tartrate solution, which becomes reduced by sugar. The reduced alkaline copper solution is treated with a standard phosphomolybdic acid solution. A blue color develops which is proportionate to the degree of copper oxide present. This is then compared colorimetrically with a standard sugar solution treated similarly as the **protein free blood filtrate**.

Reagents

(1) **Stock 1 G glucose** solution is saturated with benzoic acid (2.5 g per litre). For working prepare a solution by mixing 2 ml of the stock solution in 100 ml of saturated solution of benzoic acid (1 ml = 0.2 mg).

(2) 10% Solution of **sodium tungstate**.

(3) **⅔ N sulphuric acid.**

(4) **Alkaline copper solution**: Dissolve 40 g of anhydrous sodium carbonate in 400 ml (4 dl) of water in a one litre volumetric flask. Add 7.5 g of tartaric acid and when dissolved, add **45 g of crystalline anhydrous $CuSO_4$**. Mix and make up the volume to 1 litre.

(5) **Phosphomolybdate reagent**: Put 35 g of molybdic acid in a one litre beaker. Add 5 g of sodium tungstate and 200 ml (2 dl) of 10 per cent NaOH and 200 ml (2 dl) of distilled water. Boil vigorously for 2 hours to drive away the ammonia present. Cool; add 125 ml (1.25 dl) of ortho-phosphoric acid (89%) and make up the volume to 500 ml (5 dl).

Method

Collect 2 ml of blood from a patient before breakfast in an anticoagulant vial; keep it in the refrigerator and estimate within 4 hours; if collected in a Fluoride vial and kept at 4°C, the sample does not deteriorate even after several days (or a week).

Preparation of protein-free filtrate (Folin-Wu)

Take 7 ml of distilled water in a flask and add 1 ml of oxalated blood to it; mix by shaking, wait till the blood is hemolysed. Add **1 ml of sodium tungstate** and slowly add **1 ml of $^2/_3$ N sulphuric acid solution** shaking the flask all the time. This liberates tungstic acid which precipitates protein and a buff colored precipitate appears. If there is frothing, add **1 drop more of sulphuric acid solution**. Mix well and allow to stand for 15 minutes. Filter through **ammonia free filter paper** and collect in a dry test tube.

Test proper

Put 2 ml of blood filtrate in a **Folin and Wu tube**. In two other similar tubes put 1 ml (S_1) and 2 ml (S_2) standard sugar solutions containing 0.1 and 0.2 mg of glucose/ml, respectively. In S_1 add 1 ml of distilled water to make up the volume. Add 2 ml of alkaline copper solution to each of the tubes and place them in the boiling water bath for 6 minutes. Then cool the tubes in a water bath for 3 minutes. Add 2 ml of phosphomolybdic acid reagent and cool for 2 minutes. Then add distilled water to the mark 12.5 or 25. Put a rubber stopper and mix by inverting the tubes but without shaking. Put the solution and the appropriate standard in the colorimeter cups. Compare the color by **fixing the standard at 20 mm.**

Calculation (FOLIN-Wu)

10 ml of filtrate contains 1 ml of blood. So 2 ml of filtrate contains 0.2 ml of blood.

0.2 ml of blood contains $^S/_U \times 0.2$ mg of glucose (S_1 used as standard).

1 ml of blood contains $\frac{S_1 \times 1}{U}$ mg of glucose.

$\therefore$ 100 ml of blood contains $\frac{20 \times 100}{U}$ mg of glucose (S_1 being fixed at 20 mg).

If S_2 is used instead of S_1 as the standard, multiply by 200 instead of 100.

GLUCOSE TOLERANCE TEST

It is usually done after administration of 100 g (75 g sugar intake for the international standard) of glucose in 250 ml of water flavoured with tincture of orange. Specimens of blood are collected immediately before and after the drink and then every half an hour for blood sugar up to $2\frac{1}{2}$ to 3 hours after the drink; urine should also be examined along with it for appearance of sugar, preferably by quantitative estimation (for determining the threshold value).

Draw curves with the above data of blood sugars (study the enclosed chart).

Indications for glucose tolerance tests:

1. Persistent glycosuria, hyperglycemia and ***Syne glycosuria.**
2. To determine the **severity of diabetic** condition.
3. In individuals with quickly developing **obesity.**
4. In the event of **fasting sugar more than 120 mg % (or /dl).**
5. In persons whose **parents are diabetic.**
6. In case of **unexplained periodic weakness,** or **convulsive seizures** suggestive of hyperinsulinism.

* **Syne glycosuria**: This refers to persistent hyperglycemia and glycosuria both before (at '0' hour) and after administration of glucose. Literally **syne means 'before' or 'after'.**

CAUSES OF GLYCOSURIA WITHOUT HYPERGLYCEMIA

1. *Renal glycosuria*: It is a benign condition having **low renal threshold** for glucose where glycosuria may occur even when blood sugar is low say (60 mg).

2. *Alimentary glycosuria*: After eating a large quantity of sugar.

3. *Glycosuria of pregnancy*: This is frequently due to lactosuria. But it may be due to the presence of glucose when the **prediabetic state** may be overt **in pregnancy**. Whether lactose or glucose is present should be determined by performing an **osazone** test differentiating between **lactosazone and glucosazone crystals**. (See under Examination of urine in Clinical Pathology).

Lactosazone crystals — They assume **needles grouped in ball appearance.**

Glucosazone crystals — They assume **broom-stick appearance**.

4. *Glycosuria in advanced glomerulonephritis*: This is a rare event.

Table 13.1: Venous blood after 50 mg of Glucose orally

	Conditions	0 hr.*	½ hr.	1 hr.	1½ hrs.	2 hrs.	2½ hrs.	3 hrs.	Glycosuria after 1 hr.
1.	Normal, low (mg/dl)	80	125	135	115	80	80	80	Nil
2.	Normal, high (mg/dl)	120	160	175	150	120	120	120	Nil
3.	After mixed diet (mg/dl)	105	135	160	150	140	110	100	Nil
4.	Renal glycosuria (mg/dl)	90	130	150	145	120	120	120	Present
5.	Lag glycosuria (mg/dl)	120	180	225	120	90	90	90	Present
6.	Diabetic type (mg/dl)	160	240	300	225	225	175	170	Present
7.	Hyperinsulinism (mg/dl)	75	90	95	85	75	75	75	Nil
	Hyperglycemia & *Syne glycosria (mg/dl)	180	240	320	310	300	250	200	Present

* 0 hr. means just before the administration of glucose

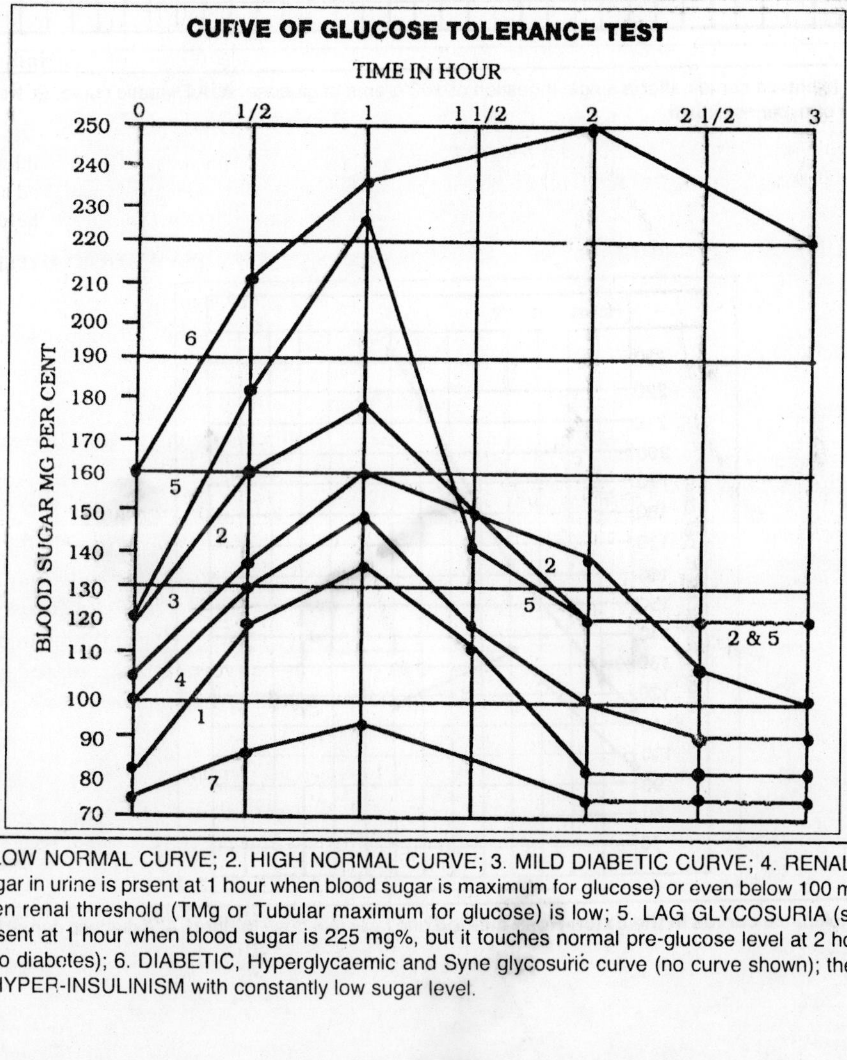

Fig. 13.1: 1. LOW NORMAL CURVE; 2. HIGH NORMAL CURVE; 3. MILD DIABETIC CURVE; 4. RENAL GLYCOSURIA (sugar in urine is prsent at 1 hour when blood sugar is maximum for glucose) or even below 100 mg%; this occurs when renal threshold (TMg or Tubular maximum for glucose) is low; 5. LAG GLYCOSURIA (sugar in urine is present at 1 hour when blood sugar is 225 mg%, but it touches normal pre-glucose level at 2 hours when there is no diabetes); 6. DIABETIC, Hyperglycaemic and Syne glycosuric curve (no curve shown); they are all same; 7. HYPER-INSULINISM with constantly low sugar level.

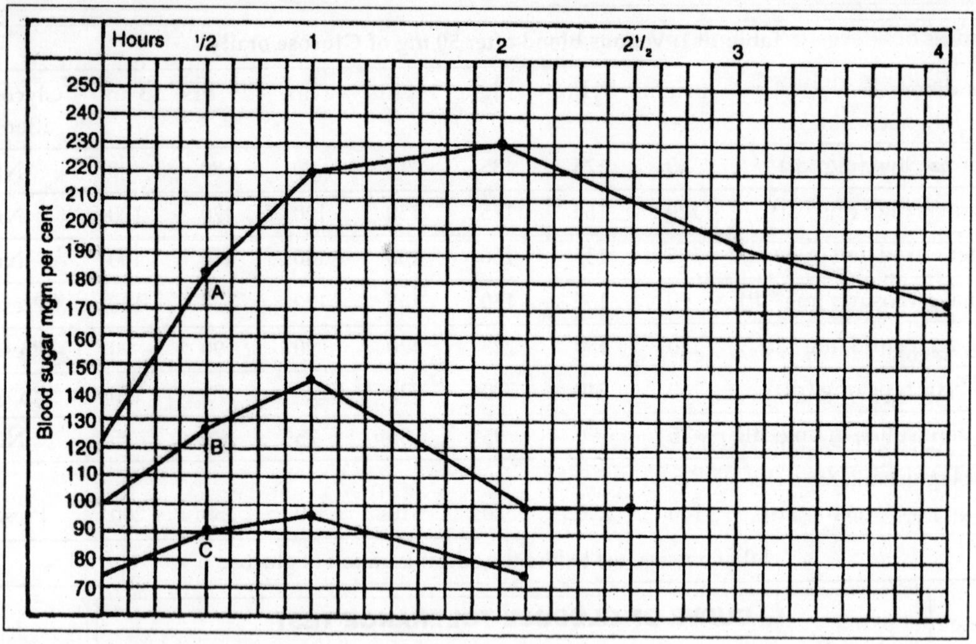

Fig. 13.2: Glucose tolerance curves after a single ingestion of 100 grams of glucose. A. A Diabetic curve, B. Normal curve, C. Curve of hyperinsulinism

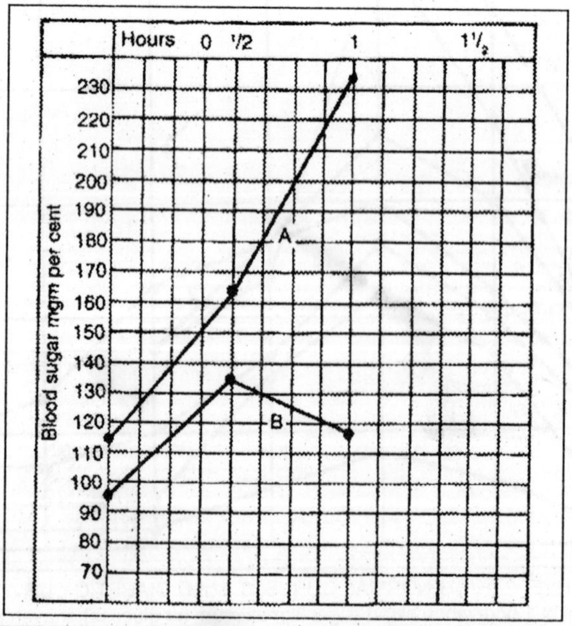

Fig. 13.3: Glucose tolerance **curves in the Exton-Rose method** one hour two dose method. A. A diabetic curve, B. A normal curve

Causes of Glycosuria with Hyperglycemia

1. **Diabetes mellitus.**
2. **Hemochromatosis (Bronzed diabetes).**
3. **Endocrinal cause:**
   (a) **Acromegaly,**
   (b) **Adrenogenital syndrome,**
   (c) **Cushing's syndrome,**
   (d) **Thyrotoxicosis (Grave's disease),**
4. **Increased intracranial tension.**
5. After ether **anaesthesia.**

CHEMICAL METHODS WITH PHOTOELECTRIC COLORIMETER (PEC)

Really speaking the instrument is an absorptiometer as the amount of light absorbed is measured in the instrument.

Essential parts

1. **Light Source.** Ideal will be a **monochromatic light.**

2. **Filters** are the means of selecting a sufficiently narrow wave band, but in some instruments there may be a ***diffraction grating,*** while in others there may be a ***prism.***

3. **Chambers** or cells to hold the final color solutions of the test.

4. **Photosensitive element** (Photo cell). There are one or two barrier layers of photosensitive cells. In the barrier layer there is a thin layer of selenium deposited on a metal disc, which is covered by a thin transparent layer of metal lacquered except for a thicker part near the periphery from where it is connected to a galvanometer (one pole). The other terminal of the galvanometer is connected to the back of the metal disc. The **light passes through the thin metal layer to the Selenium layer. Electrons** are liberated here, which pass across the barrier between the selenium and thin metal layer, that is negatively charged; the thicker uncoated metal layer becomes positively charged.

5. **Photometer.** Usually a galvanometer is used to measure the intensity of light. A variety of instruments are available depending on whether the instrument has one or two photosensitive elements and they are respectively named as '**Single cell**' or '**Double cell' Photo electric colorimeter.**

Filters

Various **filters** are used **on the basis of their spectrum band and wavelengths,** the latter may vary from 10 to 20 in different colorimeters. The specification of **Ilford spectrum filters** are mentioned below:

Table 13.2

Spectrum	Color	Wavelength
600	Deep violet	420 nm
602	Blue	470 nm
604	Green	520 nm
607	Orange	600 nm
608	Red	680 nm

GLUCOSE READING taken at 420 nm deep violet filter.

Calculation: The calculation in Photoelectric colorimeter differs from that in the visual colorimeter (see older methods). In a Photoelectric instrument the principle of calculation is as follows:

$$\frac{\text{Optical Density (O.D) of unknown}}{\text{Optical Density (O.D) of standard}} \times \text{concentration of Standard} \times \text{Original dilution of sample.}$$

Suppose, the concentration of glucose in standard solution is 10 mg % (or /dl) and the original dilution of blood is 1 : 10 (0.2 ml blood + 1.6 ml $N/_{12}$ H_2SO_4 + 0.2 ml sodium tungstate, i.e., 0.2 ml in 2 ml which is 1 : 10 dilution).

Therefore, calculation stands as

$$\frac{\text{O.D of unknown}}{\text{O.D. of standard}} \times 10 \times 10, \text{ or, } \frac{U}{S} \times 100 \text{ mg \%}$$

ESTIMATION OF BLOOD SUGAR

PRINCIPLE:

Deproteinization is done by **sulphuric acid** (acidic) and **sodium tungstate** (alkaline) and then filtered or centrifuged. **Alkaline copper reduces** the sugar present in the filtrate. **Blue color is developed by phosphomolybdic acid reagent.**

Method 1

Preparation of Reagent

1. $N/_{12}$ H_2SO_4 (Conc. Sulphuric Acid is 36 N)
2. **10 per cent Sodium Tungstate Solution.** Dissolve 10 g of sodium tungstate (Na_2 W4. $2H_2O$) in distilled water to make it 100 ml.

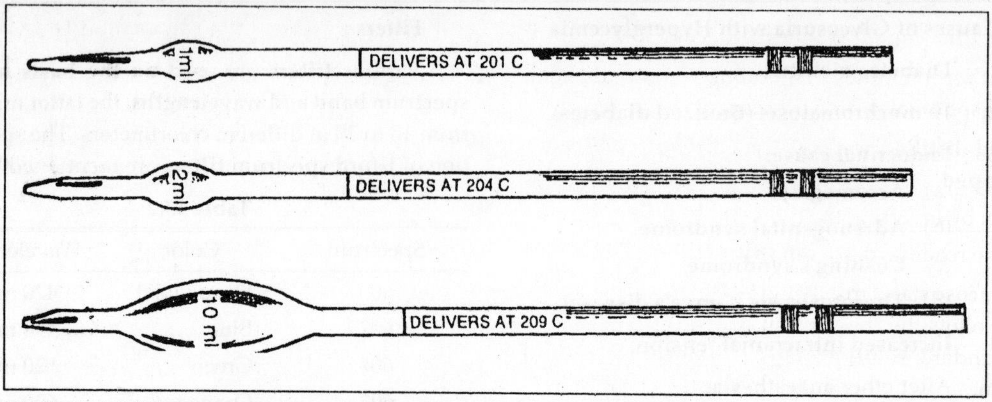

Fig. 13.4: Different sizes of Folin blood sugar pipettes

3. **Alkaline Copper Reagent (Folin and Wu.).**

Sodium carbonate (anhydrous)	... 40	g
Distilled water	... 400	ml

Dissolve. Add

Tartaric acid	... 7.5	g

Dissolve. Add the following solution

Copper sulphate (crystals)	... 4.5	g
Distilled water	... 100	ml

Dissolve, if required with gentle heat.

Make up to 1,000 ml with distilled water.

Filter the solution. Filtration of the solution every 3 months may be necessary.

4. **Phosphomolybdic Acid Reagent.**

Molybdic acid	... 35	g
Sodium tungstate (as above 2)	... 5	g
Sodium hydroxide (10%) sol.	... 200	ml
Distilled water	... 200	ml

Boil for 30 to 45 minutes to drive away the trace of ammonia impurity from molybdic acid. Now after boiling, the solution of 400 ml may be reduced to 200 ml or less due to evaporation.

Cool and transfer the solution with washing with little distilled water to a 1 litre bottle.

Add:

Ortho-phosphoric acid (This contains 89% H_3PO_4)	... 125	ml
Distilled water to	... 500	ml

Mix well and label.

5. **Working standard** by (analar) **dextrose** solution **10 mg %** in distilled water. Put some benzoic acid crystal (antifungal), shake and label. Store in a refrigerator.

Procedure

In a test tube take 0.2 ml blood, 1.6 ml $^{N}/_{12}$ H_2SO_4 and 0.2 ml 10% sodium tungstate. Mix and centrifuge. This is **deproteinization**. If a single protein particle is seen in the supernatant fluid, it may be again centrifuged to obtain a crystal clear supernate, otherwise the value increases.

Take supernate—0.4 ml in a **Folin-Wu tube** (Fig. 13.5).

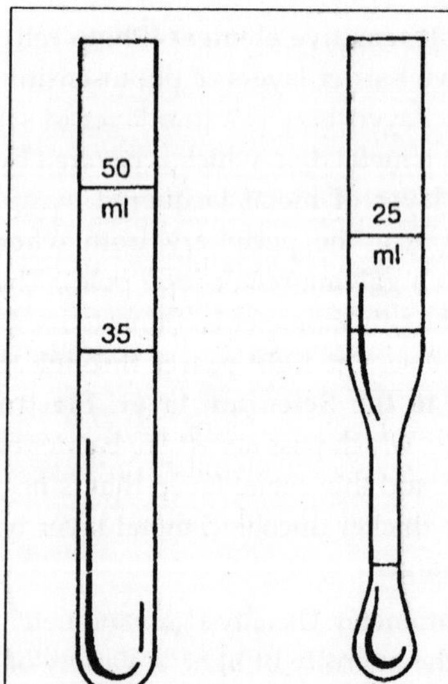

Fig. 13.5: Left: **NPN Folin-Wu digestion tube**. Right: **Folin-Wu blood sugar tube**

Alkaline copper reagent — 0.8 ml.

Boil for 8 minutes in a boiling water bath, cool, **add phosphomolybdic acid reagent — 0.8 ml.**

Add distilled water — 2 ml **after effervescence** has **stopped**.

Mix by inverting the tube.

Take reading at **470 nm (Blue filter)**.

Glucose standard: **10 mg % Dextrose** in distilled water. Follow the above technique. Instead of filtrate, take standard solution. This is **working standard solution.**

Standard reading (optical density) — Usually ranges between 0.21 to 0.32 in an **Erma (Japanese) colorimeter**.

Blank — Always blank is not necessary. Distilled water will serve the purpose.

Calculation: $^U/_S \times 100$ mg% of sugar.

Normal value: **Fasting 65-110 mg%** [Lower level has been observed by the authors in sages who maintain a disciplined regulated life with restrictions].

Post prandial (PP) — **Up to 130 mg%**.

ESTIMATION OF BLOOD SUGAR

(FOLIN-WU METHOD; See Figs. 13.4 & 13.5)

Method 2

Procedure

In a 50 ml conical flask, add 7 ml of water and 1 ml of whole blood. Then add **1 ml of ⅔ N Sulphuric acid** and mix. Then add 1 ml of **10% sodium tungstate solution shaking constantly** during addition.

Keep for some time and then filter. Take 2 ml of filtrate by a Folin-Wu pipette (Fig. 13.4) into a Folin-Wu sugar tube (Fig. 13.5), add 2 ml of alkaline copper solution and boil in a boiling water bath for **exactly 8 minutes**. In another Folin-Wu tube, take 2 ml of standard Glucose solution (working) and add 2 ml of alkaline copper solution and boil **as unknown**.

After boiling, cool the tube and add 2 ml of phosphomolybdic acid reagent mix and make the volume to 25 ml.

Compare the color in a colorimeter at 470 nm (Blue).

Calculation:

$$\frac{\textbf{Reading of the unknown}}{\textbf{Reading of the standard}} \times 100 \text{ mgm } \%$$

CAUSES OF RISE IN BLOOD SUGAR

Diabetes mellitus, diabetic coma, hyperactive thyroid, pituitary and **adrenal glands**, after administration of **hydrocortisone-like drugs**, pancreatitis, α-cell tumour of pancreas, acute infection, in conditions of stress, increased intracranial tension, etc.

Causes of hypoglycemia: Hyperinsulinism after insulin administration and **β-cell tumour** of the pancreas, hypofunction of the thyroid, pituitary and adrenal (**Addison's disease**), after severe exercise, hypoglycemic (insulin) coma, starvation, etc.

ESTIMATION OF TRUE SUGAR (GLUCOSE)

Nelson-Somogyi Method (Nelson, 1944 & Somogyi, 1945).

Principle

Blood is **deproteinized by a zinc hydroxide-barium sulfate** procedure which **gives a filtrate containing** practically **no reducing substances other than glucose**. The zinc-barium filtrate is heated with an alkaline copper reagent and then treated with a special **arsenomolybdate color reagent**. The color developed is compared with that obtained from a known amount of glucose.

Reagents required:

1. *Barium Hydroxide Solution*

Dissolve **90 g of $Ba(OH)_2 \cdot 8H_2O$** in distilled water and dilute to 2,000 ml in a graduated cylinder. Filter if cloudy. Store in well-stoppered containers (filled to capacity).

Zine Sulfate Solution

Dissolved **100 g of $ZnSO_4 \cdot 7H_2O$** in distilled water, dilute to 2,000 ml in a graduated cylinder, and mix. It is **stable indefinitely**.

It is most important that these two solutions exactly neutralize each other. Check by measuring 10 ml of zinc sulfate solution into a flask, diluting with about 50 ml. of distilled water, add 4 drops of phenolphthalein solution, and titrate with the barium hydroxide solution, slowly and with constant shaking, until 1 drop of alkali turns the mixture pink. If it requires more or less than 10.00 ± 0.05 ml of barium hydroxide, dilute one or the other solution as required and check again. Continue until the two solutions are exactly equivalent. **Protect the barium hydroxide solution** in the dispensing bottle **with a soda-lime tube in the stopper**, and test both solutions occasionally by making a trial filtrate of blood. Satisfactory solutions will give a clear filtrate, which filters rapidly and shows **little tendency to foam.**

Alkaline, Copper Reagent

Solution A

Dissolve 50 g of anhydrous sodium carbonate, 50 g of Rochelle salt (**Sod. Pot. Tartarate**), 40 g of sodium bicarbonate, and 400 g of anhydrous sodium sulphate in about 1,600 ml of distilled water, and dilute to 2 litres. Mix and filter if not clear. Store at room temperature. If a sediment forms in a few days, filter again.

Solution B

Dissolve 150 g of $CuSO_4 \cdot 5H_2O$ in distilled water and dilute to 1 litre. Add 0.5 ml of concentrated sulphuric acid, and mix.

Alkaline copper reagent (working soln.)

On the day it is to be used, place **4 ml of Solution B** in a 100 ml graduated cylinder, dilute to **100 ml** with **Solution A**, and mix.

Arsenomolybdate Color Reagent

Dissolve 100 g of ammonium molybdate in 1,800 ml of distilled water. Add 84 ml of concentrated sulphuric acid, with stirring. Dissolve 12 g of **disodium orthoarsenate** ($Na_2HASO_4 \cdot 7H_2O$) in 100 ml of distilled water and add it with stirring to the acidified molybdate solution. Place the mixture in an incubator at 37°C for 1 to 2 days. Store in a glass-stoppered brown glass bottle. This solution should be stable **indefinitely**.

Standard Glucose Solutions

Prepare a stock standard by dissolving exactly 1.00 g of higher purity anhydrous glucose in about 10 to 15 ml of 0.2 per cent benzoic acid solution, transferring quantitatively to a 100 ml volumetric flask, diluting to the mark with the benzoic acid solution, and mixing. This solution is stable indefinitely, and contains 10 mg of glucose per ml.

Procedure

A. *Deproteinization*

Place 1 ml of blood in a 50 ml flask. Add 9.5 ml of barium hydroxide solution, mixing by rotation. Add 9.5 ml of zinc sulphate solution, mixing by rotation. Shake vigorously and filter on a dry filter paper, collecting the filtrate in a dry flask.

B. *Determination of glucose*

Measure 0.5 ml of the barium-zinc filtrate into a test tube calibrated at 10 ml. Add 1 ml of alkaline copper reagent, mix by tapping, cover the top of the tube with a marble, and place upright in a boiling water bath for 20 minutes. Cool by placing the tube in water at room temperature for 1 minute. Add 1 ml of arsenomolybdate color reagent, mixing by tapping; then dilute to 10 ml with distilled water. Mix by inversion. Prepare a blank by carrying out the procedure as described on 0.5 ml of water. Set the photometer to zero density with the blank, and measure the optical densities of standard and unknown at 540 nm.

Calculation:

$$\frac{\text{Density of unknown}}{\text{Density of standard}} \times \text{mg glucose in standard} \times \frac{100}{0.025}$$

= mg glucose per 100 ml blood.

A "standard" containing 0.025 mg of glucose is satisfactory for blood samples containing up to 350 mg per cent (or /dl) blood glucose. With this standard the calculation simplifies to:

$$\frac{\text{Density of unknown}}{\text{Density of standard}} \times 100$$

= mg glucose per 100 ml (or/dl) blood.

For samples containing more than 350 mg per cent blood glucose, repeat the analysis using a smaller aliquot (fraction) of filtrate plus water to make 0.5 ml, and correct the calculations accordingly. The colors obtained by the method are said to be **stable for more than 24 hours.**

Interpretation

Normal values for "true glucose" on fasting venous blood by this method range between **65 and 100 mg** (of whole blood), with an average value of 85 mg per 100 ml.

Normal Blood Sugar: **70–110 mg/dl (%) (Fasting)**
90–140 mg/dl (%) (P.P)

ESTIMATION OF BLOOD UREA BY DIACETYL MONOXIME METHOD

Method 1: This is the best method.

Principle

Blood is deproteinized. Filtrate is treated with **Diacetyl monoxime** and **Phosphoric acid-Sulphuric acid mixture** to develop yellow color. The density of the color is measured colorimetrically.

Preparation of reagent

1. N/12 Sulphuric Acid (see reagent of blood sugar, Method). Label.
2. Sodium Tungstate Solution (10%). (See blood sugar, Method 1) Label.
3. Diacetyl Monoxime Solution (2%) in 2% acetic acid

   Add 60 ml distilled water in 2 g of diacetyl monoxime. Add 2 ml glacial (concentrated) acetic acid. Mix. Add distilled water to 100 ml. Mix well and label.
4. Sulphuric Acid-Phosphoric Acid Reagent. (**Acid Mixture**)

   Ortho Phosphoric acid (it contains 85% H_3PO_4) ... 150 ml

   Mix well. Add to this slowly

   Concentrated Sulphuric acid ... 50 ml shaking while adding.

   To this add

   Distilled water ... 140 ml

   Mix well and label.
5. Working standard solution of urea is 2.5 mg of urea in 1 ml distilled water (40%).

Take 0.1 ml of blood into a test tube in which 3.6 ml of H_2SO_4 (N/12) is taken previously, add to it 0.3 ml of Sod. Tungstate Solution (10%). Mix well, transfer to centrifuge tube and centrifuge (**For Deproteinization**).

To 1 ml of supernatant fluid, add 1 ml of distilled water, 0.4 ml of Diacetyl Monoxime Reagent (2% Diacetyl monoxime in 2% acetic acid) and 1.6 ml of Sulphuric Acid-Phosphoric Acid mixture. Place in a boiling water-bath for 30 minutes. Cool and read in a colorimeter.

Working standard solution:

2.5 mg % of urea in distilled water.

Standard

1 ml of working standard + 1 ml of water + 0.4 ml of Diacetyl Monoxime Reagent + 1.6 ml of Sulphuric Acid–Phosphoric Acid mixture; boil as in test and read in a colorimeter.

Calculation:

$$\frac{\textbf{Reading of the unknown}}{\textbf{Reading of the standard}} \times 100 \text{ mgm \% Urea}$$

Filter: **470 nm (Light Blue filter).**

Normal value of urea: 15-40 mg %.

CAUSES OF RAISED UREA LEVEL (UREMIA)

PRERENAL

In severe and protracted vomiting, pyloric or intestinal obstruction, in severe and prolonged diarrhoea, in ulcerative colitis, in hemorrhage, in conditions of chloride loss.

RENAL

In all forms of kidney disease where renal parenchyma is damaged, e.g., all types of nephritis, pyelonephritis, mercurial poisoning, polycystic disease of the kidney, etc.

POST RENAL

Obstruction in the urinary passage down the kidney, e.g., stones of the urinary passage (obstructive uropathy).

CAUSES OF LOWERED UREA LEVEL

In severe anemia, hydremia of pregnancy, etc.

Normal Range: 36–45 mg/dl (%)

DETERMINATION OF NPN (Non-Protein Nitrogen)

In present days, it has practically no value.

Principle

Protein is first digested. Then the amount of ammonia is estimated by color reaction developed by **Nesslerization**.

Take 5 ml **Folin-Wu filtrate (Fig. 13.5 left side tube)** in a hard glass test tube (8″ × 1″) and add 1 ml of ***Digestion Mixture** to it. Digest over a low flame until the solution is clear. Keep at that condition below the boiling point for another 5 minutes. Cool. Transfer the contents to a 25 ml vol. flask or measuring cylinder by repeatedly washing with small quantities of water. Then take 2 test tubes marked 'U' and 'S' and add the following:

* Digestion mixture:

5 ml	5% Copper Sulphate solution
30 ml	Orthophosphoric acid
10 ml	Concentrated Sulphuric acid

Table 13.3: PROCEDURE FOR NPN

Test tube No.	'U'	'S'
Test solution from cylinder	5 ml	0
Standard solution** [0.05 mg of $(NH_4)_2SO_4$ ml]	0 ml	1 ml
Water	0 ml	4 ml
Gum Ghatty Solution (0.1%)	0.5 ml or less	0.5 ml
Nessler's Reagent	3 ml	3 ml

Mix after each addition. Compare the color.

Filter: **Light Blue (470 nm)**.

Calculation: $\frac{\text{Reading of U}}{\text{Reading of S}} \times 50$ mg %.

Normal range: 15 to 40 mg %.

** **Stock ammonium sulphate solution**: **See Table 13.3** for this, dissolve 2.2 g of pure dry ammonium sulphate salt in distilled water to make up to a litre.

Working solution of ammonium sulphate: 5 ml of stock solution is made up to 100 ml; 1 ml of solution is equivalent to 0.05 ml of urea.

ESTIMATION OF URIC ACID

Principle

Blood is deproteinised. Urea cyanide and uric acid reagent develop the color.

Unknown tube

Filtrate (Folin-Wu)	...	5 ml
Urea Cyanide Solution (see later)	...	2 ml
Uric Acid Reagent (see later NO_2)	...	2 ml

Standard tube

Working Standard (0.4 mg %)

Uric acid solution in water	...	5 ml
Urea Cyanide Solution	...	2 ml
Uric Acid Reagent	...	2 ml

Reading: Wait for 10 minutes and compare the color.

Calculation: $\frac{\text{Reading of unknown}}{\text{Reading of standard}} \times 4$

Filter: Red (660 nm).

Normal value of serum **uric acid is 2.5-4.5 mg%**

1. **PREPARATION OF UREA CYANIDE (12%) SOLUTION:**

Purification of urea cyanide is important. **Henley's method** is given below:

High grade Urea cyanide	12	g
Distilled water ...	100	ml

Make solution

Then add Sodium bismuthate ... 0.25 g

Shake for 3 hours in a glass-stoppered flask, and leave overnight.

Filter next day.

Take the Filtrate. **Add Lithium oxalate 100 mg** and shake for 1 hour. Filter. The reagent is ready for use. Preserve the solution in an amber bottle in a dark, cool place, which keeps well for more than a year.

2. **PREPARATION OF URIC ACID REAGENT:**

A. **Sodium tungstate** A.R. (Na_2WO_4, $2H_2O$) 100 g

Disodium hydrogen phosphate (Anhydrous) 20 g

Distilled water 150 ml

Heat and dissolve.

B. **Distilled water** 75 ml

Sulphuric acid (slowly add) 25 ml

Mix.

Carefully add solution B to solution A, shaking continuously. Boil gently in a reflux condenser for 1 hour. Alternatively, a funnel may be fitted inverted on the top of 200 ml conical flask in which the solutions are gently heated, with a device to constant circulation of iced water on the stem of the funnel. The tube end of the funnel should be sealed, so that no fluid evaporates out. **The principle of a reflux condenser** is to gently heat the fluid without any loss of it, and the vapour of the fluid should be cooled down, i.e., heating and cooling of the same fluid simultaneously.

If the color of the solution becomes slightly greenish, **it will not be necessary to decolorize with bromine.**

The solution keeps well in a dark cool place for more than a year.

3. **URIC ACID STANDARD SOLUTION:**

A. **Lithium carbonate** 60 mg

Distilled water 20 ml

Dissolve by heating at 60°C.

B. Add this solution to **uric acid**—100 mg in a 100 ml volumetric flask. Dissolve by stirring and **heating if necessary**.

C. Add formalin (40%) 2 ml

Add Acetic acid (50% v/v) 1 ml

Make up to 100 ml mark with Distilled water and mix.

Preserve the solution in an amber bottle in a dark, cool place; it keeps well at least for a year.

METHOD 2 (CARAWAYS)

PTA (Phospho-Tungstic Acid) Method

In this method **sodium carbonate solution** is **used in place of alkaline sodium cyanide**. This is not poisonous. This is less sensitive but gives better reproducible color.

Procedure

Serum 0.6 ml.

Add Dilute Tungstic acid 5.4 ml slowly with constant shaking. Wait for 10 minutes.

Centrifuge:

Pipette off and mix supernatant fluid ... 3 ml

Sodium carbonate solution (10%) ... 0.6 ml

Phosphotungstic acid ... 0.6 ml

Mix well. Kept at 20°–25°C for ½ hour

Take reading at 680 to 700 nm (Red filter).

Compare with the working standard (0.5 mg %) containing 0.005 mg per ml. 3 ml of working standard is taken (like test sample), containing 3 × 0.005 mg = 0.015 mg uric acid.

1. Sodium tungstate 10%.
2. Sulphuric acid ⅔ N.

These solutions (1) and (2) will be required to prepare tungstic acid reagent (3).

3. **PREPARATION OF PHOSPHO-TUNGSTIC ACID:**

Sodium tungstate (10%; molybdate free) 50 ml

⅔ N. Sulphuric acid 50 ml

(Ortho-) Phosphoric acid 1 drop

All the above three are poured to 800 ml of water by gradual mixing and stirring. It should not be cloudy, and if so, make it fresh.

4. **SODIUM CARBONATE:**

(anhydrous) 10% solution

Keep it in a well stoppered polythene bottle.

5. **PREPARATION OF PHOSPHOTUNGSTIC ACID REAGENT:**

Stock Solution

Sodium tungstate (molybdate-free, $Na_2WO_4 . 2H_2O$) 50 g

Distilled water 400 ml

Add Ortho-Phosphoric acid (85%) 40 ml

and reflux gently in a **reflux condenser** for 2 hours. This solution should be preserved in an amber bottle. This keeps well for month at room temperature.

Working Phosphotungstic acid reagent. For this, dilute the stock solution 1 in 10 with distilled water. This also keeps well for months in an amber bottle.

6. **STANDARD URIC ACID SOLUTION:**

Stock standard:

The method of preparation is **same as in method 1. The concentration is 100 mg% (per dl)**.

Working standard solution: **1 ml** of the stock standard solution (containing 1 mg) is **diluted to 200 ml** with distilled water, containing 0.005 mg uric acid per ml, or **0.5 mg % (per dl)**.

Calculation

It has to be understood that 0.6 ml serum was taken for test. Total volume of centrifugal material was 6 ml. 3 ml of the supernatant was taken for analysis, which really contained 0.3. ml (0.6 × ½ the volume taken) of serum.

The multiplying factor for 0.3 ml of serum is 0.015 (0.005 × 3 ml of working standard).

So the multiplying factor for 1 ml of serum would be

$$\frac{0.015 \times 1}{0.3} = \frac{0.015}{0.3}$$

Therefore, the final calculation will be —

$$\frac{\text{Reading of unknown}}{\text{Reading of standard}} \times \frac{0.015}{0.3} \times 100 \text{ mg uric acid}$$

Or, $$\frac{\text{Reading of unknown}}{\text{Reading of standard}} \times 5 \text{ mg uric acid \%}$$

Normal range: 6–12 mg/dl (%).

SERUM CHOLESTEROL (Sacket's Method) [Liebermann-Burchard Reaction]

Principle

Serum cholesterol is extracted with alcohol-ether mixture. Alcohol and ether is evaporated to dryness. Cholesterol residue is colored with* **acetic anhydride-sulphuric acid mixture.**

METHOD 1

1. In a centrifuge tube with glass stopper.
2. 10 ml Alcohol-ether mixture (3 : 1; Alcohol 7.5 ml + Ether 2.5 ml) is taken.
3. Add 0.2 ml Serum and shake vigorously for 2 minutes. Stand for ½ hour. Shake occasionally. Centrifuge.
4. Pour SNF in a 50 ml Beaker.

   Evaporate to dryness at 80° – 90°C (Boiling water bath).
5. 10 ml Measuring Cylinders with stoppers—3.
6. **Blank 5 ml Chloroform.**

Test = wash with chloroform 1 or 2 ml at a time (up to 5 ml of chloroform).

Standard: Working cholesterol Standard — 5 ml (stock 200 mg % — Dilute working 1 in 25 with chloroform, i.e., **0.08 mg/ml**).

Add 2 ml Acetic anhydride-Sulphuric Acid mixture* to each (3 times inversion).

Keep in dark for 15 minutes. Take reading in the colorimeter with **Red filter (660 nm)**.

Calculation $\frac{U}{S} \times 200$ mg Cholesterol %.

* **8 ml Acetic anhydride and 0.4 ml concentrated Sulphuric Acid is required for one sample.**

TOTAL CHOLESTEROL BY FERRIC CHLORIDE METHOD

METHOD 2

Principle

Ferric chloride deproteinises the serum. Concentrated Sulphuric acid develops a brownish color which is compared with the standard in a colorimeter.

Procedure

Take one stoppered centrifuge tube and add 10 ml of Ferric chloride Solution (0.3% Ferric chloride in glacial Acetic Acid, A.R.). To it add 0.1 ml of Serum or plasma. Shake and wait for 20 minutes in the dark. After that centrifuge: **Take 2 test tubes marked: 'Test' & 'Standard'**. To test, take 5 ml of supernatant solution from the centrifuge tube, **and to standard, take 4.9 ml of the above (ferric chloride solution).** Then add to the 'Standard' tube 0.1 ml of standard cholesterol solution (100 mg %) carefully; by the side, add 3 ml of conc. Sulphuric Acid, (A.R.) to both the tubes. Shake uniformly both the tubes and wait for 20-30 minutes. Then compare the color with **green filter at 520 or 530 nm.**

Calculation: $\frac{\text{Reading of unknown}}{\text{Reading of standard}} \times 200$ mgm %

Normal value of cholesterol is 120–250 mg %.

King's Method for Total Cholesterol

Glacial acetic acid (aldehyde free)	6 ml
Patient's Serum	0.1 ml

Allow it to stand at 37°C to 50°C for 15 minutes. Centrifuge.

Take the supernatant.

***Put color reagent (H_2SO_4 + $FeCl_3$)**	4 ml

Mix thoroughly and put in dark covered space.

Take reading after 20 minutes.

Filter — Green (530 nm).

***Color reagent: Sulphuric acid** (A.R.) (36 N)	99 ml
Ferric chloride (10%)	1 ml

Always prepare it fresh. Take the required quantity of sulphuric acid first. In case of any contamination even with water, the solution becomes **turbid, when it must be discarded.**

CAUSES OF RAISED CHOLESTEROL LEVEL

Hypothyroidism, nephrotic syndrome, diabetes mellitus, hypertension, xanthomatosis, obstructive jaundice, etc.

CAUSES OF DECREASED CHOLESTEROL LEVEL

Hyperthyroidism, pernicious anemia, hemolytic jaundice, malabsorption syndrome, severe wasting, acute infections and possibly starvation, prolonged treatment with **Atorvastatin.**

ESTIMATION OF CHOLESTEROL (FREE, TOTAL & ESTERIFIED)

METHOD 3

1. **Stock Color Reagent** —2 g Ferric chloride ($FeCl_3$, $6H_2O$), dissolve in 25 ml of Glacial Acetic Acid.
2. **Working Color Reagent** — 0.5 ml of stock is taken and the Vol. is made to 50 ml with conc. H_2SO_4, A.R.
3. **Cholesterol Standard** — 100 mg/100 ml. Glacial Acetic Acid, A.R.
4. **Digitonine Solution** — 0.5 mg% in ethanol.

TOTAL CHOLESTEROL

Take 1 ml serum in 100 ml Alcohol. Acetone (1 : 1) mixture. **Boil, Cool and make volume** to 25 ml. **Filter** quickly. **Take 1 ml filtrate** in a test tube, evaporate if to dryness. Then **add 3 ml glacial Acetic Acid +2 ml color Reagent (working).**

ESTERIFIED CHOLESTEROL

Take 2 ml filtrate in a centrifuge tube, evaporate to about 1 ml. Then add 1 ml of digitonine solution. Mix and wait for 15 minutes. Centrifuge. Decant supernatant fluid, add 2 ml Acetone, centrifuge again and drain acetone. Semi-dry the ppt. and add 3 ml of Glacial Acetic Acid + 2 ml color Reagent.

Standard: 0.1 ml standard solution + 2.9 ml Glacial Acetic Acid + 2 ml color reagent (**Blank** – 3 ml acetic Acid + 2 ml color reagent).

Calculation:

Total Cholesterol —

$$\frac{\text{Reading of unknown}}{\text{Reading of standard}} \times 125 \text{ mg \% (/dl)}$$

(**TOTAL CHOLESTEROL – ESTERIFIED CHOLESTEROL**) = FREE CHOLESTEROL.

Filter — Green 530 nm.

ESTIMATION OF TRIGLYCERIDES (TG)

Take 0.5 ml of plasma in a **25 ml vol. flask**. Add exactly 16 ml Chloroform. Then the vol. is made up to **25 ml with methanol**, mixed and filtered.

20 ml filtrate is transferred to a separating funnel and shaken vigorously with 40 ml saturated solution

Table 13.4: Procedure for TG [Triglyceride (Old Method)]

Test tube No.		S	*SB	T	**TB
Filtrate	...	0	0	1 ml	1 ml
Working standard	...	1 ml	1 ml	0	0
Methanol	...	0.5 ml	0.5 ml	0.5 ml	0.5 ml
KOH (25%)	...	2 drops	0	2 drops	0
Water	...	0	2 drops	0	2 drops
The contents of the tubes are dried by water suction, and after drying add Sulphuric Acid 6.56%	...	1 ml	1 ml	1 ml	1 ml
M-Per iodate Solution	...	0.1 ml	0.1 ml	0.1 ml	0.1 ml
(Wait for 10 minutes). Then add Sodium Arsenite Solution (6.5%)	...	0.1 ml	0.1 ml	0.1 ml	0.1 ml
Chromotropic Acid Solution	...	5 ml	5 ml	5 ml	5 ml

* Standard blank, ** Test blank

of **Sodium chloride**. Kept for 1 hour for separation. Heat for $\frac{1}{2}$ hour in dark at 100°C, cool, compare the color.

The lower Chloroform layer is transferred to a stoppered cylinder through a funnel fitted with, absorbent cotton. To the filtrate few grams of **Silicic Acid** is added by spatula and shaken.

The clear fluid is filtered and kept for estimation.

Standard used is a **standard Fat solution (500 mg coconut oil in 100 ml chloroform).**

Heat for $\frac{1}{2}$ hour in dark at 100°C, cool, compare the color.

Filter — Blue 470 nm.

Calculation:

$$\frac{T - TB}{S - SB} \times 160.25 \text{ mg \% of triglycerides.}$$

Normal value 140 mg %.

It is advisable to do serum triglyceride by one step Enzymatic Method by chemical Kit available.

1. **LIPID PROFILE**

This includes:

(1) Total Cholesterol **150–240 mg/dl**

(2) Triglyceride (TG) up to **180 mg/dl**

(3) HDL Cholesterol **(HDLc-good cholesterol) 40–60 mg/dl**

(4) LDL Cholesterol **(LDLc-bad cholesterol)** up to **360 mg/dl** and

(5) VLDL **36 mg/dl**

HDLc is High Density **Lipoprotein.**

LDLc is Low Density **Lipoprotein.**

VLDL is Very Low Density **Lipoprotein.**

HDL is directly estimated.

VLDL is $\frac{1}{5}$th TG.

LDL is: **Cholesterol – (HDLc + VLDL)**

2. **ATHEROGENIC INDEX IS:**

$$\frac{\text{LDL} - \text{VLDL}}{\text{HDL}}$$

Index below 2.6 indicates little chance of intravascular thrombosis.

TOTAL PROTEIN, ALBUMIN AND GLOBULIN IN BLOOD (Biuret Method)

Principle

Serum is treated with biuret reagent. Light absorption of the colored Solution at **530 nm** is compared with that of a **standard albumin (3 mg per cent)** solution treated similarly. By suitable fractionation albumen is determined separately. **The value of albumen is subtracted from the value of total protein which will give the value of globulin.**

For Blood Proteins

Serum	0.3 ml
23% Sodium Sulphate Solution	5.7 ml

Shake and take immediately 1 ml of mixture in a test tube (T).

Table 13.5: Set up for Serum Protein Estimation

For Serum		T	A	S	B
Biuret Reagent	...	4 ml	4 ml	4 ml	5 ml
Serum Solution	...	1 ml	1 ml Ether extract	0	0
Water (Nil)	...	0	0	0	0
Standard Protein Solution	...	0	0	1 ml	0

Table 13.6: Set up for CSF Protein Estimation

For Cerebrospinal Fluid (CSF)		B	S	Test	
Water	...	1 ml	0	0	
Standard Protein (300 mg%)	...	0	1 ml	0	Mix
CS Fluid	...	0	0	1 ml	
Biuret Reagent	...	4 ml	4 ml	4 ml	

Then mix equal vol. of ether to the balance in the same centrifuge tube and mix thoroughly. Then centrifuge.

After centrifugation take 1 ml from the bottom and take in another tube (A).

BIURET REAGENT (Weichselbaum): Rochella salt (**Na-K-tartarate**); 45 g N/5 sodium hydroxide — 400 ml; copper sulphate — 15 g; stir and dissolve, **Add potassium iodide — 5 g; N/5 sodium hydroxide up to a litre Rochella salt (Na–K–Tartarate).**

Standard Protein: 3 mg/ml of Bovine albumin in normal saline.

Take 5 ml biurette solution in Tube B.

Mix and **take reading after 10 minutes** with **green filter (530 nm)**.

Calculation (Blood Proteins): $\frac{U}{S} \times 6$ G %

Wait for 10 minutes and then reading is taken.

Calculation (CSF Protein): $\frac{U}{S} \times 300$ mg %

BIURET REAGENT

1. **Stock Solution:**

A.	Sod. Pot. tartarate (Rochella)	45 g
	Pot. Iodide	5 g
	Sod. Hydroxide	8 g
	Water	600 ml
B.	Copper Sulphate	15 g
	Water	100 ml

Mix (B) to (A) slowly with constant stirring and make the volume to 1,000 ml. This is **STOCK BIURET SOLN.**

2. **Working BIURET Solution:**

Stock Biuret Solution	200 ml
NaOH	6.4 g
KI (Pot. iodide)	4 g
Water to make volume	1,000 ml

Normal value of total blood protein is 6–8 g/dl (%), of which Albumin is 3.5–5.6 g/dl (%) and Globulin is 1.5–3.5 g/dl (%).

T + Total Protein; A = Albumin;
S = Standard; B = Blank.

NORMAL VALUE OF PROTEIN IN CSF IS 12 to 40 mg% (/dl).

ESTIMATION OF SERUM BILIRUBIN (King: Mallory & Evelyn, 1937)

Principle

Diluted serum is acted upon with methanol in such a way that it is insufficient to precipitate proteins but sufficient to permit all bilirubin to react with diazo reagent which gives coloration to bilirubin. The color is compared to a standard solution. **It is a diazo reaction.**

Total Bilirubin

Take 3 Test Tubes — B, T, S.

Test:

Take 0.2 ml **serum**

Add 1.8 ml **distilled water** and mix.

Add 0.5 ml **Diazo mixture***, mix

Add 2.5 ml **Methanol,** mix

Wait for ½ hour.

Control (Test Blank):

Take 0.2 ml serum

Add 1.8 ml distilled water; mix

Add 0.5 ml ** Diazo Blank, mix

Add 2.5 ml Methanol, mix

Wait for ½ hour.

Standard:

Take 0.2 ml Stock standard bilirubin (10 mg %)

Add 1.8 ml Distilled water, mix

Add 0.5 ml Diazo mixture, mix

Add 2.5 ml Methanol, mix

Wait for ½ hour.

Control (Standard Blank):

Same as standard, put **Diazo blank** instead of Diazo mixture.

Calculation:

$$\frac{\dagger (T - TB)}{(S - SB)} \text{ or } \frac{U}{S} \times 10 \text{ mg bilirubin}$$

---

* **Preparation of Diazo Mixture:**

1. **DIAZO 'A': Mix I G Sulphalinic acid + conc. HCl — 15 ml, water up to 1 lt; 10 ml Diazo 'A' + 0.3 ml Diazo 'B' mix.**
2. **DIAZO 'B' (0.5% Na-Nitrite Solution in distilled water)**

** **DIAZO Blank: 1.5 ml conc. HCl to 100 ml of distilled water**

† **U = T — TB.**

Normal value: 0.2 to 0.8 mg % (/dl).

CONJUGATED BILIRUBIN (Conjugates with Glucuronic acid to form Bilirubin Mono- and Diglucuronide)

Method is same as Total bilirubin excepting using distilled water instead of Methanol in T & B tubes. Standard for above will do.

Calculation is same as above.

TOTAL SERUM BILIRUBIN RANGE: 0.2 mg to 0.8 mg/dl (%)

UNCONJUGATED BILIRUBIN (Not conjugated with Glucuronic acid)

Total bilirubin—Conjugated bilirubin = Unconjugated bilirubin.

Take reading in **Green Filter at 530 nm.**

ESTIMATION OF CHLORIDE (Schales and Schales, 1941)

Principle

Protein free filtrate (see in blood sugar) of blood or cerebrospinal fluid (CSF) is titrated with mercuric nitrate solution.

Reagent:

1. **Mercuric nitrate solution**: Dissolve 3.0 grams mercuric nitrate in 300 ml of distilled water. Add 20 ml of 2 N nitric acid (**Conc. HNO_3 is 16N**) and make up to a litre with water.

2. **Diphenyl carbazone indicator**: Diphenyl carbazone in 100 ml of 95% alcohol; keep in the dark in a refrigerator. The solution fades in light within a few days and cannot be used. **Prepare freshly, once a month.**

3. **Standard chloride solution**: (See below).

Technique:

Use 2 ml of **Folin-Wu filtrate**, or 0.2 ml of plasma + 1.8 ml of water. Add **0.06 ml of the indicator** and titrate with the mercuric nitrate using a microburette (or pipette) calibrated to 0.01 ml. The end point is better with protein-free solutions which give an **intense violet blue color** when the first drop of excess mercuric nitrate solution is added. A sharp change to pale violet denotes the end point. Carry out the titration on 2 ml of the standard chloride solution.

Standard Chloride Solution:

This is a solution of 585 mg or 100 MEq of **sodium chloride** dried at 120°C, in water and made up to 1 litre.

Calculation:

Hg. chloride per 100 ml plasma or CSF =

$$\frac{\text{ml mercuric nitrate solution required for the unknown}}{\text{ml mercuric nitrate solution required for the standard}} \times 585$$

This method is applicable for whole blood, plasma, serum and CSF. If the **result to be given in MEq/Lt., multiply by 5.85 instead of 585.**

CAUSES OF DECREASED CHLORIDE LEVEL IN CSF; I. Tb. Meningitis and Fungal meningitis shows value of 600 mg/dl

NORMAL VALUES:

Whole blood — 450–510 mg/dl (%) or 77–87 MEq/Litre.

Serum/Plasma chloride — 560–620 mg (%) or 95–106 MEq/Litre.

CSF chloride—700–785 mg/dl (%) or 120–131 MEq/Litre.

METHOD OF ESTIMATION OF SODIUM

Principle

Sodium and the serum proteins are precipitated together **by magnesium uranyl acetate reagent** and it is centrifuged to remove the precipitate. Then sodium in the precipitate is **determined colorimetrically by measuring the loss in concentration of the original reagent solution.**

Take 3 stoppered centrifuge tubes marked as under and add the following:

Table 13.6A: Set up for Sodium Estimation

TUBES →	*T(Test)*	*S (Standard)*	*B (Blank)*
Magnesium Uranyl Acetate Solution	5 ml	5 ml	5 ml
Serum	0.1 ml	—	—
Standard Solution	×	0.1 ml	—

Standard Solution: 500 mg % (/dl) Sodium chloride solution is used. Dissolve 1.271 g of dry sodium chloride dried (in water moistured) and make up to 100 ml.

Agitate vigorously by blowing through the pipette.

Then add water 0.1 ml.

Stopper and wait for 5 minutes to form ppt.

Then shake for ½ minute and centrifuge.

Take 2 ml supernatant fluid in two 100 ml Volumetric flask and add **8 ml 1% Acetic Acid** Solution;

add **4 ml of Pot. Ferrocyanide Solution** and make the Volume to 100 ml with 1% Acetic Acid Solution.

Mix and **read within** next **10 minutes**.

Filter — Violet (420 nm).

Calculation: $\dfrac{\text{Reading of unknown}}{\text{Reading of standard}} \times 200 \text{ MEq/L}$

N.B. Dilute the Glacial Acetic Acid 1 ml to 100 ml with water to make 1% Acetic Acid Solution.

NORMAL VALUE OF SERUM SODIUM is 306–336 mg/dl (%) or 135–150 MEq/Litre.

To convert mg% (/dl) into milliequivalents/Litre, it is necessary to multiply by 10 and divide by equivalent weight.

PRINCIPLES OF FLAME PHOTOMETER FOR ESTIMATION OF Na, K, Li

For estimation of serum **Sodium, Potassium, Lithium and Calcium**, Flame photometric method is best and ideal. Different dilutions of a particular substance in milliequivalent are prepared and is inserted into a flame photometer (Dilution range in milliequivalent) which are used as standard for comparison. The sample is then inserted after dilution and is compared with the standard, and calculation is made accordingly. The intensity of the emitted color at the wavelength is specific for a given ion, e.g., Na^+, K^+, Ca^{++}, etc. 'D' line for Na^+ is 589 nm. For Sodium and Potassium estimation flame photometry is best and convenient.

METHOD OF ESTIMATION OF POTASSIUM

Principle (see Table 13.7)

Potassium is precipitated from serum by sodium cobaltinitrite as a double salt. After suitable washing by water and alcohol the amount of cobalt in the precipitate is determined colorimetrically.

Procedure

Take 3 centrifuge tubes marked as under and add, the following:

Read in a colorimeter.

Filter — Orange 620 nm.

Table 13.7: Set up for Potassium Estimation

Technique		T (Test)	S (Standard)
Serum	...	0.1 ml	0 ml
Standard Solution (Working)	...	0	1 ml
Sodium Cobaltinitrite Solution	...	2 ml	2 ml
While adding Cobaltinitrite Solution shake continuously, Then wait for 45 minutes.			
Then add water	...	2 ml	2 ml
Mix and centrifuge only the T (test) tube			
Remove the supernatant fluid by inverting the tube and allowing to drain on a filter paper for a short time.			
Add again			
Water (without disturbing ppt.)	...	1 ml	1 ml
Centrifuge again, invert and drain as before,			
Then add 70% alcohol only in T (test) tube	...	2 ml	2 ml
Mix with glass rod, centrifuge again, invert and drain.			
Repeat the washing with 70% alcohol.			
Then add water	...	2 ml	2 ml
Boil for 10 minutes in a boiling water-bath to dissolve the ppt. Allow to cool and add—			
1. **Choline Chloride Solution**	...	1 ml	1 ml
2. **Sodium Ferrocyanide Solution**	...	1 ml	1 ml
Water	...	2 ml	2 ml

NORMAL VALUE: 15-22 mg %(/dl) or 3.9-5.6 MEq/ Litre.

N.B. To prepare Sod. Cobaltinitrite Solution take 2 g of Sodium Cobaltinitrite and add 4 ml of water; mix.

SERUM CALCIUM (COLORIMETRIC METHOD)

Principle

Calcium is made to react with **chloranilic acid.** It is then titrated. Color is compared.

1. Chloranilic Acid or Sodium chloranilate.
2. Isopropanol.
3. EDTA — **Tetra Sodium salt.**
4. Ferric chloride.
5. Calcium Standard — **10 mg %(/dl) Calcium carbonate solution** in water.

Procedure

1. Transfer 0.5 ml of serum to a 15 ml **conical centrifuge tube** and add 0.25 ml of Sodium Chloranilate Solution to it.
2. Mix properly and allow to stand for 30 minutes at room temperature. Then centrifuge rapidly for 10 minutes and decant the supernatant fluid carefully.
3. Permit the tube to drain on filter paper for approximately 5 minutes but do not allow to dry.
4. Add by a forced jet (stream) 8 ml of 50% isopropanol into the precipitate. Centrifuge again and drain as before.
5. Add 0.1 ml of **EDTA Tetra-Sodium Salt** solution and break up the ppt. by tapping the tube against a rubber stopper or by mixing.
6. Add 5 ml of Ferric Chloride Solution (Working) and mix well by invertion. All the ppt. must be dissolved.
7. Filter — After 5 minutes read through blue filter at **470 nm.**
8. Report the same procedure with 0.5 ml of Calcium Standard (Working).

Calculation: $\frac{\text{Reading of unknown}}{\text{Reading of standard}} \times 10 \text{ mg \%(/dl)}$

NORMAL VALUE: 9-11 mg/dl (4.5–5.5 MEq/Lt.)

ALKALINE PHOSPHATASE ESTIMATION

Principle

Disodium Phenyl Phosphate (common substrate) is hydrolyzed by the phosphatase present in serum with liberation of phenol, and sodium phosphate. The amount of phenol so formed is compared with phenol standard solution colorimetrically. **It is common for both the phosphatases.**

Procedure (see Table 13.8)

Take 4 test tubes marked as under and add the reagents as given below, mixing after each addition. Mix after each dilution. Then compare the color.

Table 13.8: Set up for Alkaline Phosphatase Estimation

		Test	T. Blank	Standard	S. Blank
Buffer solution for Alkaline phosphatase (see later)	...	1 ml	1 ml	1.1 ml	1.1 ml
Substrate for Alkaline phosphatase Disodium Phenol Phosphate (Mix and keep 3 mins. in a bath at 37°C) then add	...	1 ml	1 ml	0	0
Working Standard (same for both) **Phosphatases** (See Phenol standard in Acid phosphatase)	...	0	0	1 ml	0
Water	...	0	0	0	1 ml
Serum (Incubate at 37°C for 15 mins).	...	0.1 ml	0	0	0
Then add **0.5 N Sodium Hydroxide** solution **for Alkaline phosphatase**	...	0.8 ml	0.8 ml	0.8 ml	0.8 ml
Serum	...	0	0.1 ml	0	0
0.5 N Sodium Bicarbonate solution **for Alkaline phosphatase**	...	1.2 ml	1.2 ml	1.2 ml	1.2 ml
Color Reagent for Alkaline phosphatase	...	1 ml	1 ml	1 ml	1 ml
Pot. Ferricyanide solution for Alkaline phosphatase	...	1 ml	1 ml	1 ml	1 ml

Buffer Solution for Alk. Phosphatase:

Sodium Carbonate (Analar)	...	6.36 g
Sodium Bicarbonate	...	3.36 g
Water to	...	1000 ml

Calculation:

$$\frac{\textbf{Test—Test Blank}}{\textbf{Standard —Standard Blank}} \times \textbf{10 K–A units}$$

Filter—Orange (620 mm).
Working standard to be prepared freshly (see later in Acid phosphatases later):

1 ml of stock solution in dilution with water to 100 ml.

NORMAL VALUE: **3–13 K–A units.**

ACID PHOSPHATASE ESTIMATION

Buffer Soln. for Acid Phosphatase:

Citric Acid	....	42 ml
(N) NaOH	...	376 ml
Water to	...	1000 ml

(same for both phosphatases)

Substrate for Phosphatases:

Disod. Phenyl Phosphate	...	2.18 g
Water to	...	1000 ml

Just boil and cool.

Phenol Standard (Stock) – 1 mg/ml in-N/10 HCl.
0.5 N. NaOH Solution 2 g/100 ml.
0.5 N. $NaHCO_3$ Solution 4.2 g/100 ml.
Color reagent (same for both phosphatases):

1. 4-Amino Antipyrin — 0.6 g/100 ml Water
2. **Pot. Ferricyanide Solution — 2.4 g/100 ml water.**

SERUM AMYLASE TEST

Principle

Amylase present in serum **breaks down starch,** when iodine no more **reacts** with the solution.

Reagents Required

1. Starch Solution — **75 mg starch** is mixed with 80 ml of 312 mg % NaCl or **250 mg NaCl. in 80 ml boiling water**. Cool. Make up to 100 ml (2 ml contains 1.5 mg of starch). Keep this at 4°C.
2. **Gram's iodine** — (Modified)
   Iodine — 1 g
   Potassium iodide (KI) — 2 g
   Water 300 ml
   This is **0.005 N Iodine Solution.**
   Dilute: 1 ml + 4 ml water (for working).
   Set up 11 tubes each containing 0.2 ml of this iodine solution.

Procedure

2 ml of Starch Solution (No. 1) is kept at 37°C for 5 minutes + 0.5 ml of serum or plasma. Start the stop watch.

Take out **0.2 ml of this serum starch solution** at ½ **minute, 1, 2, 3, 4, 6, 8, 10, 13, 16 and 21 minutes. This is t.**

This is King's close approximation to **Somogyi Unit (SU). One Amylase unit is defined as** the amount **of amylase which digests 1.5 mg of starch in 8 mts.**

$$\text{Amylase} = \frac{8}{t} \times \frac{100}{0.5} \text{ or } \frac{8 \times 200}{t} = \frac{1600}{t} \text{ units/100 ml}$$

NORMAL SERUM: AMYLASE LEVEL is upto 1–70 Somogyi units.

AMYLASE ACTIVITY IN URINE

Reagents Required:

1. **Starch Solution** — (0.2% w/v).
   0.5 g (500 mg) starch is mixed in 200 ml boiling water. Cool. Make the volume to 250 ml. Keep at 4°C.
2. **Gram's Iodine** — (Modified)
   Iodine (I_2) — 1 g
   Potassium iodide (KI) — 2 g
   Water — Up to 300 ml

Specimen: Fresh urine or urine with 5 ml of toluene in 24 hours' urine. Use Acetic Acid to make the **pH of urine between 5–7**. Isolated sample of urine will also do.

Table 13.9: Set up for Amylase

t	1/2	1	2	3	4	6	8	10	13	16	21
Amylase	3000	1500	1000	500	400	300	200	150	125	100	75

Take **9 test tubes.**

'5' '10' '20' '50' '100' '150' '300' '600' '1000'.

Add water **3.2 ml to '5'**, and **2 ml to each** of the other tubes.

Add **0.8 ml urine** to '5' and mix thoroughly. Transfer 2 ml. fluid from Tube '5' to the next tube. Mix thoroughly. Again transfer 2 ml to the next one, and so on, finally discard 2 ml.

Add **1 ml of starch solution to each tube**, mix. Stopper the tubes.

Incubate at 37°C for 30 minutes.

Add 1 drop of Gram's iodine to each tube from '1000' to the descending order up to tube '5'.

The **amylase content** of the urine is given by the first tube showing no blue or violet color is numerically equal to the serial number of the tube.

These are given in **Wohlgemuth (W) Units**. The unit is defined as the **number of ml of 0.1% starch solution is completely digested by 1 ml of urine at 37°C in 30 minutes**. Report the result **as Urinary Diastase** — .... Units/ml of urine. In case of 24 hours collection, report as Urinary Diastase — ... units/.... ml. (Put urine volume in 24 hours in ml).

NORMAL VALUE: 5–50 W. units/ml in fresh urine, but 5–20 units/ml of 24 hours' specimen.

ESTIMATION OF SGOT (AST) AND SGPT (ALT)

SGPT is Serum Glutamic Pyruvic Transaminase or **Alanine Transferase**. SGOT is **Aspartate Transferase (AST).**

Incubate these tubes in a bath at 37°C for 30 minutes and add 1 ml **DNPH solution**. Leave in the ordinary temperature for 20 minutes. Then add 10 ml 0.4 N Sod. Hydroxide Solution and read in the colorimeter with **Green Filter (530 nm).**

Table 13.10: Set up for SGPT and SGOT

Test Tube No.	Control	Test
Substrate (SGPT or SGOT)	1 ml	1 ml
Serum	0 ml	0.2 ml
Incubate at 37°C		
Remove from the bath and then add:		
DNPH reagent	1 ml	1 ml
Mix and then add Serum	0.2 ml	0 ml
Wait for 20 mins. and then add **0.4 N Sod. Hydroxide** Solution	10 ml	10 ml
Mix after each addition.		

Read at **520 or 530 nm (Green Filter).**

International Units may be obtained directly from the graph (See Result).

DNPH is Dinitrophenyl Hydrazine.

Result

As much reading in Transmission is seen so many international units (I.U.) is the result.

Or, **Calculation for SGOT:**

$$\frac{\textbf{Test reading – Control reading}}{\textbf{Standard reading – Blank reading}} \times 67\mu \textbf{ Mole.}$$

Blank (B) is distilled water.

Calculation for SGPT: $\frac{T-C}{S-B} \times 133\mu$ **Mole.**

Conversion Table of μ Mole to International unit. (See at end of the chapter). If the reading is more than 60 I.U./Lt., the test should be repeated with less serum (0.1 or 0.05 ml), or allowing less time for incubation (half or less the total time).

Table 13.11: Estimation of S.G.P.T and S.G.O.T; and plotting for Graph

To Prepare Curve		1	2	3	4	5	6	7
Substrate (ml)	...	1.0	0.95	0.9	0.85	0.8	0.75	0.7
Pyruvate standard (ml)	...	0	0.05	0.1	0.15	0.2	0.25	0.3
Phosphate Buffer (ml)	...	0.2	0.2	0.2	0.2	0.2	0.2	0.2
Pyruvate Unit/100 ml(/dl)	...	0	50	100	150	200	250	300
International Unit	...	0	8.3	16.7	25	33.3	41.7	50

Preparation of Phosphate Buffer for SGOT *AST & SGPT **ALT

Solution (1):

Disodium hydrogen phosphate		
(Na_2HPO_4, $2H_2O$)	11,876	g
Distilled Water	1,000	ml

This is $^M/_{15}$ **disodium hydrogen phosphate solution.**

Solution (2):

Potassium dihydrogen phosphate	9.078	g
Distilled water	1,000	ml

This is $^M/_{15}$ **Potassium dihydrogen phosphate solution.**

Take: Solution 1	825	ml
Solution 2	175	ml

Mix. and adjust **pH 7.45**, if required, with **N/10 NaOH or** $^N/_{10}$ **HCl.**

Substrate for GOT (AST):

L–Aspartic acid	2.66	g
α-Oxoglutaric acid	30	mg
Phosphate buffer	20	ml
N. NaOH solution	0.5	ml

Gentle warmth of the substrate may be necessary. Make the volume up to 100 ml with Phosphate buffer.

Substrate for GPT (ALT):

d-l-Alanine	1.78	g
α-Oxoglutaric acid	20	mg
Phosphate buffer	20	ml
N. NaOH solution	0.5	ml

Make up the volume up to 100 ml with phosphate buffer.

Preserve the substrate in the refrigerator. A drop of chloroform may be added. This will keep the substrate for a few months.

Preparation of DNPH (Dinitrophenyl Hydrazine) Reagent Solution

2, 4-Dinitrophenyl hydrazine	200	mg
Hot Hydrochloric acid	100	ml

Dissolve, and make the volume up to 1000 ml with the acid.

Preparation of 0.4N Sodium Hydroxide Solution

Calculating on the basis of atomic weight, Normal solutions are made. **Atomic weight of sodium is 23,** that of **oxygen and hydrogen is 16 and 1**, respectively. So **23 + 16 + 1 or 40 g of NaOH** crystals with 1000 ml distilled water will make 1 Litre of **N. NaOH** solution. So, for 1 Litre 0.4N.NaOH the ingredients will be $2\frac{1}{2}$ times less.

NORMAL VALUE of **SGOT is 10-40 I.U.** and for **SGPT is 9–32 I.U.**

N.B. For Standard solution, Pyruvate solution should be prepared just before preparation of curve by adding exactly 100 ml of Phosphate Buffer solution to 22 mg of sodium pyruvate powder.

Table 13.12

The relation of the μ mole of pyruvate per minute per litre in the colorimetric reaction to **International Units (I.U.)** determined **spectrophotometrically** or **by autoanalyser** at 25°C.

Calculated pyruvate (μ mole per min, per litre)	GOT result in I.U.
2	2
4	3
6	5
8	6
10	7
12	9
14	11
16	13
18	15
20	17
22	19
23	20
24	21
26	23
28	25
30	27
32	29
34	31
36	33
38	35
40	37
42	39

Contd.

* AST is **Aspartate Transferase**

** ALT is **Alanine Transferase**

Table contd.

44	41
46	44
48	47
50	51
52	55
54	60*

* Denotes highest normal limit.

Table 13.13

The relation of the μ mole of pyruvate per minute per litre in the colorimetric reaction to **International Units (I.U.)** determined **spectrophotometrically** or **by autoanalyser** at 25°C.

Calculated pyruvate (μ mole per min, per litre)	GOT result in I.U.
2	1
4	2
6	2
8	3
10	4
12	4
14	5
16	6
18	7
20	7
22	8
23	8
24	9
26	9
28	10
30	11
32	12
34	13
36	14
38	15
40	16
42	17
44	18
46	19
48	20
50	21
52	22
54	23

Contd.

Table contd.

Calculated pyruvate (μ mole per min, per litre)	GOT result in I.U.
56	24
58	25
60	26
62	27
64	29
66	30
68	31
70	33
72	34
74	35
76	36
78	37
80	38
82	39
84	40
86	42
88	44
90	46
92	48
94	50
96	52
98	54
100	56
102	60°

° Denotes highest normal limit.

DETERMINATION OF INORGANIC PHOSPHATE (KING)

Take 1 ml serum or plasma in 9 ml of **Trichloracetic Acid Solution 10%**; mix and then filter.

Table 13.14

Test tube No.	Unknown	Standard
Filtrate	5 ml	0 ml
Standard (working)°	0	5 ml
Molybdate II Reagent	1 ml	1 ml
Ascorbic Acid Solution (2 mg %)	0.4 ml	0.4 ml

° Stock Standard of Phosphorus: 2.194 g KH_2PO_4 in 500 ml water = 1 mg of Phosphorus per ml.

Working Standard: 2 ml stock-standard in 100 ml water = 2 mg%.

Ascorbic Acid: 50 mg in 25 ml water.

Wait for 10 minutes and read in a colorimeter.

Filter — Red 660 nm

Calculation: $\frac{\text{Reading of unknown}}{\text{Reading of standard}} \times 4 \text{ mg } \%$

NORMAL VALUE: In children : 4–6 mg %
In adults : 2.5–4.5 mg %

PROTEIN-BOUND IODINE (PBI)

Principle

Serum proteins are precipitated and mixed with potassium carbonate. This is incinerated in a muffled furnace at 600°C to produce potassium iodide. It is dissolved in acid; the iodine content is determined by the **ceric-arsenite reaction.**

GLYCOSYLATED HEMOGLOBIN

Estimation by GHB Ion-Exchange Resin Method (using the Kit)

Glycosylated Hemoglobin (GHb) Kit is intended for *in vitro* quantitative determination of GHb% in whole blood.

Explanation of test

Glycosylated Hemoglobin (GHb) is a normal adult hemoglobin (**HbA**) which is covalently bound to a glucose molecule. GHb concentration is dependent on the average blood glucose concentration. It is formed progressively and irreversibly over a period of time and is stable till the life of RBC.

A single glucose determination gives a value which is true only at the time the blood sample is drawn. GHb on the other hand is unaffected by diet, insulin or exercise on the day of testing and thus reflects the average glucose level over the last several weeks. Hence, **it reflects on the long term metabolic control of glucose in individuals.** GHb is now widely recognized as an **important test for** the diagnosis of **Diabetes mellitus** and is a reliable indicator of the efficacy of therapy. Abraham et al reported excellent correlation between HbA concentration and diabetic control, and concluded that the determination of HbA, rather than **HbA_{1C}** or **HbA1C** (fraction of HbA) to be used for clinical purpose.

There are several acceptable methods of GHb measurement like **electrophoresis, ion-exchange chromatography, affinity chromatography, HPLC and colorimetry**. Stangen GHb Kit is based upon the property of **non-glycosylated hemoglobin to bind with a weak cation-exchange resin leaving GHb free in the supernatant.**

Principle

Whole blood is mixed with lyzing reagent to prepare a **hemolysate.** This is then mixed with a weakly binding **cation-exchange resin.** The **non-glycosylated hemoglobin binds to the resin leaving GHb free in the supernatant.** The GHb percentage is determined by measuring the **absorbance of the GHb fraction and that of the total Hb.**

Table 13.15: Reagents and accessories provided in the kit

	10 Tests	25 Tests
1. Lysing Reagent	5.0 ml	12.5 ml
2. Resin Tubes	10 × 3 ml	25 × 3 ml
3. Control (Lyophilized)	0.5 ml	0.5 ml
4. Resin Separators	10 nos.	25 nos.

Reagent storage and stability

All reagents are stable at 2–8°C till the expiary date mentioned on the label. Do not freeze at 0°C.

Specimen

Whole blood collected with EDTA/Heparin. GHb in blood is found to be stable for one week at 2–8°C.

Equipment required

1. Spectrophotometer/Photocolorimeter
2. Test tubes
3. Vortex mixer
4. Pipettes & Micropipettes
5. Waterbath at 23°C/30°C
6. Timer

Reagent preparation

Dissolve the control (3) with **0.5 ml** of deionized water by inverting/swirling. Do not shake vigorously. **Reconstituted control is stable for** only 30 minutes at ***R.T. (Room Temperature) or 15 minutes at 20°C.**

* R.T. = Room Temperature

Precautions

1. Ion Exchange Resin is pre-pipetted and securely sealed to ensure accuracy and reproducibility of results. Do not use Resin Tube in case of visible significant leakage.

2. Ensure constant assay temperature (preferably 23°C) of Resin during **Step II** of the assay.

3. Initial use of control is advised to check test system performance within assay limits for the particular new kit.

Procedure:

Assay Temperature: 23°C/30°C ± 1°C

Wavelength : **415 nm (Hb 405 nm)**

STEP 1: HEMOLYSATE PREPARATION

1. Pipette 0.5 ml of Lysing Reagent (1) in a test tube
2. Add to it 0.1 ml of well-mixed sample/control
3. Mix well and allow to stand at R.T. for 5 minutes.

STEP 2: GHB (HbA_{1c}) SEPARATION AND ASSAY

1. Bring a Resin Tube (2) to assay temperature by incubating the tube in a waterbath.
2. Add to it 0.1 ml of hemolysate (from Step 1).
3. Position, a Resin Separator in the tube, so that the rubber sleeve is at the upper mark of tube (approximately 3 cms above the Resin level).
4. Mix the contents on Vortex mixer intermittently for 5 minutes.
5. Allow the Resin to settle at assay temperature for 5 minutes. Push down the Resin Separator in the tube until the Resin is firmly packed.
6. Pour the supernatant directly into a cuvette and measure the absorbance against deionized water.

STEP 3: TOTAL HEMOGLOBIN (THB) ASSAY

1. Pipette 5.0 ml of deionized water into a test tube.
2. Add to it 0.02 ml of hemolysate by using a 0.1 ml or 0.2 ml pipette or a **Hb pipette** (from Step 1).
3. Mix and read absorbance against deionized water.

Calculations:

$$\text{GHb\%} = \frac{\text{A* of GHb}}{\text{A* of THb}} \times 10 \times \textbf{Temperature factor}$$

***A = Absorbance**

For assay **at 23°C, TF = 1.0; at 30°C, TF = 0.68**

Example:

The assay is performed at 30°C, hence **TF** = 0.68

A of GHb = 0.720; A of THb = 0.670

$$\text{GHb\%} = \frac{0.720}{0.670} \times 10 \times 0.68 = 7.31\%$$

Quality control

It is recommended that a control of a known patient's sample be included in each set of assays. Factors which might affect the performance of this test other than **reagents** include **temperature, proper instrument** function, **cleanliness** of glassware, **accuracy** of sample and reagent **pipetting** and **meticulous adherence to the assay procedure.**

Expected results of GHb (HbA_{1c})

Table 13.16

Non-Diabetic (Normal)	4.5%	to	8.0%
Good Control	8.0%	to	9.0%
Fair Control	9.0%	to	10.0%
Poor Control **(Highly diabetic !)**	**10.0%**		and above

N.B. 1. Interference due to aldimine fraction is eliminated. However, in uncontrolled diabetes very high aldimine fraction may be present. In such cases, the hemolysis time (Step 1) should be increased to 15 minutes to ensure the elimination of interference due to aldimine fraction.

2. Hemolytic anemia, presence of HbS, HbC and other hemoglobinopathies may produce low GHb values.

3. **High fetal hemoglobin (HbF) and lipemia, as well as iron deficiency anemias** may result in high GHb values.

Performance:

Linearity : Upto 20% GHb

Accuracy : Accuracy is found satisfactory.

Precision:

The coefficient of variation is 1.9% (n = 20) for normal, and 1.6% (n = 20) for abnormal samples.

Clinical significance

Elevated GHb (HbA_{1c}) levels are found in badly (worst) controlled diabetic patients. Traditional urine, plasma/serum glucose determinations, though useful, fail to give the clinician all the informations **necessary to assess carbohydrate control.** In contrast, GHb measurement offers a more accurate and

convenient measure of the overall glucose metabolism of patient.

GHb correlates well with glucose tolerance test (GTT) in patients with either juvenile or maturity onset diabetes. Hence, **GHb** measurement **(HbA_{1c})** **provides** a convenient **alternative for GTT**.

The unique ability of **GHb** to retrospectively **meausre the patient's mean plasma glucose concentration for the previous 6-8 weeks** also makes it a **useful indicator in evaluating glucose metabolism during pregnancy.**

CHROMIC ACID CLEANSING FLUID FOR GLASSWARES

Potassium dichromate	...	100 g
Sulphuric acid	...	250 ml
Distilled water	...	750 ml

Mode of Preparation

Grind the potassium dichromate to a fine powder with a pestle and morter. Measure the distilled water into a heat resistant flask and add the powdered dichromate. Pour the powder in the acid slowly and with great care; the heat evolved serves to hasten dissolution of the potassium dichromate. Bottle and label with the words "ACID"—DANGER.

N.B. (a) Chromic acid cleansing fluid should be handled with great caution. When using the fluid, it is advisable to wear protective clothing (thick rubber gloves).

(b) The color of the fluid turns dark green after repeated use. When this occurs the fluid should be discarded and replaced with a fresh batch.

SPECIFICATION OF COMMON ACIDS AND ALKALI

Table 13.17

Acid/Alkali	**Specific gravity**	**Normality of Conc.**	**Ml. of Conc./Lt to make normal acid or Alkali**
Acetic Acid	1.05	**17 N**	58
Ammonia	0.88	**17 N**	109
Hydrochloric Acid	1.18	**11 N**	90
Nitric Acid	1.42	**16 N**	63
Perchloric Acid	1.54	**9 N**	57
Sulphuric Acid	1.84	**36 N**	27.8 ml

Diagrams/Notes

Diagrams/Notes

Diagrams/Notes

Diagrams/Notes

PART SIX

Automated and Semiautomated Methods in Pathology

CHAPTER 14

QUANTITATIVE ASSAYS IN CLINICAL FIELDS

QUANTITATIVE ASSAYS IN CLINICAL FIELD

Quantitative Assays involved the use of laboratory methods for analysis of biological samples. An analysis may be —

1. **Qualitative**
2. **Semi-Quantitative**
3. **Quantitative**

Qualitative analysis indicates just the presence or absence of a substance in a sample, e.g., Benedict's Qualitative Test for sugar done by Benedict's Qualitative Reagent.

Semi-Quantitative method is to compare the amount of substance in a sample with the amount in a **Reference Sample**, and to report the presence of the substance in increased or decreased quantities. Often **Chromatographic and Electrophoretic methods are interpreted in a Semi-Quantitative Basis.**

Quantitative analysis involves expression of the **presence of a substance in a sample in meaningful units of measurement** which is **statistically significant** (one-or a few hundred normal samples done where there should be a variation within normal limits, and this is called Statistical significance or Statistical assessment).

An **outline of the whole concept of Analysis** will be stated.

I. **The selection of a valid method of Analysis**

INSTRUMENTAL METHODS

This involves

(a) **Identification** of a substance in a sample

(b) **Quantitation** of the substance.

Formerly, many complex reagents were designed to specifically react with particular test substances which effected in color formations. The colors were measured by visual comparators. With this method some interference was the **main handicap.**

To overcome the problem of interference, an analysis is divided into two parts :

(1) **Preparatory step** — effecting **partial purification** of the sample.

(2) **Quantitation step** — The **real specific test** procedures.

Such two steps led to the development of methods whereby both steps are attained simultaneously by a single procedure in one shot, like **Gas Chromatography** and **Liquid Chromatography**.

Table 14.1

Hormonal substance	Parameter measured	Analytical method	Animal system used
ACTH	Plasma Cortisone	Chemical	**Rats**: Hypophysectomized
FSH	Weight of Ovaries and Uterus	Gravimetric	**Female Mice**: Hypophysectomized
LH	Testosterone production	Chemical	**Mouse**: Cell suspension of testes
TSH	Loss of RA Iodine from Thyroid	Radiochemical	**Female mice**: Thyroid

Physiological methods (biological assay)

Chemical substances can be practically measured by their response in animals physiologically. This method is known as **Bioassay**. For example, some important **peptide hormones** are measured by **Bio-Assay in different systems of various animals** as shown in **Table 14.1**.

For this method, **dose and response relationship** for different samples should be plotted in a graph. This graphical and statistical methods should necessitate the **use of logarithm of the amount to produce a straight line rather than a curve**. This is to confirm the validity of using purified synthetic preparations as standards in quantitative methods.

II. Variability in data of analyses (Analytical data)

In an experiment or analyses, some variations occur due to the following reasons:

1. ***Random Error**: It can be reduced by careful technique (experimental hand)*: It is due to **error of procedure**. This reflects to random error and **magnifies total error**.

2. ***Systematic Error***: It is due to **error of procedure**. This reflects to random error and magnifies total error.

3. ***Instrumental Error***: (a) **Componental error** (some parts go wrong). (b) **Designing error** — faults in design leading to **drift in the readings**.

4. ***Methodical Error***: Many of the methods suffer from more or less **some extent of interference**. The best example is **that test for reduction of sugar where interference is maximum, with the presence of some other reducing substance**, like ascorbic acid, pyridoxin (in Vit. B complex). In this instance, patient should be instructed accordingly.

5. ***Operational Error***: This is more or less **similar to** that of **instrumental error and systematic error**. It does not mean that there is a mistake in the operation of the instrument, but, **unnecessary use of instruments should be avoided**. The number of manipulations in a test should be **kept minimum** and should be **done with great care**.

III. Assessment of Analytical Methods

This is based on the following:

1. ***Precision***: The precision of a method is defined as the proximity or closeness of a number of replicate measurements (value of test samples) and is affected mainly by the random error.

Precision may be expressed in terms of **standard deviation** of a large number (above 30) of replicate measurements.

2. ***Accuracy***: Accuracy may be defined as the proximity of the mean of replicate analyses to the true value of the substance in a sample. After assessing the accuracy of one method related to another method, the so-called **true mean value** of the substance is attained in general; true for that particular substance in any sample in a population. 't' test of statistics is necessary to compare and corelate the means of replicate analyses (value of test samples).

3. ***Sensitivity***: Sensitivity is the ability to detect small amount of the test substance present in a sample.

4. ***Specificity***: Specificity is the ability to detect only a substance in a sample under test (qualitative term). **FALSE POSITIVITY** of results occurs **due to lack of specificity** in a qualitative test; in a similar situation, the results will be more by quantitation. This is due to the presence of allied interfering substances.

When sensitivity of a test is reduced to avoid interferences, **the test may not detect the desired substance in a sample due to its presence in trace amount**. In such a situation, **FALSE NEGATIVE RESULTS** are obtained. Hence, optimum sensitivity of a test has to be found out and employed in the analyses.

Hence, the analytical methods should be **precise, accurate, sensitive and specific**. After trying all methods for analysis of a substance, a consistent method which should fulfil all these criteria to maximum has to be followed.

IV. Expression of data and choice of units

For expression of the test result, different units have been used. Formerly there was no confusion regarding expression of the result in any unit one liked to use. To bring about a consistency in the procedure of analyses and expression of their results, an **International conformation** of ideas was laid down in 1960, and results are since expressed in **SI units**. The full name SI is derived from Le Systeme International d'unites. This is an **universal system of units**, where **1 unit is used for any physical quantity**.

The basic units (See **Table 14.2**): There are seven basic units which are independent of one another.

Table 14.2: Showing Basic Units

Physical Data	Abbre-viation	Expression in SI Basic Unit
Time	s	**Second**
Length	m	**Metre**
Mass	kg	**Kilogram**
Amount of a substance	mol.	**Mole**
Luminous intensity	cd.	**Candela**
Thermodynamic temperature	K	**Kelvin**
Electric Current	A	**Ampere**

Derived units (See **Table 14.3**): These units can combine in very many ways to give rise to certain units, called derived units, as the units are derived from the basic units.

In the derived units, coherence is well maintained as no conversion factors are involved.

Multiples and Submultiples of units: In order to provide units of convenient size for various applications, a series of standard prefixes are used.

Table 14.3: Showing Derived Units

Physical Data	Abbre-viation	Expression
Velocity	ms^{-1}	Metre per second
Area	m^2	Square metre
Volume	m^3	Cubic metre
Substance concentration	mol. m^{-3}	Mole per Cubic metre
Density	kg m^{-3}	Kilogram per cubic metre
Force	kg m s^{-2} (Newton)	Kilogram metre per second
Pressure	N m^{-2} (Pascal)	Newton per square metre

These prefixes are multipliers used with coherent units to obtain units of alternative size.

One prefix can be used at one time (**see Table 14.3, 14.4**).

In order, to avoid some confusions and for better understanding, Kilogram of derived units are not used for multiple units. So, it was conformed, all multiples of mass would be called in terms of Gram.

Table 14.4: Different Methods of Analysis

The major manipulative steps in a generalized method of analysis	Examples of specific methods	
Purification of the test substance	Determination of pH using a glass electrode	Determination of glucose using a fully automated analysis system
Development of a physical characteristic by the formation of a derivative	↓	Dialysis ↓ Production of a color using a specific reagent
Detection of an inherent or induced physical characteristic	Potential difference between two electrodes	Photoelectric detector
Signal amplification	↓	(Electronic)
Signal measurement	Voltmeter	Galvanometer
Computation	Calibrated scale on meter	Electronic calculator
Presentation of result	Visual	**Print-out**

So also for the unit of volume, instead of Cubic metre (m^3), it is called **1 litre (10^{-3} of a cubic metre)**. So 1 L. can also be expressed as 1 cubic decimetre. Now, once the term Litre is accepted and taken in multiple units, the submultiple units to express becomes easier as $^1/_{10}$ Litre or 10^{-1} Litre may also be called 1 dL. (deci-Litre), i.e., 100 ml.

SI unit of enzymes is expressed in Katal. One Katal is defined as the amount of enzyme which **catalyses the conversion of 1 mole of substrate in 1 second.**

Katal is a very large unit; **Nanokatal** is conveniently used to express the enzyme activity.

International Unit of Enzyme Activity which is **1 micromole per minute** is not an acceptable SI unit, but frequently used. Always interconversion between I.U. and S.I. can be done as **1 Nanokatal** is equivalent to 0.06 I.U.

Table 14.5: Units of Multiples

Multiples	Abbreviations	Prefix
10^1	da	Deca-
10^2	h	Hecto-
10^3	k	Kilo-
10^6	M	Mega-
10^9	G	Gia-
10^{12}	T	Tera-

Table 14.6: Units of Submultiples

Submultiples	Abbreviations	Prefix
10^{-1}	d	Deci-
10^{-2}	c	Centi-
10^{-3}	m	Milli-
10^{-6}	μ	Micro-
10^{-9}	n	Nano-
10^{-12}	p	Pico-
10^{-15}	f	Femto-
10^{-18}	a	Atto-

I. INSTRUMENTS

- **Photometer**
- **Spectrometer**
- **Spectrophotometer**
- **Photo-Electric Colorimeter**

A **Photometer** is an instrument designed **to measure the intensity of a beam of light**, in comparison to the intensity of some reference source of radiation.

A **Spectrometer** is an instrument capable of **splitting the incident radiation into a spectrum**, used to **identify the individual wavelengths**.

A **Spectrophotometer** is an instrument which **combines the functions of Photometer and Spectrometer**. Precisely, a **Spectrophotometer is capable of producing radiation of defined wavelength** characteristic from a mixed source of radiation and subsequently **measuring the intensity of the radiation**.

Principles of a Spectrophotometer

1. There is a radiation (light) source controlled by shutter system or operating voltage controller.
2. The geometrical linear path of light is controlled by a series of lenses or focusing mirrors. The **light passes through a monochromating device.**
3. That light is measured by suitable Photoelectric detection.

A **Photo-Electric Colorimeter** is a simple type of Photometric instrument for measuring the density of a liquid in the visible region of the spectrum which relies on colored filters of different wavelengths with the help of a simple **Photo-Electric Detector (Photo-cell)**.

Barrier Layer or Solar Cell: Such Photometers (Photo-electric Colorimeter) operating in the visible region requires only a barrier layer or solar cell (photo-cell). But a spectrophotometer operating in the ultraviolet (invisible) region requires **Photo-emissive tubes, capable of greater Photosensitivity** and better **precision**.

The Barrier Layer: It is an iron plate acting as one electrode, on which a semiconductor (Selenium) is deposited.

This whole thing (Selenium coated iron plate) is covered with an extremely thin transparent layer of gold or silver, which acts as an **electron collector**.

When the light (Radiation) strikes the selenium-gold or selenium-silver, **electrons are released**. Electrons (by nature of selenium) pass to the silver, but not to the iron plate. Consequently, a small limited voltage is generated, which is proportional to the Incident Radiation (Light). Such a current which is generated is too small to amplify due to low internal resistance of the photo-cell. Hence such photo-cells are not so sensitive.

Single electrode and an electron collector in a 'P-E' Colorimeter

So, it is found in a photo-electric colorimeter that **there is a single electrode, and an electron collector**.

In a spectrophotometer, multiple photoemissive tubes are set in.

Photo-emissive tube in a Spectrophotometer

A Photo-emissive tube consists of two electrodes in vacuum. One electrode is the cathode, coated with an alkali metal, which maintains a potential difference of approximately 100 volts from the anode, which is a simple silver wire acting as an electron collector.

In a powerful spectrophotometer, a photomultiplier device is designed, consisting of a series of 10 electrodes or so, of which the first one is a **Photo-emissive electrode** (see above), and the rest ones are **electron multiplier electrodes**. Light falling on the **first electrode** releases electrons. Electrons are collected in the **next electrode**, which is held at a slightly higher positive charges. Hence, the electrons stimulate the release of 4 to 5 times more electrons from this higher-positively charged electrode. Voltages of successive electrodes increase in steps of approximately 100 volts. This results in amplification of the initial current, several million volt, causing the photo multiplier tube (electrodes) highly sensitive and making it a very **sensitive Photoelectric instrument**. However, overall device requires a very **high voltage stable power supply**.

Most of the biochemical analyses are done by the above mentioned instruments.

The dispersion of a spectrum is defined as linear spread of radiation per unit distance, which is expressed in nanometres per millimetre spread.

More improved instruments are provided with **internal built-in prismatic systems** which alters or accommodates the light wavelengths and linear dispersions. Some **linear dispersion and wavelength ranges are shown below (Table 14.8)**.

FLUORIMETRE AND FLUORIMETRIC METHODS

Fluorimetric techniques has the advantage over colorimetric or Spectrophotometric methods, that it provides a greater degree of specificity than **molecular absorption spectrophotometric methods** — due to the following facts:

1. Some **compounds absorbed in the ultra-violet rays do not fluoresce**, hence they interfere in **absorptiometry (Spectrophotometry)**.
2. Such interference is **not seen in fluorimetry**.
3. Another advantage in fluorimetry is that very small **measurements and traces of substances** in a sample can be **measured by a Fluorimeter down to the level of 1 ng or 10^{-9} G quantity**.

Cortisol thus can be effectively detected and measured by a Fluorimeter.

Principles of Fluorimeter

The principles of a fluorimeter is the same as that of a spectrophotometer with the following differences:

Flourescent light rays are emitted in all directions, but by moving the detection system at right angles to the cell, the fluorescent fraction of the light only is detectable by a fluorimeter. This is the key point of its precision and advantage over spectrophotometer.

SPECTROFLUORIMETER

In a Fluorimeter when secondary monochromator is not constituted by mere filters, but is built up by **True Optical Monochromators**, the **instrument attains a very high precision** and is termed as **Spectrofluorimeter**.

Disadvantages of a Fluorimeter: A wide variety of substances and wide range of conditions suppress emission of fluorescent light. As such emission may not be suppressed. But, many excited molecules lose their molecular energy by **molecular collisions** resulting in the **rise of temperature**.

On the other hand, cold or frozen samples show intense emission than the ordinary samples.

So also, **low pH of a sample reduces intensity of fluorescence due to the binding of protons by the non-binding of electrons**.

Some compounds, like **Carboxylic compounds, AZO compounds** and **Halogen compounds suppress the fluorescence** to some extent **due to** their possession of **electrophilic groups**. Presence of these compounds in trace amounts even can also reduce the intensity of fluorescence emission significantly. Hence, the **highest grade of purity of the reagents**

Table 14.7: Showing atomic absorption and flame emission lines with suitable flame sources

Elementary metals	W/L suitable for atomic absorption	W/L suitable for flame emission	Flame source suitable for:	
			Atomic absorption	*Flame emission*
Calcium	423 nm	423 nm	*A + AC**	†N + AC
Copper	325 nm	325 nm	A + AC	N + AC
Iron	248 nm	372 nm	A + AC	N + AC
Lanthanum	550 nm	579 nm	†N + AC	N + AC
Lead	283 nm	406 nm	A + AC	N + AC
Lithium	671 nm	671 nm	A + AC	N + AC
Magnesium	285 nm	285 nm	A + AC	N + AC
Mercury	254 nm	254 nm	A + AC	N + AC
Phosphorus	214 nm	526 nm	N + AC	A + H††
Potassium	767 nm	767 nm	A + AC	A + AC
Sodium	589 nm	589 nm	A + AC	A + AC
Zinc	214 nm	214 nm	A + AC	N + AC

(*) A + Air; (**) AC = Acetylene; (†) N = Nitrous Oxide; (††) H = Hydrogen

used in Fluorimeter and its cleanliness are the prime **important factors to get the best** successful **result** of such a very highly sophisticated instrument.

Fluorimeter Lights: High intensity of Light (radiation), chiefly in the 'uv' region can be attained by using an ARC lamp. Though by the usage of mercury vapour lamp, high energy concentration into a few sharply defined lines is achieved, yet it (**Mercury Vapour Lamp) offers intense** (relatively) **monochromatic light** which is **selected by filters** within limited wavelengths **for excitation of the electrons causing** scanning of the **excitation spectrum**.

For certain particular **analysis like Cortisol, Zinc emission light** at **472 nm** (4,720Å), and for **Oestrogen estimation, Thallium emitting light is used at 538 nm**.

Xenon Arc Lamp is of lower cost and **repetitive flash. It has** a high intensity source of illumination of **220 nm wavelength** and was originally **developed for Search Light used during the IInd World War.**

ATOMIC SPECTROSCOPY METHODS

In Atomic Spectroscopy, light emission occurs by the atoms of about a dozen of elementary metals by the use of **wavelength of emission for qualitative analyses** of metals, while the **intensity of light emission** is required for the **quantitative analyses** of those metals.

Atomic Spectroscopy is the basis of **flame emission photometry** which is **restricted to the visible wavelengths region** of the spectrum and used for the detection of only those elementary metals which are **easily excited at a temperature of a simple flame (Table 14.7)**. Such excitation of metals can also be attained by a **high voltage Arc (like Xenon Arc)** which is stuck between the two electrodes. This method is often used in **spectrographic analyses of metals**.

Higher the temperature is raised for excitation of metal atoms, **higher sensitivity** levels of the analysis is achieved. At present a **temperature of 10,000°C produced by argon plasma discharger** has been achieved. But such a method of high temperature emission with higher sensitivity is often not suitable for biochemical analyses.

However, **flame emission techniques are more sensitive** than atomic absorption technique for the elementary metals for analyses.

FLAME EMISSION PHOTOMETRY

In a flame photometer, **two events** occur,

(a) **Excitation of atoms,**

(b) Subsequent **measurement of the intensity of the emitted light (radiation).**

A **monochromating system is the absolute requirement for a flame photometer to differentiate** between:

(a) The **light emission** of the elementary metal and (b) **Radiation** (light) arising from the flame. Hence, the flame is the sum total of the source of light (radiation) as well as the atomized sample.

The flame temperature must be enough high to excite the atoms of the metal under investigation (e.g., **Na^+, K^+, Ca^{++}**). The more hot the flame is, greater proportion of atoms will be excited. So, the temperature should be optimally regulated (built-in with the instrument). **As excessive heat may raise the atoms to a very high energy levels,** when electrons become altogether removed ***resulting in total ionization***.

Principles of a Flame Photometer

I. ATOMIZATION IN AN ATOMIZER

1. The testing sample (serum) is converted into **aerosol in an atomizer.**

2. **Aerosol passes through an expansion chamber where the gas pressure falls.** At the expansion chamber the larger particles (droplets) settle out before passing to the burner flame.

3. The **aerosol solvent evaporates** in no time, while the **atoms are left behind as** a finely distributed **gas**.

4. **Atoms** bound in molecules in the sample are **decomposed at the flame temperature** very very **quickly producing the same effect as aerosol atoms.**

Because of the larger drop size of the atoms (which are settled out as mentioned above) 95% of the sample cannot reach the burner to produce emission of the test element. Also it is a fact that in **low temperature flames, one sodium atom amongst 60,000 atoms only is excited. Despite** such apparently low efficiency, the **technique is a very very sensitive one.**

II. MONOCHROMATING SYSTEMS

1. Any of the monochromating systems mentioned for **absorptiometers** may be used. If specific filter systems are used instead of the monochromatic optical systems, the price of the instrument may be brought down. But for wavelength interference very dense filters are the remedies. The use of **interference filters improves the specificity of analysis and precision of the instrument.**

2. High concentrations of some other elements if present in the samples, they cause suppression of light emission by the metal atoms under test.

This is called **Matrix effect**, or **Matrix phenomenon**, or **Matrix interference effect.**

The left out molecules (larger droplet molecules) can also interfere if they are somehow absorbed in the burner flame from the expansion chamber. This is called **molecular absorption interference effect.**

It is said that both Matrix interference and molecular absorption effects may be eliminated when standard solutions are prepared which also should contain equivalent amounts of interfering elements. Other **interfering agents are**:

(i) **Proteins,**

(ii) **Various anions** like phosphates and aluminates which complex the cations **giving falsely low readings.**

These may be **avoided by** using **organic chelating agents,** like **EDTA** or **citric acid which** themselves **bind cations** and are readily **decomposed in the flame.**

The use of **Lanthanum Chloride** and/or **Strontium Chloride** may be conveniently **used for the anionic interference by phosphates and albuminates, chiefly for estimation of Calcium and Magnesium.**

These cations bind the interfering anions which are precipitated at the time of aerosol formation in the atomizer.

However, the interferences and problems described above are more disturbing (or interfering) element in case of an **atomic absorption spectroscopy** than the **flame emission spectroscopy (photometry).**

For all the above reasons considered together, flame emission photometry can be commented as "not absolute" a method. Hence, it is absolutely essential to construct calibration curves for analysis.

Procedure of recording the reading in a flame photometer

Light emitted by the flame on spraying pure solvent is set at Zero (Null point) of the instrument. When highest concentration of the standards is sprayed, it gives the maximum reading which is recorded and plotted.

Now, **different concentrations of standard solutions are sprayed**, the **flame emission readings noted** and accordingly **plotted on the Graph Paper and a standard curve obtained**.

With many samples of close range of concentrations, the **LINEARITY OF THE 'LOGIT' CURVE BECOMES MORE ACCURATE**. The minimum concentration may be taken as 0.25 m.mol./Lt. while maximum is 25 m.mol./Lt.

DUAL-FLAME PHOTOMETER SUITABLE FOR LITHIUM ESTIMATION

For quantitative lithium estimation, a Dual-channel flame photometer is ideal, which is capable of recording both the test as well as reference readings simultaneously. Both the readings are unaffected by flame fluctuations.

ATOMIC FLUORESCENCE FLAME PHOTOMETRY

In this, the method is essentially an emission technique. Atoms are excited by absorption of radiation (light) which cannot be seen by detector.

Light emitted from excited atoms is viewed at a right angle to the exciting beam, as in case of a fluorimeter.

Principles of an Atomic Fluorescence Flame Photometer

In this, some of the excited atoms emit the resonance wavelength by returning to the ground state and also, to metastable state, resulting in either **loss or gain of energy by collision with gas molecules in the flame**. This causes **emission of quanta of larger or smaller sizes than the resonance quantum**.

Advantages

1. The fluorescence intensity is derived from a high energy source, a microwave discharge lamp or a continuum. **Sensitivity is higher when the energy source is higher**.

2. Sensitivity is also increased by **directly amplifying** more, **the detector signal**. These are also found in Fluorimeters.

3. Burners are simple and optical **alignment of the beam with the flame length is easier**.

4. **More choices of fluorescent wavelengths** can avoid some interference problems.

Disadvantages

1. Sensitivity varies with little change in radiation intensity.

2. **Scattering of light** by particles in the flame increases the background noise.

ATOMIC ABSORPTION SPECTROPHOTOMETRY

When atoms are dispersed in a flame, a small proportion of them are thermally excited leaving the others in the ground state as mentioned in atomic fluorescent flame photometer. Those which remain in the ground state and when a beam of white light is passed through a flame, they will then absorb the appropriate wavelength of radiation (light) for each element. A series of absorption bands may be demonstrated in such transmitted radiation. The absorption bands correspond to the excitation of valence electrons. The energy levels result in **very narrow absorption bands** to the extent of **0.001 nm**. For ordinary **metals and semi-metals**, it is used at a low range of radiation at **levels of 200 to 900 nm.**, but **for the non-conducting** insulating elements very high energy level is necessary to the extent of **ultra-violet (UV) and X-rays regions**.

The proportion of the incident light absorbed by the **atoms in the flame or vapour is measured** and is **related to the number of atoms in the flame** as in the case of **molecular absorption spectrophotometry**.

Design of Atomic Absorption Spectrophotometer

Incident light should have correct wavelength and an appropriate band-width and intensity. Usually a lamp is used in which the cathode is coated with atoms of element under investigation, and which emits light of the same wavelength as that, which will be absorbed by **nonexcited (ground state) atoms** of the same element in the flame.

The Cathode Lamp

A hollow cathode lamp comprises two electrodes sealed in a glass jacket filled with inert gas, like **argon and neon**. The end window of the lamp is made of quartz or silica in order to transmit the emitted light. The **cathode of the lamp is cup-shaped made of the desired element** or coated with that element whose spectrum is to be found out. The high voltage of the light should have a potential of **300 to 400 volts**

required to excite the atoms to get the proper light (radiation).

Electrodeless Discharge Lamps (EDL)

For detection of certain elements electrodeless discharge lamps are used where **excitation** of atoms is **achieved by radio frequencies inducing resonance effects**. The energy thus liberated causes vaporization and excitation of the element.

Double Beam Atomic Absorption Spectrophotometers are also available but not in much use for **no blank sample can be put for flame techniques.**

Pye Unicam is a double beam instrument which is **capable of operating** in many ways like **electro-thermal atomization, microsampling, emission spectrophotometry and automatic curvature correction.**

Atomizer: The method of atomized spray production is important and the design of an atomizer is similar to that in flame emission photometer. This involves spraying the sample in air or an oxidant gas (see before; **Table 14.7**).

Optical monochromating system: A high quality of Monochromating Systems are necessary to select out the required emission line of element from the gas emission lines present in the lamp. Atomic emission lines have very narrow spectroscopic bands. So, for this reason it is not sufficient only to select out the specific wavelength alone by the monochromator scale. The 'peaking up' procedure also has to be included in the machine. This offers monochromating systems in such a fashion that there is maximum response obtained from the detector.

There occurs lots of interferences by using normal flame techniques especially working with small quantity and/or solid samples. To avoid these problems, an improved technique termed **electrothermal atomization** has been developed. **Electrothermal is a flameless atomizer** which contains an electrical **heating device instead of Light or Radiation energy. This produces atomic vapour in the atomizer.**

The cuvette used in this instrument **is a graphite tube** which has a small injecting part drilled on the top surface. The graphite tube is held between the electrodes, which supply **electrical energy for heating,** as well as **energy for cooling down the tube quickly to normal temperature after atomization.**

Test procedure

1. The sample is introduced into the cuvette by a micropipette very very carefully.

2. **Ashing Temperature: Heat the sample to ash** (ashing) **to remove the solvents,** and **destroy** the **stroma** and all **matrices of the sample solution.**

The generated **carbon particles** arising out of organic materials **have to be driven** out **without the loss of solvents** or **more volatile metals, like lead** and **mercury**. Otherwise the carbon particles should interfere in absorbance. Hence an ideal instrument should have these devices.

3. **1000°C above ashing temperature**: After completion of ashing, the temperature of the cuvette is quickly raised to about 1000°C higher than that of the ashing temperature **to attain the atomizing temperature.**

Once that high temperature is attained, vapourization of the sample occurs, which results in transient increase in absorbance (2–5 Secs.). A good instrument has the ability to detect and record the maximum absorbance value.

Cleaning of the cuvette: Further increase of temperature — the cuvette is automatically cleaned by raising the temperature further to several hundred degrees higher. In case of samples containing more proteins and organic materials, repeated heating and mechanical clearing is necessary.

Further **development of both Flame and Flameless (Electrothermal) Atomic Absorption Spectrophotometer has been achieved,** which is a **hybrid microsampling system** known as **Delve's Cup**. In this the **atomic vapour is trapped** in the tube for a little longer time **upto 10 seconds,** when the **absorbance measurements are made.**

Further modification to overcome matrix interference effect in **Atomic Absorption Spectrophotometry** are alike that in **Flame Emission Photometer** has been achieved by the use of **Ionized Lanthanum** and **Caesium mixture** in the diluting fluid in which the samples are prepared.

THE MAGNETIC RESONANCE SPECTROSCOPY (Imaging) (MRI)

Atomic principle: Two electrons when present in the same atomic orbital, they shall have opposite rotations. So, they shall effectively **neutralize all magnetic effects** that each of the electrons possess.

Similarly, a pair of protons in the Atomic Nucleus **do not show any overall magnetic effect**. But an unpaired proton or electron imparts a magnetic moment to a species just like a magnet, and interacts like an applied magnetic field. Such interactions are the basis of magnetic resonance spectroscopy.

The unpaired proton means the nucleus contains an odd number of protons. When an External Magnetic Field is applied, that unpaired proton either lies in the same direction as the Magnetic field (indicating a **low energy state**), or, lies against or directly opposite the magnetic field (indicating a **high energy state**).

The difference in energy levels depends on :

(a) **Character of the Nucleus**, and

(b) **Magnitude of the applied External Magnetic Field**.

In such a situation, most of the Nuclei lie in a low energy state, but the real equilibrium proportions depend on the difference of energy levels between two energy level states.

Transitions can be imposed between these two states of energy levels by absorption of radiation from the short wave radio region of the spectrum. This is the basis of **Nuclear Magnetic Resonance (NMR) spectroscopy**. For the NMR studies the solvent used should be absolutely free from protons. So in place of ordinary water (H_2O), **deuterated water (D_2O)** is used.

In Nuclear Magnetic Resonance (**NMR**) Spectroscopy, the sample is suspended **between the poles of an electromagnet** and quickly rotated to get an average absorption effect. When a specific radio frequency is applied, the magnetic field is gradually increased. The radio signal is detected and recorded.

Absorption of radiation occurs on the basis of strength of the magnetic field, which is the characteristic of a nucleus.

ELECTRON SPIN RESONANCE (ESR) SPECTROSCOPY

ESR spectroscopy is in some way comparable to the **NMR spectroscopy**. ESR Spectroscopy depends on an **unpaired electron** (instead of unpaired proton in NMR spectroscopy), which **provides the magnetic moment**.

Electrons are much smaller than protons, the **former causes greater magnetic moment**. For inducing transitions also, **high energy microwaves are required for ESR spectroscopy**, rather than **Low Energy short waves or radio waves required for NMR spectroscopy**.

ESR spectroscopy though more specific, yet more difficult to interprete.

Both NMR spectroscopy and ESR spectroscopy are **employed in Radio Isotopic Studies of metals and non metals**.

THE AUTOMATED METHODS OF ANALYSIS

More developments of analyses and increased demand for investigations have led to the invention and introduction of new machines and equipments.

Automated system performs a required work at a predetermined point in its process (computerised). Further the system has a self-acting and self-regulating performance. Intervention of the analyst is not required. The system today is incorporated with a **microprocessor** or **computer capable of auto-controlling, auto-performing and auto-monitoring the analyses**. Auto-analyzers require very small volumes of samples and reagents. They show high levels of sensitivity, specificity and suffers only minimal Interference effects. **Centrifugation** or **Separation processes** of protein (from the samples for any estimation other than proteins) are all **"built-in" within the instrument**.

The **mechanized analyzers** were used as early as in 1950. It was very rudimentary and did not fulfil much requirements. Later in 1957, a step forward towards the advancement of "**continuous flow**" automated analysis was developed. This was a single channel instrument capable of measuring only one constituent, say, **Sugar**, or **Urea**, or **Cholesterol at one time**.

Still later **multichannel instruments** were developed which dealt **with various measurements** of a single sample simultaneously at one time, e.g., one sample of blood where **Sugar, Urea, Cholesterol, SGOT, etc. are done in one shot**.

At present multichannel machines have been developed of both '**discrete**' as well as "**continuous flow" automated analyzer types containing microprocessors and computers**. These are the bases of a

multichannel computerised automated instruments. The operator sets the optimum conditions for analysis for each different assay, and give instructions regarding the acceptable limits of the results for standard concentration samples. Having this information, the computer is capable of continual self evaluation of the performance of the analyzer, and accordingly the quality of results are produced. All necessary calculations are done, before the concentration of each **sample is printed out**. However, sometimes the **printer of the computer is instructed to produce the results and data in the form of different varieties of graph and histograms.**

The results of **single channel instruments** are presented as list numbers with their corresponding concentrations.

Whereas, multichannel analyzers require all the data for each sample collected together, before they are printed out. For this, each sample has to carry its own identification, which the computer can recognize.

An extension of Automated Analyzers in some means of data processing, which can handle all the results, generated by the computer has been devised. This is just like the central computer which accepts information from Different Automated Analyzers for an useful presentation.

Procedure for working in a computer: The **identification of a sample**, and the **tests performed** from the sample, are all **typed together by the use of key board**. The **informations** are all collected, **computed**, and results are assessed statistically. Further, the informations are stored for future references which can produce in no time through a **Visual Display Unit (the computer screen)**.

Deciding factors to have an auto-analyzer or a computer:

1. The facility, the work-load, and the money involved will be worthwhile or not, are the prime factors. The efficiency and High Grade Result production of the machine has to be considered.

2. Initial cost of buying the instrument is the second consideration.

3. Running cost (in terms of the reagents and personnels) and servicing cost and servicing facilities have to be deeply considered.

4. Reliability and life-expectancy are also important considerations.

5. In many countries, there is neither much fuel available to run generators, nor the electric power is adequately available, where **such a machine** cannot be run smoothly, and there is every chance of such a sophisticated machine to **go out of order**, whereby the problems and points for buying such a costly machine should always be thought repeatedly prior to its purchase.

Basically, there are two varieties of analyzers:

Discrete analyzer: (1) Discrete analyzers, of which the efficient variety is the **centrifugal fast analyzers.**

Continuous flow analyzer: (2) Continuous flow analyzers which may be — (a) **Single channel** instruments (b) **Dual channel** instruments.

THE DISCRETE ANALYZERS

These are analyzers handling each specific sample at a time separately in individual containers.

All discrete analyzers have a basic design which includes a built-in

(a) **Pipette system**

(b) **Spectrophotometric detector**, and

(c) **Microprocessor**

CENTRIFUGAL FAST ANALYZER

This is a step forward in the development of the old type of Discrete Analyzers in late 1960s which has led to the invention of centrifugal fast analyzer. The prototype of the instrument was named **GeMSAEC (General Medical Sciences Atomic Energy Commission).**

Transfer and mixing of solutions (Sample + Reagent): In this, batches of samples are treated in parallel. Centrifugal force is applied to transfer and mix the solutions, while the **reactions are continuously monitored photometrically**.

Photometric monitoring: They are also capable of analyzing variety of different types of analysis, when the reagents should be changed in the dispensers. With changing of reagents, the spinning programme (rate and time) has also to be adjusted.

Advantages of discrete centrifugal fast analyzer

1. Reagents required are of small volumes.
2. So, running cost is minimized.

3. Advantage of analyzing with micro volume samples.

Working with a centrifugal fast analyzer: Analysis is done in a circular disc named transfer disc or a motor built of inert material like teflon or acrylic possessing least surface liquid adhesion property. The transfer disc has radially arranged sets of grooves or cavities, and each set comprises 2 or 3 cavities which are interconnected; one for the **sample** and other one or two for the **reagents**.

Before spinning or centrifugation: Before centrifugation sample and reagents remain in separate compartments.

One type of analysis for different samples: A number of samples can be done at a time, while the reagent being the same (only one type of analysis say for **sugar only**, or **urea only** can be done at a time for different samples).

'Automatic pippetting': Small measured volumes of different samples, but the same or only one type of reagent is delivered in amount of 5 to 200 ml by automated pipetting into appropriate wells.

The reagent blank: One set is used for reagent blank. After switching on the machine, **during acceleration, mixing** of the sample and the reagent occurs, and the chemical reaction starts in no time.

Minitoring of absorbance applicator: After a while, the Absorbance applicator is monitored, no matter if the transfer disc is still engaged in spinning (centrifuging).

At this stage, there are two ways to take reading:

One system of machine: In some systems of machines, there are optical cuvettes, one for each sample, i.e., each set of wells. The cuvettes are incorporated at the periphery of the transfer disc for the purpose of **absorbance reading, which are taken** as they pass a **vertical light beam**.

Other systems of machines: In other systems of machines, the finally processed fluid is expelled into individual cuvettes with built-in arrangement inside the centrifuge.

The whole process takes about 2 minutes. Almost simultaneously, the transfer disc is cleaned and dried; ready for the next lot of samples.

Built-in computer: The "**Assay Temperature Controls**" and the "**Spinning Programme Controls**" **are controlled by a built-in computer. The spinning** (centrifuging) programme **includes 2 things:**

(a) **The speed of centrifugation**

(b) **The duration of spinning**

Programme is pre-set in the computer: The spinning programme and the reaction stages are pre-set in the machine with the aid of the computer.

Calculation in the computer: The computer also calculates the concentrations of test samples, comparing the respective absorbance readings with that of the respective standards.

Utility of centrifugal fast analyzers

1. For **all end point analysis** of biochemical samples.
2. **Enzymatic analysis** is done.
3. **Enzyme immuno-assays** (EIA) are very suitable and ideally performed.
4. Very suitable for **kinetic assays** for continuous monitoring capability of the instrument.

CONTINUOUS FLOW ANALYZERS

The earlier description for continuous flow analysis was described by **Prof. Skeggs** as early as **1957**. Such an autoanalyzer is marketed by **Technicon Instruments Company Ltd., Basingstoke, U.K.** Further developments led to the invention of **sequential multiple analyzers with built-in computers**. These sequential analyzers analyze many constituents of **many samples at a time**. Such capacities **depend on the number of channels present in the machine**. The **channels** may **vary from 12 to 20**, in the more developed analyzers.

Working principle of Continuous Flow Analyzers: The samples and reagents are pumped through a tubing system (instead of their being retained in separate containers) to different units of the analyzer.

Unlike the Discrete Analyzer or the normal methods, though absolute volumes are not pipetted, yet the constituents of Reagents are mixed in precisely controlled proportions. Such **unique controlled proportions are dependent on the various internal diameters of the delivery tubes, with a constant speed pump**. This is a vital factor, involving different rates of flow for different reagents, and this governs the necessary ratio of the reagents. The different rates of flow are calculated **in millilitres per minute** (ml/min) or (dl/min) within the tubes.

At first air bubbles are introduced into the flowing reagents. This results in a reaction stream. The reaction stream is interspersed by those air bubbles at regular intervals.

The samples are then aspirated in sequence into the analyzer through the tubing system with a small volume of demineralized water, which separates one sample from the other. In order to maintain a regular bubble pattern under normal operating conditions, an **inert wetting agent** is usually applied, like **Brij 35** in the liquid streams **to alter the highly charged surface of the non-wettable polyvinyl connecting tubing**.

The liquid-air has also a special importance in that it serves the purpose of a visual check on the flow rate of the samples and reagents and also the functioning of the analyzer. Any problem in the flow of liquid can be readily and promptly recognized by watching the Liquid-Air pattern.

Air bubbles are vital and very fundamental for the continuous flow type analyzers. Functions of air bubbles are laid down as follows:

Functions of air bubbles

1. Air bubbles fill the tubing system completely, preserving the integrity of each individual aliquot (proportionate ratio) of liquid (reagents) by providing barriers between aliquots of liquid concerned in the reaction.

2. Air bubbles reduce contamination amongst sequential samples by their air pressure against the inner wall of the tubing, which wipes away any droplet contamination of the previous sample and saving the next sample from any such mixing contamination. That means there is a shorter water wash occurring simultaneously, which saves a lot of time.

3. Even with low liquid flow, **air bubbles actually provide turbulent flow**, which **results in thorough mixing of the individual liquid**.

Attainment of perfectly homogeneous mixture

When **two (liquid-air-segmented) streams are brought together at a junction**, one liquid segment is derived. To attain this, the liquid stream is passed through a glass made horizontal mixing coil, whose internal circumference is 3 times greater than the horizontal length of the liquid column. Each fluid segment is repeatedly inverted and with this, the viscous fluid layers pass through the lighter fluid layers, ensuring a thorough mixing.

Advantages of Continuous Flow Analyzers

A continuous flow analyzer can perform all the basic steps involved in a **quantitative colorimetric procedure** which consists of:

Sample and reagents pipetting.

Mixing

Heating at specific temperatures, like 37°C and 100°C.

Recording of the result.

Presentation of the result.

In addition, the **following facilities** are also offered by the Continuous Flow Analyzers:

Sample digestion

Solvent extraction

Separation and removal of interfering substances

Phase separation

Dialyzing performance

Refractive index determination

Radiochemical studies

Electrochemical works

Fluorimetric studies

Nephelometric (turbidometric) determinations

Flame photometric purposes

Single or monochannel system

The original technicon is AAI which is single-channel, comprising a few inter-connected units. These interconnected units are called modules. The liquid streams flow through the modules. Each module (interconnecting unit) has a different analytical function, e.g.,

(a) Sampling of test

(b) Sampling of standards

(c) Addition of reagents

(d) Incubation and/or heating

(e) Detection

(f) Recording, and so on.

The more developed later analyzers, **AAII**, instead of having **separate analyzing modules (units)** have **analytical cartridge**. The analytical cartridge associates **a number of** the above **functions in one unit as a whole**.

Dual or double channel analyzers

They are basically the same as single-channel analyzers, but they analyze each sample for 2 constituents simultaneously.

The sample stream is divided into two equal fractions, each one flowing independently through its (each fraction's) own tubing system in the analytical cartridge.

The proper corresponding reagents for each constituent to be analyzed are added.

Each channel engaged in estimating each constituent of the sample possesses a separate and specific **detector**.

For investigation of 2 constituents, the results are displayed on a **dualpen recorder**, using different colored ink to avoid any confusion.

Multi Channel Analyzers

Just like dual-channel analyzers, at present **multi-channel analyzers have been in use**, where, instead of performing tests for 2 constituents, about **50 constituents can be done simultaneously** in such a huge **multi-channel fully automated computerized continuous flow analyzer**.

The result displayed should be on a multiple-pen recorder, using multiple colors.

Parts of a Continuous Flow Analyzer:

1. **Proportioning pump**: It is a speed pump comprising **a constant speed roller bar peristaltic pump**.

Sufficient air is forced through the pump to produce air bubbles as described above.

Twenty standard pump tubes or manifold tubes which deliver 0.015 to 3.9 ml/minute. They are **color-coded** for identification.

The **reagent pump** tubes are connected by flexible tygon tubing to appropriate reagent bottles. The sample tube is connected to the probe on the sample module. The air pump tubes are open to the atmosphere.

2. **Manifold**: Manifold refers to the **assembly of pump tubes** together with glass and plastic fittings used to **join the liquid and air streams**, the glass mixing coils, and the interconnecting tubing.

Distinctive manifolds are used for each analytical method and designed for the fastest sampling rate, consistent with required sensitivity, accuracy and precision.

3. **Sampler**: Sampler unit holds a tray or a plate which can be loaded upto 40 cups each containing an individual sample. Each sample is aspirated in turn when a narrow bore metal probe connected to the **sample pump** tube on the manifold, **dips into it for some specific period**.

The volume of sample delivered into the analyzer is dependent on the **internal diameter of the sample pump tube**, and the **dwell (dipping) time** of the probe. For this, the probe should have a quick dipping action.

In between samples the probe aspirates demineralised water from a small container. The length of time for aspiration of the sample and water (wash) is set by selecting an appropriate can which fits into the center of some sampler units. It may also be set by setting proper dials. However, this synchronizes the movement of the probe and the tray, so that each sample is in turn presented to the probe.

4. **Separation modules**: The separation steps like **filtration, digestion, extraction, distillation, phase separation or dialysis can all be performed within the analyzer. For each** of the above processes, **a separate module is built in the analyzer**.

The dialyzer module comprises a thermostatically controlled water bath which houses a matched pair of spirally grooved plastic or **lucite plates**, clamped together with a **semi-permeable cellophane membrane** stretched between the plates. This forms a narrow tube about 2 metres long divided lengthwise by the membrane. **Air segmented sample** which **is the donor**, and **saline or reagent is the recipient**. So, both donor and recipient streams, flow side by side along the semi-circular channels. Small analyte molecules diffuse across the membrane into the recipient stream.

The rate of dialysis is dependent on the concentration of dialyzable molecules, provided other factors affecting dialysis are constant.

The dialyzer is incorporated in the analytical cartridges offering high sensitivity by the use of thinner cellulose membranes and lesser dilution of samples.

5. **Heating bath**: Heating is accomplished by inclusion of single or double mixing coils in the mani-fold, or spiral glass coil enclosed in a **thermostatically controlled oil bath** permitting a selected temperature between 37 degree and 95 degree. For further higher temperatures, **thermostable silicon oil** is to be used.

An analytical cartridge is provided with a small metal electric heating block having a sightly wound glass coil inside it offering a rapid rise (of temperature) and effective control of temperatures.

6. **The detection systems**: The detection system is capable of continuously monitoring the reagent stream linked to multi (colored) pen recorder. The height of the peaks of the samples in trace is converted to high concentration by comparing with the peak heights of standards of respective tests, either by plotting a calibration curve, or by the use of a computer.

At the outset, a set of standards should be analyzed and the detector is adjusted accordingly to produce the required response.

7. **Other miscellanies**: The component parts are usually used for this purpose:

(i) A combined **de-bubbler** and

(ii) A flow-through cell

To remove air bubbles efficiently, and **to draw the sample stream through the flow cell, a recycle pump tube is used** for a suitable flow rate. The flow rate should be little less than the total liquid flow (not the air) which reaches the flow cell. Slight **resulting back pressure makes the de-bubbling system more efficient**.

Diagrams/Notes

Diagrams/Notes

PART SEVEN

Preliminary Experimental Pathology

CHAPTER 15

EXPERIMENTAL SERIES

EXPERIMENT I

Animal Inoculation

1. Subcutaneous, intramuscular and intracutaneous injections into guinea-pig.
2. Cardiac puncture in a guinea-pig (for **obtaining complement**).
3. Intravenous injections in:
   (a) Ear vein of rabbit.
   (b) Tail vein of mice and rats.
   (c) Paw or penile vein of guinea-pigs.
4. Intraperitoneal inoculation into mice.

GUINEA-PIG

Subcutaneous injection into Guinea-pig

Purpose: Pathogenicity test of *C. diphtheriae* or *Myco. tuberculosis*.

Requirements: Male **guinea-pig,** weighing 250-300 g, sterile 5 ml **syringe, needle** of suitable size, tincture of **iodine, alcohol, cotton wool**, etc.

Material for inoculation, Culture of ***C. diphtheriae*** *or suptum for testing of* ***Myco. tuberculosis***.

Method

1. The infection is made under the skin of the flank. **Paint the area with tincture of iodine** to disinfect the skin and iodine is removed in its turn by alcohol.
2. The animal is held conveniently by assistants who grasps it by the shoulder in one hand with thumb curved round the neck so that it **rests on the lower jaw**, and the **flank is presented for injection**. The hind legs are secured with the other hand.
3. For injection the **skin of the flank of mid or lower abdomen is pinched with** the help of the **thumb and index finger** of the **left hand**.
4. The needle is introduced into the base of the fold and pushed down in the subcutaneous tissue till it reaches the groin, where the material is injected.

An amount of 2.5 ml can be injected in the subcutaneous tissue. This method obviates superficial ulceration when tuberculous material is injected.

Intracutaneous inoculation

Purpose: For the virulence test, neutralising action of diphtheria **toxin-antitoxin mixture** (L-dose), etc., (see authors' **Bacteriology book**).

Depilate a white guinea-pig (300–400 g) on a previous day in the flank, side or back of the animal (see **authors' Bacteriology**) and inoculate next day on a healthy skin. Excoriation if any is avoided.

Requirements: Depilatory paste, which contains: **Barium sulphide** (commercial)—7 parts, **flour**—7 parts, **talcum powder**—7 parts, **castile soap** powder—1 part and water q.s. to make a smooth paste to apply on the flank; tincture of iodine, absolute alcohol, **tuberculin syringe with 25–26 S.W.G.** (stainless steel wire gauze) needle as used for **Schick or Dick test**, cotton wool, etc.

The areas of inoculation are now marked with ink or dye of 1 inch in diameter after inoculations are made. Take the rectal temperature of the animal*.

* **The normal temperature of the animal is 99.6° (35°C) to 102°F (36°C).**
To ascertain the animal's temperature, a clinical thermometer with a small round bulb, smeared with vaseline, is gently inserted into the rectum of animal.

The **skin is now pinched with thumb and forefinger**, the **needle is inserted** in the centre of the marked area at the base of the fold with the level of the needle towards the surface of the skin. The **needle** should pass **only into the dermis** as near the surface as possible and **not subcutaneously. Wheal** forms in a successful case.

0.2 ml is the amount usually used and when several tests are done, the injections should be at least one inch apart and not too near the middle line of the abdomen or back.

Not more than totally 10 injections are to be made in each animal.

Results are read 24-48 hours later for the reaction.

Intracardiac Puncture

Purpose: For collection of complement (Serum) for complement fixation test.

Requirements: At least six guinea-pigs (Male), 5 ml sterile syringe, fitted with 16 gauge needle, sterile test tubes, tincture iodine, alcohol, etc.

Procedure: The animal is tied by 4 limbs to an animal board. The apex bit of the **heart is felt with the index finger of left hand.** The **needle is inserted** through the intercostal space **at that point first directly backwards and then slightly upwards**, to a depth of about **one inch (2.5 cm)**. The **blood** is now **drawn with gentle suction** and **3 ml** of blood is safely collected from a guinea-pig at a time. **Blood** from several guinea-pigs is **pooled for complement. Light ether anesthesia** may be used by a beginner.

RABBIT

(*Chiefly for preparation of antibodies*)

Intravenous Injection in Rabbits

Purpose: For introducing material directly into circulation, e.g., Friedman's test for pregnancy or for **immunizing rabbit with sheep cells for hemolysin** or for preparing other antibodies, etc.

Requirements: Rabbit, 2 kg in weight, sterile **all-glass** 5 ml syringe fitted with a medium sized No. 20 or 22 needle, sharp safety-razor, xylol, methylated spirit, cotton wool, etc.

Procedure: The **marginal ear vein** is selected for the purpose. The rabbit is held by an assistant in a box or towel and one ear is dry-shaved. The vein is engorged by several taps with finger followed by rubbing with a piece of cotton wool soaked in xylol which makes the vein more clear and prominent. The **ear is held horizontally with the left hand** and the **needle is introduced parallel with the vein towards the head** of the animal. The needle is felt free in the vein and the **material is slowly introduced**. The needle is withdrawn after completion of the injection. The part (vein) is **pressed with** a piece of cotton wool soaked in **methylated spirit** and **compressed between** the **thumb and the finger**.

MOUSE

Intraperitoneal Injection:

Purpose: To study **pathogenicity test of pneumococci**, effects of various chemical substances, like carbon tetrachloride, **tumour implantation**, studying of various **phases of inflammatory phenomena**, to study the **pathogenicity test of mycotic material** from clinical cases, etc.

Requirements: White mouse — 20 g in weight, 2 ml sterile syringe, medium-bore needle 20 or 22 SWG, tincture iodine, alcohol, cotton wool, etc.

Procedure: The **animal is held by the** assistant at the **nape of the neck on the loose skin** with the **left hand** and **the root of the tail by the right hand**, with the **ventral aspect forward and head downwards** so that viscera are away from the site of **puncture** in the **lower abdomen in the middle line**. The abdominal skin is pinched and valve-like puncture is made first puncturing the skin and introducing the **needle to subcutaneous tissues and then downward through the abdominal wall into the peritoneal cavity**. Not more than **2 ml** should be **injected.**

RAT

Intravenous Injection

For introducing (drugs) directly into the circulation.

Requirements: A small cylindrical cage to hold the rat securely with its tail protruding out, sterile syringe to hold the solution, a small medium sized hypodermic **needle No. 20–22**, cotton wool, xylol, alcohol, etc.

Procedure: The rat is held by the loose tissue at the nape of the neck and put in the cylindrical cage with the tail protruding. The **tail is gently pulled out** and the **vein at the root of the tail** along its course is dilated by rubbing with a piece of cotton wool soaked with xylol. The needle gives a free feel when inside the vein. The injection is introduced into the prominent and dilated tail vein.

EXPERIMENT II

Koch's Postulates

Robert Koch postulated that, to **call an organism** (isolated from a lesion) **to be pathogenic**, i.e., causing disease, the following criteria should be fulfilled.

1. The **organism** must be present **in the exudate**, diseased **organ** or **tissue**.
2. It must be **isolated in pure culture**.
3. The **organism thus isolated** must be capable of **causing disease in a susceptible** experimental **animal**.
4. The **organism** must be **recoverable from** disease caused in experimental **animal**.

A **fifth postulate** can be added as a corollary, i.e., it must be **able to provoke specific antibodies** like **agglutinin, precipitin** or **complement fixing antibodies**, etc., in the affected person in response to the infection.

Requirements: Pus from a case of abscess or purulent lesion, materials for making culture and the identification of the organism isolated, culture media, platinum loop, gas or spirit lamp.

1. **Make a smear** of the material and stain by **Garm's stain**, study **morphology** of the organism **Gram positive or negative, cocci** or **bacilli**.
2. Selected suitable media accordingly for culture. Take an **isolated colony for sugar reaction** and further detailed study. Finally **confirm by agglutination**, if necesary.
3. **Pathogenicity test** in a number of guinea-pigs is undertaken, **from** broth or slope **culture** in a sterile, saline suspension and **lesion produced locally or in viscera**.
4. The **organism** may be **further cultivated** from the animal, **isolated and identified**.

Different groups of students can deal with different organisms.

> **N.B. Tuberculous** material (AFB) can be **stained with Ziehl-Neelsen stain, cultured in Loewenstein-Jensen's medium and inoculated** into the thigh of a guinea-pig intramuscularly.

It is to be noted that **leprosy bacillus**, though an AFB, fulfils the first postulate only and not the others all the time.

EXPERIMENT III

Study of the Inflammatory Phenomena

Requirements: Rats, Copper disc, gas flame, forceps, etc.

Purpose: To **prove cardinal signs** and to study increased permeability and vascularity that occurs in the tissues during the inflammatory process.

Heat (physical): Shave the skin of the rat on the flank and inject 2 ml of 1 per cent sterile solution of **Trypan blue**. A copper disc is heated to 55°C and applied to the shaved skin for 20 seconds. The change in the skin color is noted by naked eye and histologically.

Bacterial inflammation *caused by Staphylococci.*

Inject 0.5 ml of 24 hours broth culture of Staph. aureus subcutaneously on the thigh of each of the experimental rats on three successive days. Local inflammatory changes will be observed and noted daily. When the abscess is produced, skin with the subcutaneous tissue is taken from the area and histological section may be studied including a control of normal skin from the other thigh.

EXPERIMENT IV

Study of Phagocytosis

Purpose of Study: To find out the **role of histiocytes in removing foreign bodies** from blood, that is injected subcutaneously.

Requirements: Rats—5; human blood with anticoagulants; syringe with needle; **stains of different types (H & E, Toluidin blue, Pearls' Prussian Blue)**, and hyalase (material used for tissue spreading factor), etc.

Procedure: Human blood mixed with anticoagulant will be injected subcutaneously on the thigh of rats in a dose of 3 ml. The gross changes of the hematoma will be observed. Subcutaneous tissue round the hematoma are studied for 2 weeks (3, 7, 10 and 14 days) in different rats.

EXPERIMENT V

Determination of Opsonic Index

Purpose: To **find out the phagocytic activity of leukocytes** and **resistance of the human patient** against the organism.

Requirements:

1. Leukocytes collected from the buffy leukocytic zone of a normal blood and washed with saline.
2. Normal serum.
3. Patients serum.
4. Suspension of organism in normal saline.

Test:

1. Take **equal parts of bacterial suspension, leukocytes** and **normal serum** on a slide. Mix it with a Pasteur pipette and after mixing draw a part of it in capillary portion and **seal it by melting in a flame**.
2. As in (1) take bacterial suspension, leukocytes and patient's serum mixed and drawn in a capillary pipette and seal it.

Incubate both the capillary pipettes for 15 minutes at 37°C.

Smears are then prepared and obtained on two separate slides (a and b), stained with Leishman's stain. **Count 500 leukocytes** under oil immersion lens. Take the average number of organisms per leukocytes calculated in each instance.

Opsonic index is calculated as $\frac{(a)}{(b)}$

Unity (1) is the normal figure — but the opsonic index of the serum may be that the **index is greater** or **less than unity** (1) according to the **opsonic power of the serum.**

EXPERIMENT VI

Production of Foreign Body Granuloma

Purpose: To study the changes in the tissues when **aseptic foreign bodies are introduced into the body**.

Requirements: Adult **albino rats** — 5, sterile lycopodium powder, **sterilized instruments** for an aseptic operation.

Procedure: Five rats are taken in the experiment. They are operated under **ether anesthesia. Lycopodium (10 g) powder** is introduced **into the peritoneal cavity,** and the **abdominal wall is stitched**. Animals are sacrificed at intervals of 2, 7, 14 and 22 days after the operation. Changes at the site of foreign body (introduced) will be studied microscopically after **H & E staining**.

EXPERIMENT VII

Experimental Anaphylaxis (in a Guinea pig)

Requirements: For pairs of **healthy guinea-pigs 250 g each** serially numbered, horse serum (fresh), tuberculin syringe with a 20-22 gauge needle, instruments for animal autopsy, etc.

Procedure: Animals are selected in 4 groups, 2 in each.

Sensitizing (initial) dose: All the animals are injected with 0.1 ml of horse serum by subcutaneous injections on the flank. The animals are kept for 3 weeks and the animals are injected as follows with 0.4 ml of horse serum except the last group (**Group IV**).

Group I (1 and 2)—**Subcutaneously**.

Group II (3 and 4)—**Intraperitoneally**.

Group III (5 and 6)—**Intravenously in the paw vein, or dorsal vein of the penis or by intracardiac route**.

Group IV (7)— Kept as control.

In all the animals, anaphylactic shock is studied and noted.

Results: Group I & II will escape or show aborted shock but **Group III will show typical anaphylactic shock** — for details consult authors' Bacteriology book; immediate symptoms of shock lasts for 2 minutes and the animal dies. For type of reaction, carry out the autopsy immediately. **Gross and microscopic studies** of organs are done.

Lungs: Voluminous—distended with air, marks of ribs on the lung surface are prominent in the case of guinea-pig.

In case the animal does not die it becomes desensitized and refractory.

EXPERIMENT VIII

Study of Chemically Induced Diabetes

Requirements: Rabbits — 8, alloxan — 5 per cent in normal saline, spirit, syringe, needles, cotton wool, vaseline, oxalated tubes, normal saline, metabolic cage, etc.

Purpose of study: To study biochemical and histopathological **changes in alloxan-induced diabetes mellitus in rabbits.**

Procedure:

1. Group I— Two rabbits to act as control.
2. Group II — Two rabbits to receive 50-75 mg of alloxan/kg body weight, intravenously once a week.
3. Group III— Four rabbits to receive 25 mg of alloxan/kg body weight intravenously daily for 6 days.

Group I (Control group):

1. Fasting blood sugar levels will be estimated. They will receive 1 ml of N. saline intravenously per kg body weight.
2. The animals will be kept in metabolic cages.
3. The quantity of water taken and the amount of urine excreted will be noted.
4. Urine will be tested for albumin, sugar, acetone and examined microscopically.

In Group II, blood sugar will be examined at 2 hours, 24 hours and 72 hours after injection of alloxan.

In Group III, blood sugar estimation will be done twice a week or earlier if indicated by urine examination.

Histological examination of various tissues are done after the death of the animal or at an autopsy. Examination shows progressive **MICRO-ANGIOPATHIC changes**.

EXPERIMENT IX

Preparation of Agglutinins

H (Flagellar) and **O (Somatic) High Titre Sera.**

Organism: *Salmonella typhi* H & O suspension used as antigen. **H** suspension is **formalized** and **O suspension** is alcohol treated.

Purpose: **Production of specific antibodies** against the particular antigen of *Salmonella typhi*.

Requirements:

1. Male healthy rabbits—8, each weighing 2 kg.
2. Suspension of H and O antigen of ***Salm. typhi*** containing ***100 million organisms*** per ml. Two rabbits are used (for H & O) for each group of students who perform the experiment.
3. Alcohol.
4. Cotton wool.
5. Xylol, etc.

Method:

Inject into the ear vein of the rabbit at intervals of 5 days in doses given below.

Table 15.1

Dose	Day/s	Volume
1	1	0.1 ml
2	6	0.2 ml
3	11	0.3 ml
4	16	0.4 ml
5	21	0.5 ml
6	26	0.6 ml

Seven days after the 6th (last) injection trial **bleeding is done from the marginal ear vein.**

Separate the serum. **Dilute serum 1 : 10** initially and perform **H and O agglutination tests by Dreyer's method**; find out the titre of agglutinin and dilute it **[Rabbit serum (agglutinin)]** to give a titre of 1 : 250, to **use it as high titre serum to agglutinate *Salm. typhi*.**

Compare the result of each group of students with that of the other and present the result to the whole class.

N.B. Make special note of weight of the rabbit and diet, to observe the highest titre.

In the same way, *Salm. paratyphi* A and B high titre antisera may be prepared.

Diagrams/Notes

PART EIGHT

Postmortem Methods

CHAPTER 16

AUTOPSY METHODS

PRELIMINARIES AND GENERAL RULES

Autopsy means postmortem examination.

No autopsy should be undertaken without the written permission of the person in charge of the body.

The prosector should put on a pair of thick rubber gloves and an apron. There should be arrangements for smears, cultures and fixatives.

1. In all cases, thorough examination of the whole body must be carried out to reach an honest opinion as to the cause of death.
2. Record the observations as dictated by the prosector as he proceeds on with the autopsy.
3. Anatomical diagnosis should bear the opinion of the prosector.
4. Gross materials of interest should be saved for museum specimens.
5. Slices of tissue from organs are preserved in **Zenker's fluid**.
6. Smears and cultures should be collected properly with asepsis.
7. Autopsy report should bear the results of these bacteriological and histological investigations.
8. The body should be reconstituted after the postmortem is finished.

Note: Name, age, sex, religion, etc., ward, date and time of admission, cause and time of death.

Date and hour of autopsy, clinical diagnosis and anatomical diagnosis of the prosector.

1. **External examination of the body**: **Height** and general **nutrition**. Presence of discoloration, jaundice or pigmentation, edema and subcutaneous emphysema should be noted. Presence of any **external** wound or other **signs of violence** (together with marks of burns) and presence of **deformity, hernia,** etc. are noted.

Condition of the **eyes, pupils, nose, mouth, ears, urinary meatus, anus, umbilicus, vagina** and **hymen** are examined.

2. **Internal examination of the body**: **Stand** on the **right side of the body, extend the chin, make a medial incision** just **above the prominence of the thyroid cartilage,** carry the incision **downwards to symphysis pubis.**

In the neck, the skin and the subcutaneous tissues should only be divided: Over the sternum the **incision should go down to the bone.** Reflect the **chest muscles towards the axillary line on each side.**

The **peritoneal cavity** should be cautiously **opened by nicking through the peritoneum at the lower third of the abdomen,** extending the incision **down to the pubis and above to xiphisternum.** Inspect the contents of the peritoneal cavity **and the** pelvis in situ. The fluid, if present, **may be cultured** and then measured.

3. **Removal of the thoracic organs**: Open the **thorax by cutting through the costal cartilages** and **also the sterno-clavicular** joint. The **sternum** and the **costal cartilages can** thus be **removed in one piece.** Examine the anterior mediastinum and pleura. Note the presence of **fluid, gas, adhesions** or amount of **retraction of the lungs. Pass the hand over the whole surface of each lung** and **bring it forward** breaking down any adhesion.

Open the **pericardium** and examine the same. **Measure the pericardial fluid**, if any, make an inspection of the heart for adhesions, etc. **Cut** through the **vessels from below upwards**, namely **inferior vena cava**, the **pulmonary veins, superior vena cava, pulmonary artery and aorta**. Take the **weight of the heart.**

Open the heart with a straight scissors **placing it on the table** with the **anterior surface up**. The **right auricle is opened by the superior vena cava**, and the **right ventricle by extending the incision along** the **right margin** of the heart. **From the apex**, this **cut is extended upwards to the pulmonary** artery, keeping **close to the inter-ventricular septum**. The **pulmonary artery** should be **examined for** any antemortem **thrombus** and postmortem clot.

Examine the **tricuspid valve** and estimate with finger tips, **whether its orifice is dilated or narrowed. Open** and examine the pulmonary valves. **Open the auricular appendix**. Remove all clots and **inspect the mitral orifice** from above. It should **admit two fingers. Cut** through the **mitral ring along the left border down to the apex** of the left ventricle.

Palpate the **aortic valve** with your fingers and then **cut upwards from** the **apex** of the left ventricle, keeping **close to the interventricular septum towards the aortic opening**. Pass one blade of the scissors through the opening and **extend it**, cutting **across the pulmonary artery** just **above the pulmonary vein. Cut open the aorta** above and below the thoracic part. **Examine the walls of** the aorta and the **great vessels. Introduce a probe into** the **coronary** arteries. Lay them open and inspect the interior by putting a longitudinal incision.

Examine the interior of the **left ventricle** after removing all clots. Incise the wall of the myocardium and note its color, consistency and thickness. **Examine** the **thyroid, the thymus** and **lymph nodes at the bifurcation of the trachea**. Examine the **tongue** and the **soft palate**.

Both the **lungs** are **removed at their roots**. Open the lungs by a **long deep incision from the apex** to the **base**. Examine for any pathological manifestations. Small **pieces** should be **thrown into water**: they will **float unless collapsed** or **consolidated**. Examine the lungs also for any pale area in the inflated lungs, which will be due to **minute infarcts**.

Slit open the larynx, trachea and the main **bronchi**.

4. **Removal of abdominal organs**: The abdominal viscera are now examined.

Put ligatures and cut at the junction of the **Jejunum** and **duodenum**, and also at the junction of the **sigmoid colon** and the **rectum**. Remove the **small intestine** and open it in a sink along the line of mesenteric attachment. The *ileo-cecal valve* and the *appendix* should be carefully examined. The wall of the gut should be cleansed with running water, palpated and inspected along the whole extent.

The *stomach* is **opened along the greater curvature** and spread out. Look for any **helminths, ulcer or neoplasm**.

Spleen: The spleen is examined for **adhesions, enlargement**, and **weighed**. It is incised along its **long axis towards the hilum**. The cut surface of the spleen is examined.

Liver: The liver is removed and examined; **weigh, inspect** and **palpate** it. **Turn the liver upside down**. Take a **culture from the gall-bladder. Slit** the gall-bladder **lengthwise**. Wash out and examine the mucus membrane. Examine for any **enlarged lymph nodes at the portal fissure. Cut** the liver now (placed with its convex surface upwards) with the incisions **parallel to the falciform ligament** (an inch apart). These **should not completely divide** the liver.

Examine the duodenum *in situ*. See the **pancreatic ducts** by passing a probe.

Pancreas: The pancreas should next be incised and its main duct opened.

Next examine the **pelvic viscera**. The position, mobility and the condition of the vessels and ureters are noted before their removal from the body.

Kidney: Remove the kidneys and **separate the suprarenal glands**; weigh. Examine kidney surface and **incise from the convex border to hilum in one sweep** of the knife. Along the cut surface of the kidney the capsule is stripped off with forceps. Note the surface, adhesion, decortication, color, and measure the **ratio of cortex to medulla** and measure the thickness of each.

Remove the abdominal aorta and examine for any dissecting aneurysm. The condition of the **urethra, penis** and **scrotum** are investigated *in situ*. The testes can be drawn up out of the scrotum by dissection, examined and removed. The presence of **hernial** sacs and congenital anomalies should be noted. **Catheter** should be passed **into the bladder** and any urine present is drawn out for analysis.

Pelvic Organs: The **bladder, prostate, seminal vesicles, urethra** and **rectum** should be examined in order. ***In the female,*** it is advisable to remove the **uterus, tubes and ovaries** and incise them carefully after removal. Also examine for signs of recent delivery.

5. **Removal of brain and spinal cord**: **Incise the scalp down to bone in a line joining the mastoid processes over the vertex.** Reflect the scalp into anterior and posterior flaps.

The **parotid glands** may be examined by continuing the **coronal incision downwards in front of the ears.**

Remove the **skull cap by sawing** and using chisel and hammer. Care must be taken not to damage the meninges. The **dura is incised** along the line of the saw cut, starting at the frontal region, **detaching the falx cerebri from the crista galli** and turning the dura back over the posterior scalp flap. If the dura is so adherent, as to prevent the skull cap being lifted off, it (dura) should be carefully incised and removed with bone. **The skull cap** should be **examined**, then the **dura, subdural** and then **arachnoid spaces.**

The **Brain** is removed by raising it gently from the **frontal lobes backwards**, dividing the nerves successively as they appear and **incising** the **tentorium cerebelli** along its attachments.

The **spinal cord** is removed after **cutting through** the **soft parts in the midline.** Expose the laminae and then saw through them. The ensheathed cord is then separated from all connections from below upwards and lifted from its bed.

It is often advisable to delay the examination until the material has been fixed in formol-saline for some days.

Examine the base of the skull and the ends of the nerves. Lay **open** the **cranial sinuses** by incisions through the dura; strip off the dura from bone. The pituitary should be **removed** by cutting away the posterior clinoid processes with the chisel. Carefully dissect the **pituitary** gland out of the fossa.

Cut-section of the brain

After examining the vessels, nerves, etc., at the base of the skull, **place the brain with base downwards** and gently separate the cerebral hemispheres. **Divide the corpus callosum transversely** throughout its length, first on one side and then on the other. The point of the knife should slant slightly upwards so that the **lateral ventricle is opened** and both **anterior and posterior horns** can be **inspected** including the **choroid plexus.**

Table 16.1: Average size and weight of Adult organs

	Male	Female	Remarks
1. Heart	Wt. 250–300 g	230–280 g	
2. Lungs	Wt. Rt. 625 g Lt. 567 g		
3. Liver	Wt. 1,500–1,800 g In proportion to body wt. 1 : 37	1,300–1,600 g 1 : 43	
4. Brain	Wt. 1,400–1,600 g	1,200–1,400 g	
5. Kidney	Length: 11 cm Breadth: 6 cm Wt. 150–170 g Thickness 3 cm	 115–155 g	
6. Spleen	Length: 12 cm Breadth: 7 cm Thickness: 3–4 cm Wt. 150–200 g	 150 g	Tends to diminish in size and weight with advanced age

Basal ganglia can be examined by making a series of parallel incisions transversely across the floor of both lateral ventricles. The incision should be a quarter of an inch apart and should extend almost, but not quite to the basal surface of the brain. **Split the cerebellum in the middle**. Examine the third and the fourth ventricles. **Examine the cerebellum,** the **pons** and the **medulla** by a series of transverse cuts at intervals of ¼ inch. The **spinal cord is examined.**

In case of anemia, a **femur** should be removed and the **bone marrow cavity exposed** by sawing the bone longitudinally. Incision should extend to the shaft of the femur. **Remove a portion of the sternum as well.**

Bacteriological

Culture and smear from the involved area should be made aseptically. **Blood** can be obtained from the right **atrium** using a glass pipette with rubber teat. As soon as the pericardium has been opened and the surface of the heart examined, a hot spatula is placed for a moment on the right auricle. The pipette is plunged through the wall and the fluid (blood) withdrawn. It is then squeezed out of the pipette into a sterilized test tube containing **trypsin broth**. Obtain a smear also from the same material.

The **surface** of the solid organ like **liver** or **spleen is touched with a hot spatula and an incision is made** into that area with a sterile scalpel and a quantity of the juice removed with a platinum loop to make **direct films and plate, smear and culture respectively** in suitable media.

Special tests used in postmortem examination:

1. **Lugol's iodine**: It will stain the **amyloid substance "mahogony brown"**.

   If iodine **treatment** is followed **by 1% H_2SO_4**, the brown color will turn blue. This method is used to determine the presence of amyloid in an organ.

2. Hemosiderin gives a **Prussian blue (Pearl's) reaction** for iron with Pot. ferrocyanide and HCI. These methods may be employed for gross appearance in cut sections to find out the evidence of **hemosiderosis.**

Diagrams/Notes

PROTOCOL FOR POSTMORTEM-RECORD

P.M. No. .... Serial No. ....

Date .... and Time .... (of holding P.M.)

Hours Postmortem ....

Name .... Age .... Religion .... Sex ....

Restriction (Partial / Complete)...

Clinical Diagnosis ....

Anatomical Diagnosis ....

Signature of Prosector ....

External Examination:

PRIMARY INCISION

PERITONEAL CAVITY

PLEURAL CAVITIES

MEDIASTINUM

PERICARDIAL CAVITY

HEART: Weight

Valves:	T.V.	M.V.	A.V.	P.V.
Measurements:	L.V.	Rt.V.	L.A.	Rt.A.
	(Ventricle)		(Left atrium)	

MUSCLES (Myocardium):

VESSELS:

Aorta:

Portal veins and tributaries

LUNGS: *Weight*: R L

Spleen:

Wt. Size Cut surface

ORGANS OF NECK:

Tongue: Appearance (description) Larynx: Appearance

Tonsils: Appearance Trachea: Appearance

Salivary glands: Appearance Thyroid: Appearance; presence of any nodules, hemorrhage, necrosis, etc.

LYMPH NODES: Enlargement; Evidence of any metastasis

ALIMENTARY TRACT: Pharynx

Esophagus:

Stomach:

Small intestine:

Appendix:

Large intestine:

Rectum:

PANCREAS:

LIVER:

Weight g Size

Cut Surface:

GALL BLADDER: BILE DUCT

KIDNEYS:

Weight { Rt.: / Lt.:

ADRENALS:

Weight: Rt. Lt.

PELVIC ORGANS: Urinary Bladder

MALE:	FEMALE:
Prostate:	Ovaries:
Testes:	Uterus, cervix and vagina:
Spermatic cords	Fallopian tubes:

BONES: Ribs:

Vertebrae:

Sternum:

Pelvis:

Femora:

BRAIN: Weight

Pituitary:

Middle ear and mastoid processes:

Air sinuses of skull:

SPINAL CORD:

Relevant Microscopic Findings:

Chemical and Bacteriological Investigations:

Clinical Summary:

Pathological Summary:

Clinicopathological correlations:

MEDICAL AUDIT:

CHAPTER 17

MUSEUM SPECIMENS

I. CARDIOVASCULAR SYSTEM

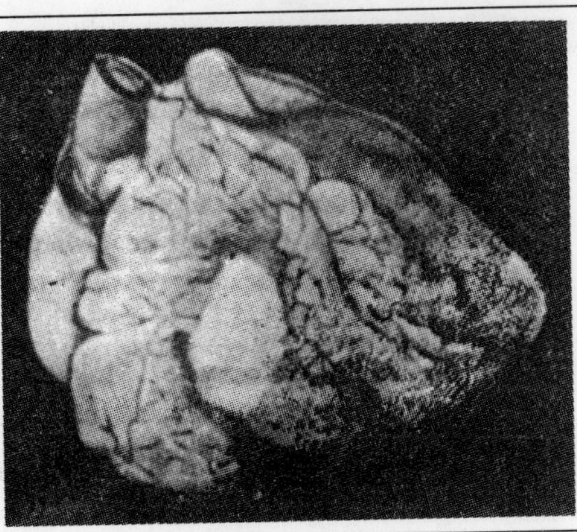

Fig. 17.1: Milk spot

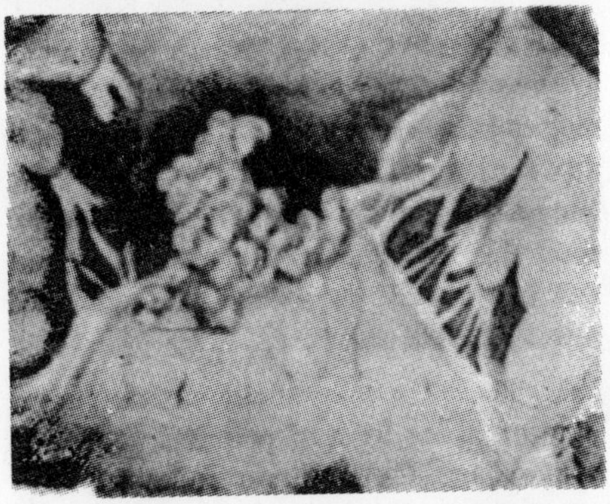

Fig. 17.2: Subacute bacterial endocarditis, showing vegetations on mitral valve

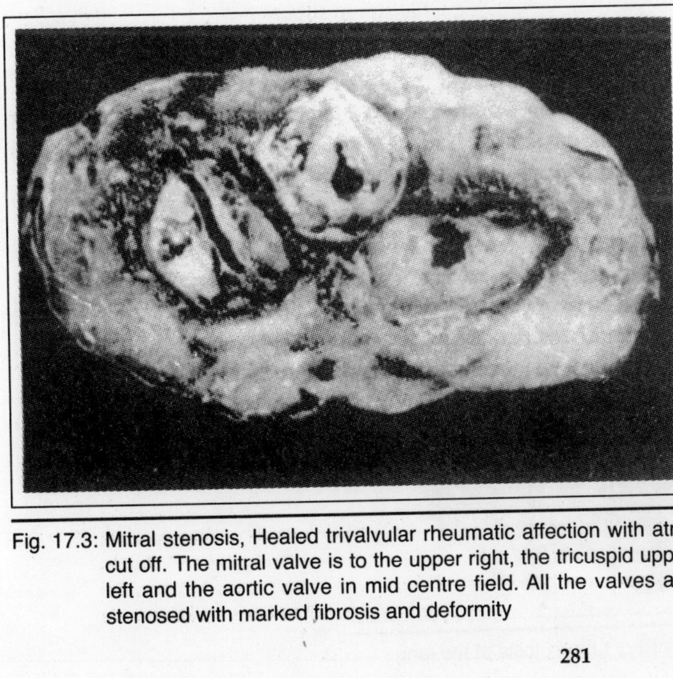

Fig. 17.3: Mitral stenosis, Healed trivalvular rheumatic affection with atria cut off. The mitral valve is to the upper right, the tricuspid upper left and the aortic valve in mid centre field. All the valves are stenosed with marked fibrosis and deformity

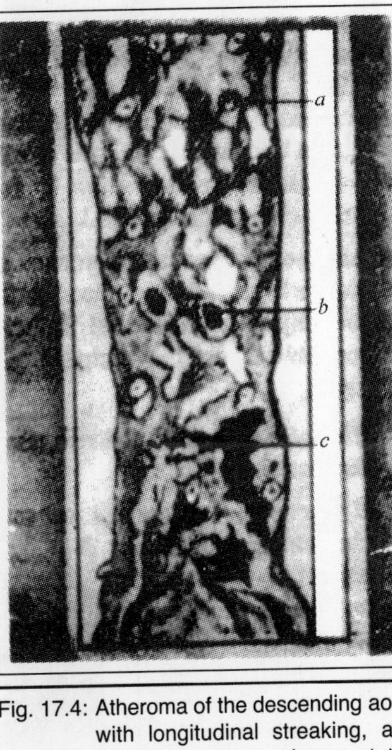

Fig. 17.4: Atheroma of the descending aorta with longitudinal streaking, and (a) atheromatous plaque at the branching of the artery; (b) ulcer; (c) ulcer with calcification, with deformity of the intima and a mural thrombus

II. RESPIRATORY SYSTEM

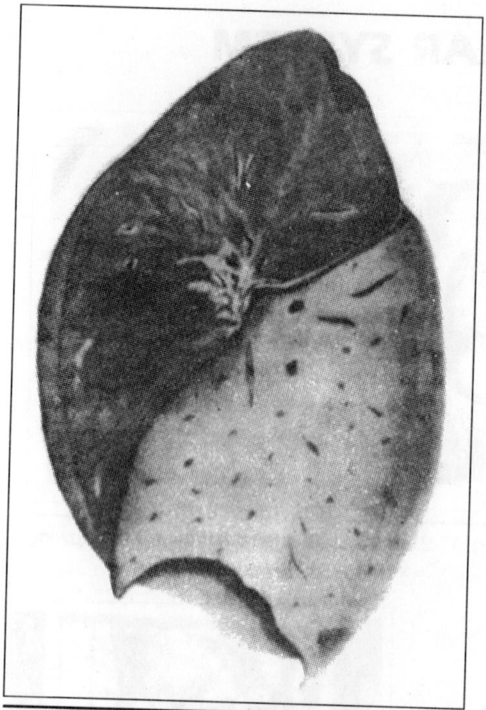

Fig. 17.5: Acute lobar pneumonia in the stage of grey hepatisation, showing massive consolidation of the lower lobe

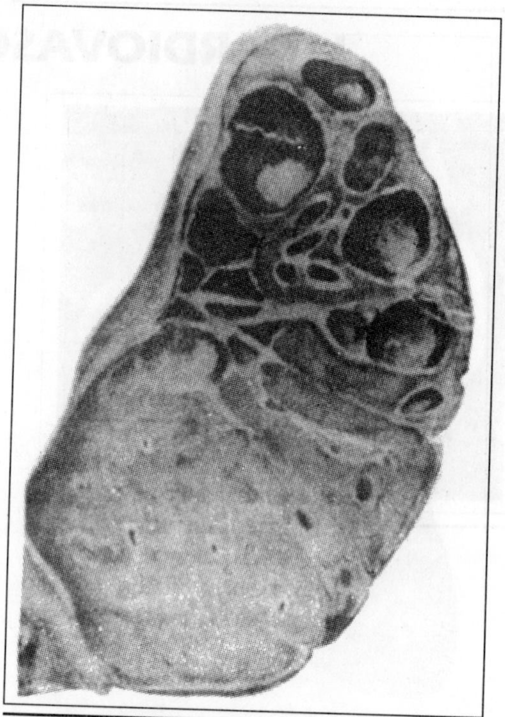

Fig. 17.6: Fibrocaseous tuberculosis of the lung in a young adult

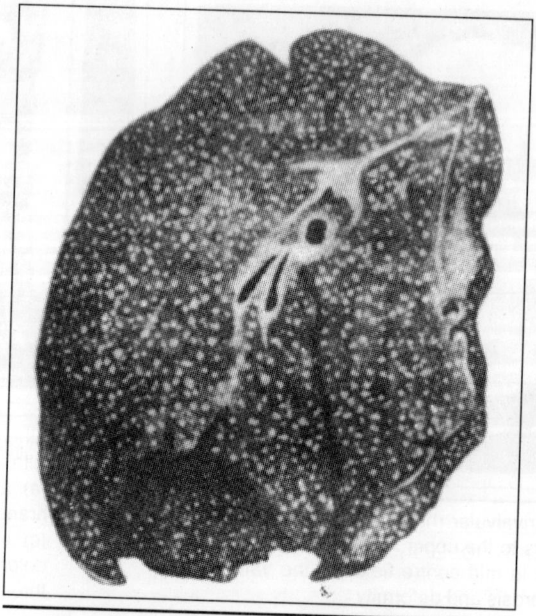

Fig. 17.7: Acute miliary tuberculosis of the lung

II. RESPIRATORY SYSTEM Contd.......

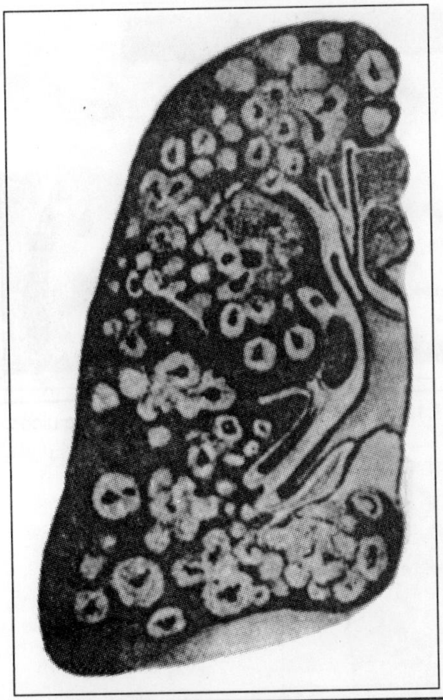

Fig. 17.8: Bronchopneumonic type of Tb. spreading all over the Lung

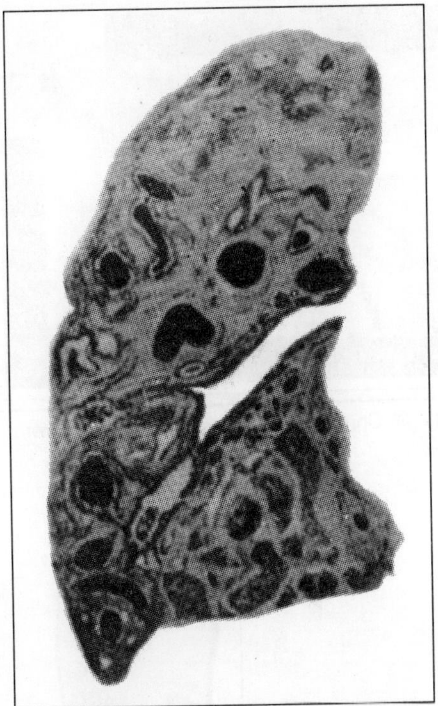

Fig. 17.9: Bronchiectasis of the lung

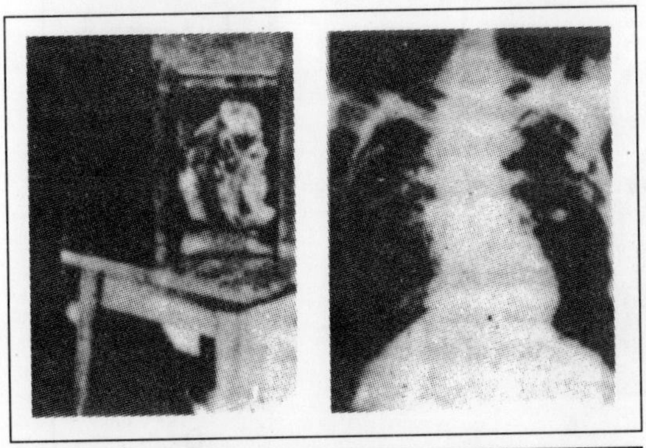

Fig. 17.10: Bronchogenic carcinoma producing Pancoast's syndrome. *Left*: the tumour affecting the right apex; *Right*: X-ray picture of the same

III. DIGESTIVE SYSTEM

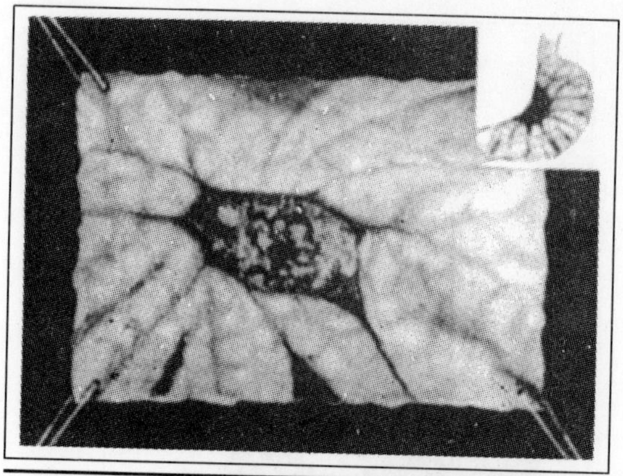

Fig. 17.11: Chronic gastric ulcer (*lesser curvature*)

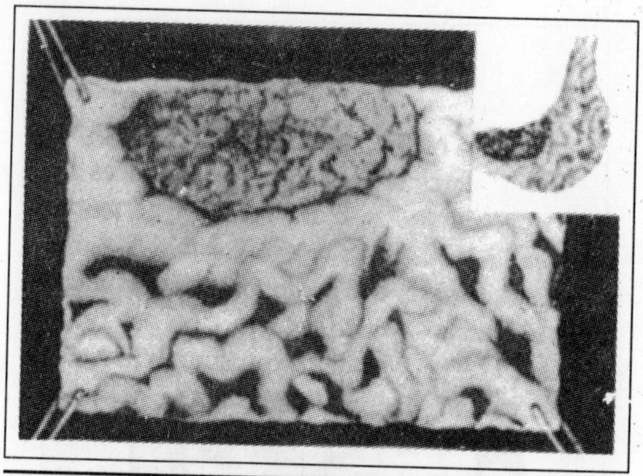

Fig. 17.12: Malignant change in chronic gastric ulcer

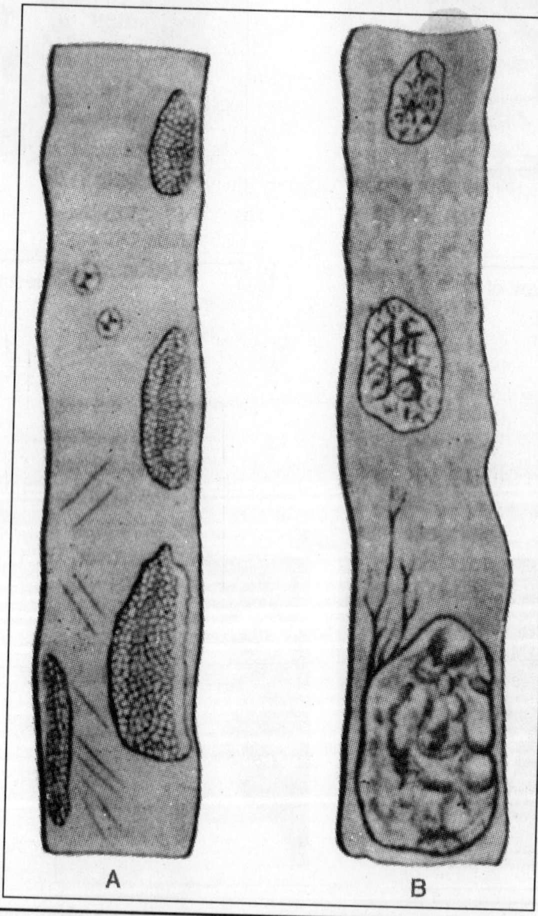

Fig. 17.13: A. Hyperemia and Hyperplasia of Peyer's patches; B. Stage of necrosis in the second week of typhoid fever (Thyroid ulcer). The ulcer occurs along the **longitudinal** axis of the bowel, unlike Tb. ulcer (along the **transverse axis**)

III. DIGESTIVE SYSTEM Contd.......

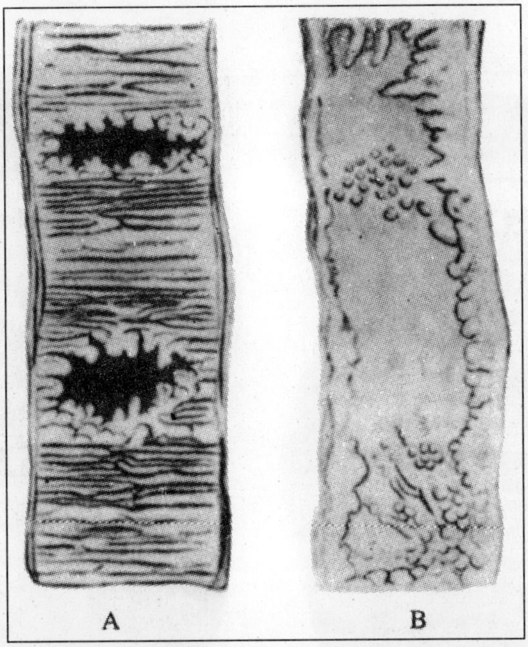

Fig. 17.14: A. TUBERCULOUS ULCER of the small intestine; B. Tubercles on the peritoneal surface

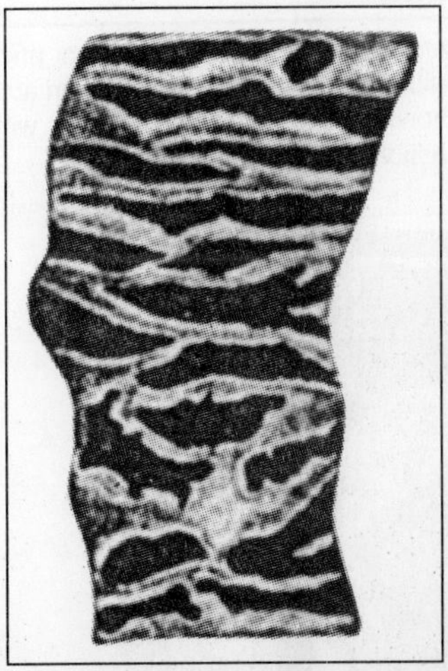

Fig. 17.15: Sigmoid colon in a case of bacillary dysentery caused by *Sh. dysenteriae infection.* Note necrosis at the summit of the rugae. Rugae disappear and look like a piece of leather

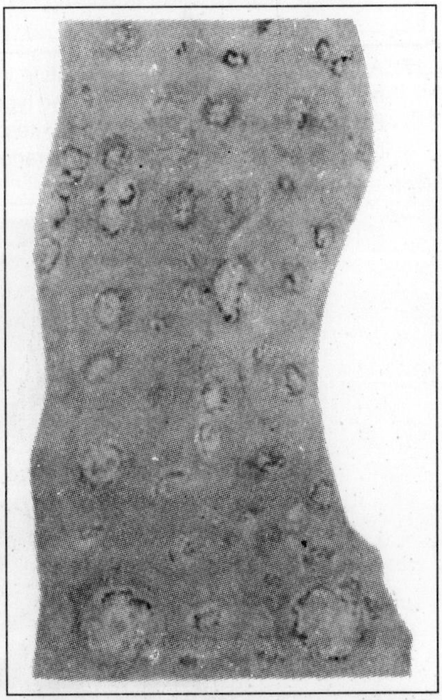

Fig. 17.16: Amoebic ulcer of the rectum

IV. AMOEBIC ULCERS

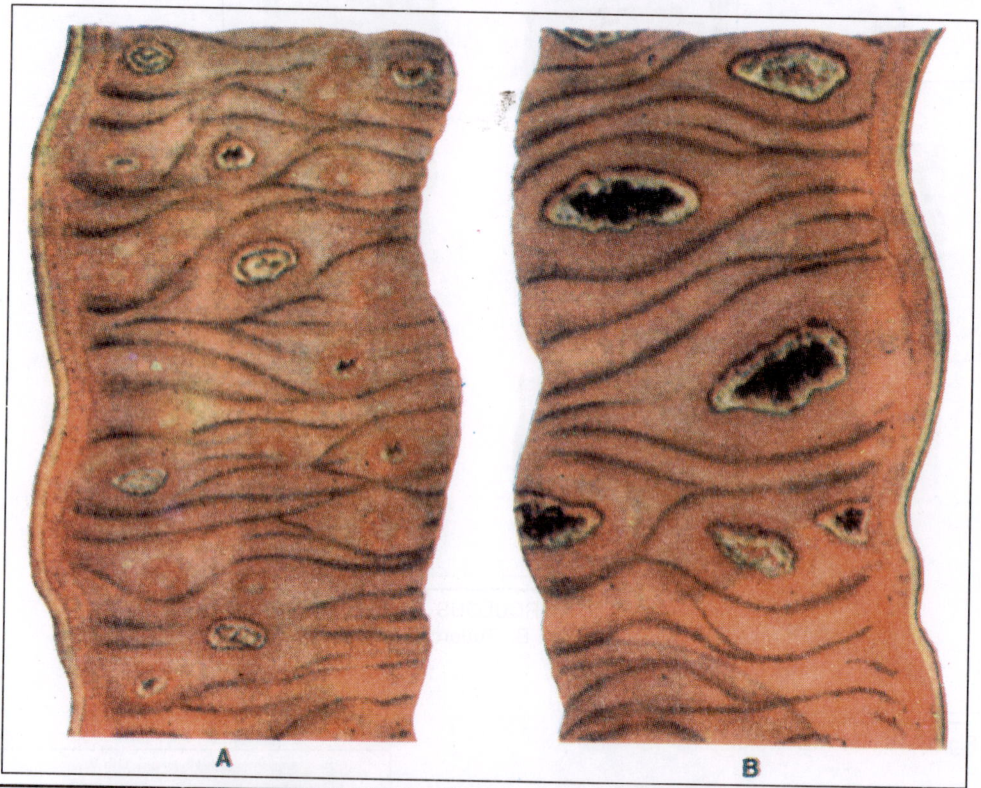

Fig. 17.17: A. Early lesions of the large intestine in Acute amoebic dysentery showing nodular elevation, and acute and subacute ulceration (of flask shaped type with undermine edge) with areas of marked congestion around ulcers; B. Advanced lesions of the large intestine in amoebic colitis showing chronic amoebic ulcers with brownish black slough having shaggy appearance within Moderate congestion seen round the ulcers

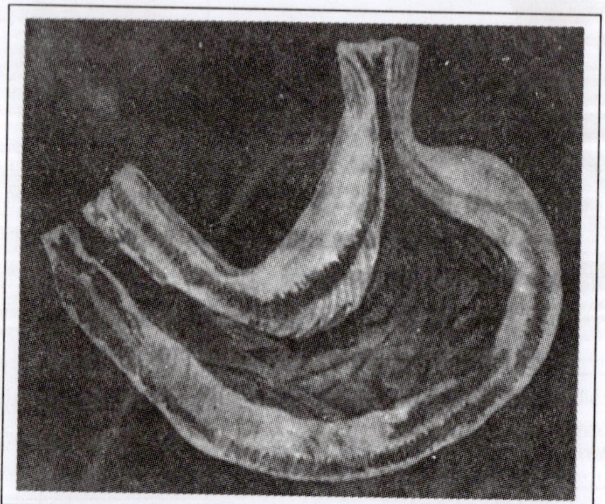

Fig. 17.18: Scirrhous carcinoma stomach

V. LIVER

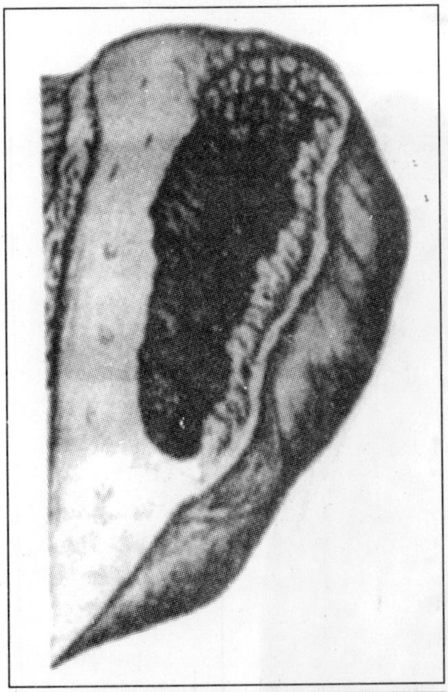

Fig. 17.19: Amoebic liver abscess (*Solitary*)

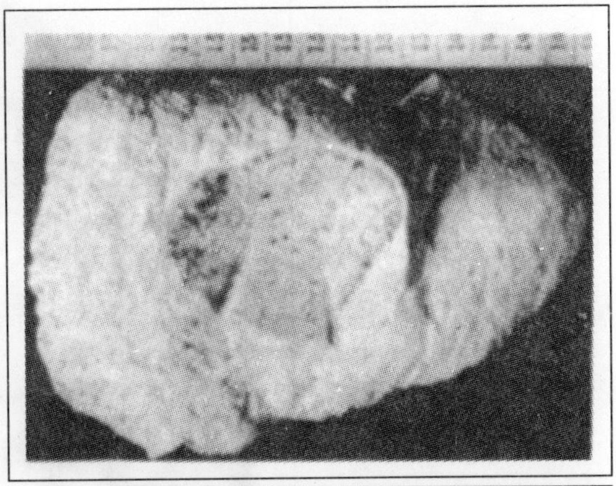

Fig. 17.20: Portal cirrhosis of liver with diffuse, small nodules, 2 cm or less (micronodular type)

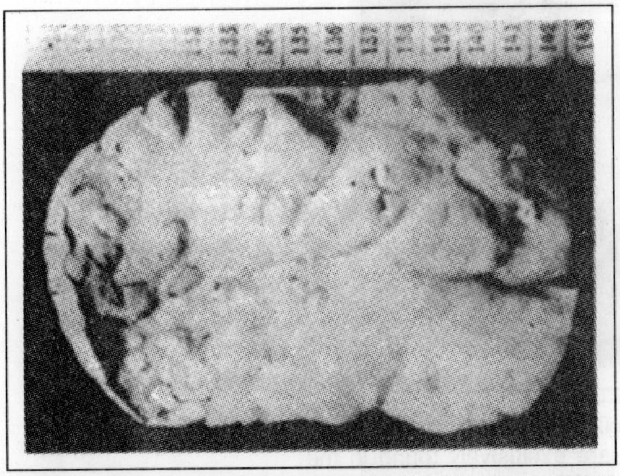

Fig. 17.21: Posthepatitic cirrhosis with diffuse small nodules (2.5 cm)

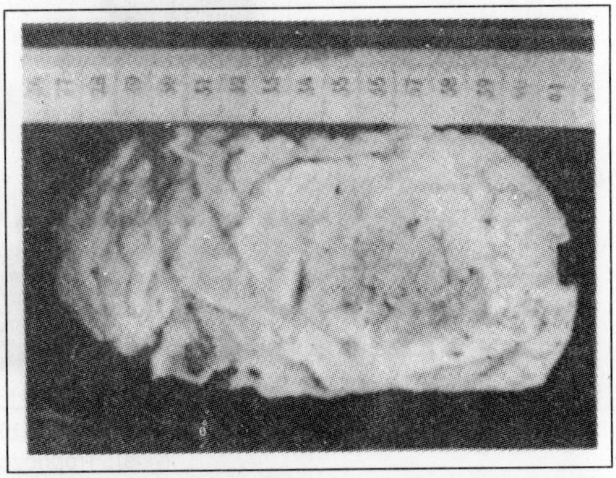

Fig. 17.22: Postnecrotic cirrhosis with large nodules (2.5–5 cm) after (Post-) viral hepatitis

V. LIVER Contd.

TROPICAL AMOEBIC, SOLITARY (or MULTIPLE) LIVER ABSCESS

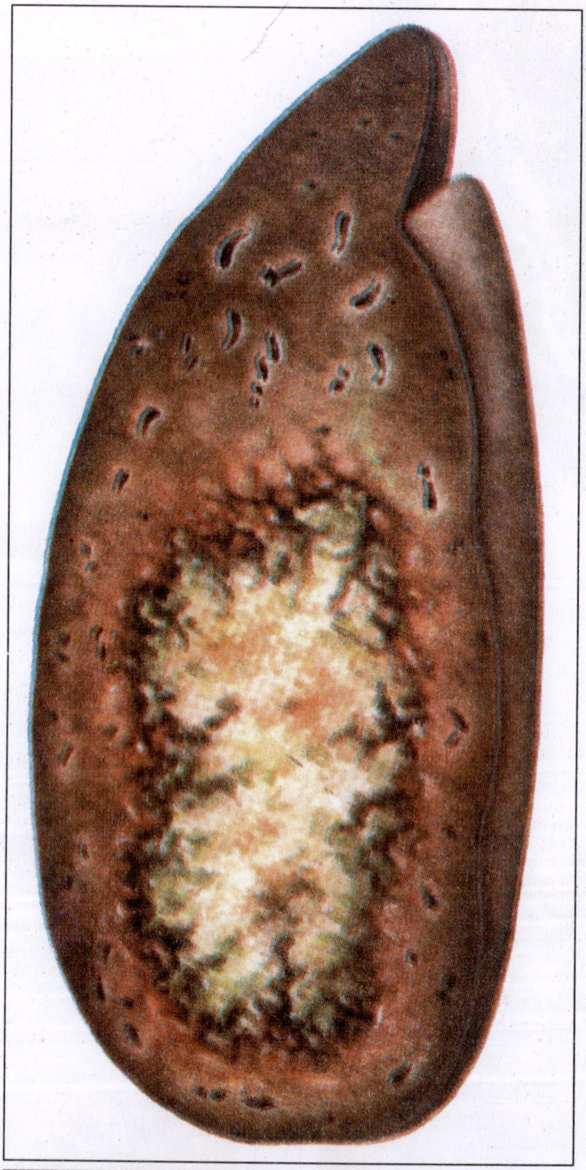

Fig. 17.23: Liver showing big, solitary area of necrosis (Histolysis): Trophozoites are exclusively found in the abscess wall scrapings. It is a pseudoabscess; Pus is formed by cytolysis of liver cells. Pus cells are not present; **inflammatory exudate is absent**

VI. KIDNEY

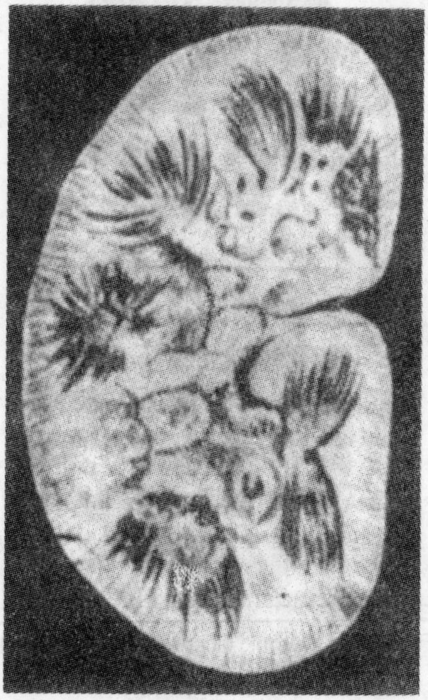

Fig. 17.24: Section of a large white kidney **(Rapidly progressive GN)**

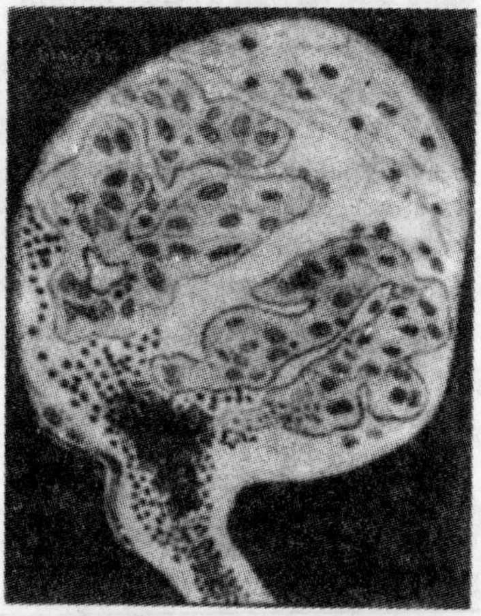

Fig. 17.25: Glomerulus in RPGN (older subacute glomerulonephritis), showing hypercellularity of the tuft and epithelial crescent formation

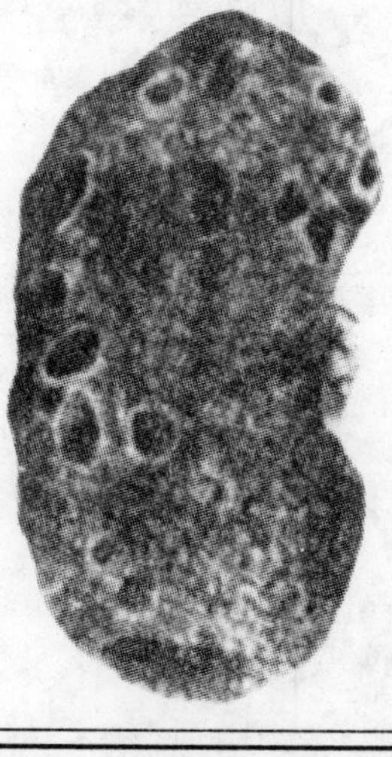

Fig. 17.26: Granular contracted kidney with cysts on the surface (end stage kidney of chronic nephritis)

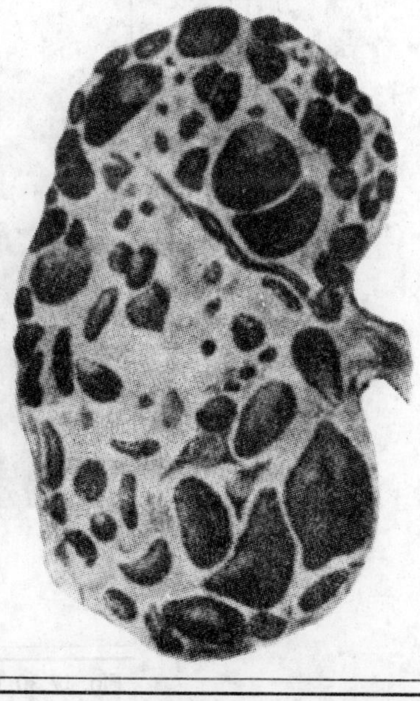

Fig. 17.27: Cut section of a polycystic kidney

VI. KIDNEY Contd.

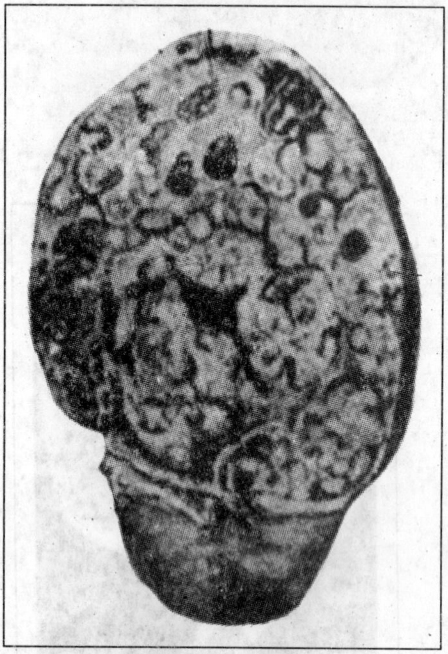

Fig. 17.28: Cut section of renal (clear) cell carcinoma (hypernephroma) with kidney pushed to lower pole

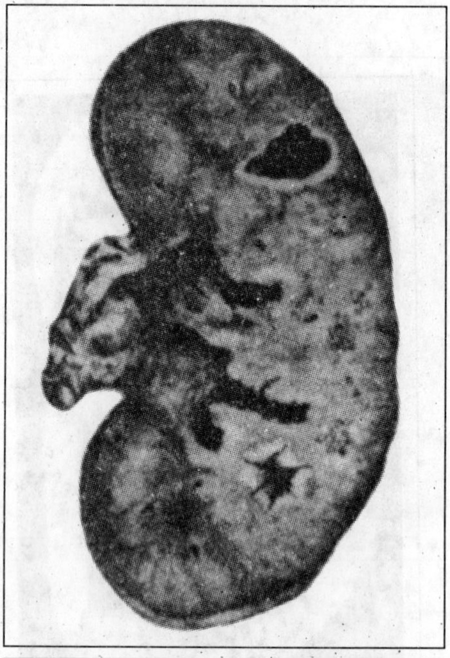

Fig. 17.29: Chronic ulcero-caseous tuberculosis of the kidney

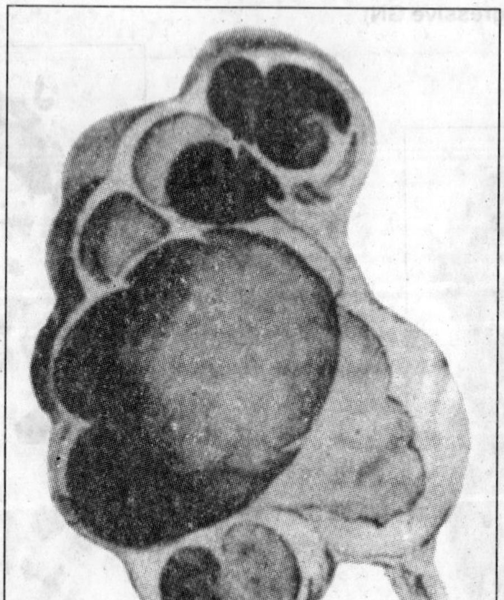

Fig. 17.30: Hydronephrosis of the right kidney

VII. FEMALE GENITALIA

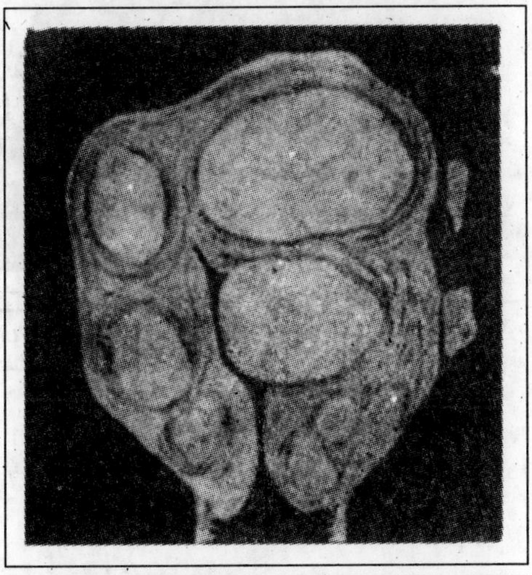

Fig. 17.31: Various types of fibroid in one uterus

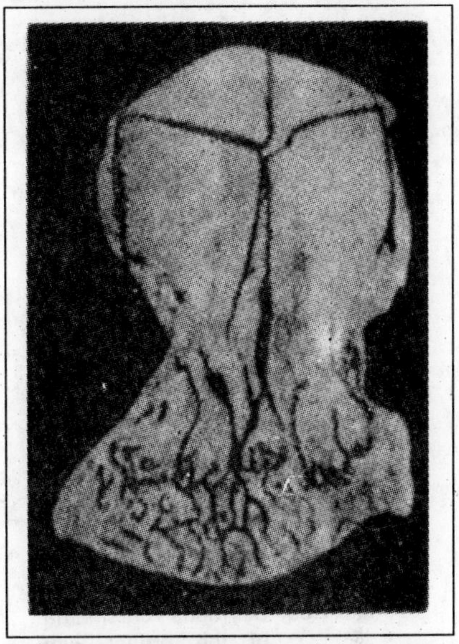

Fig. 17.32: Carcinoma, cervix uteri

VIII. BREAST

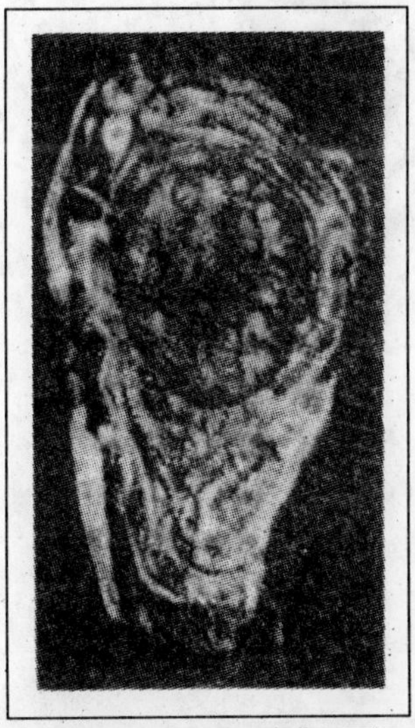

Fig. 17.33: Cut section of intracanalicular fibroadenoma of the breast

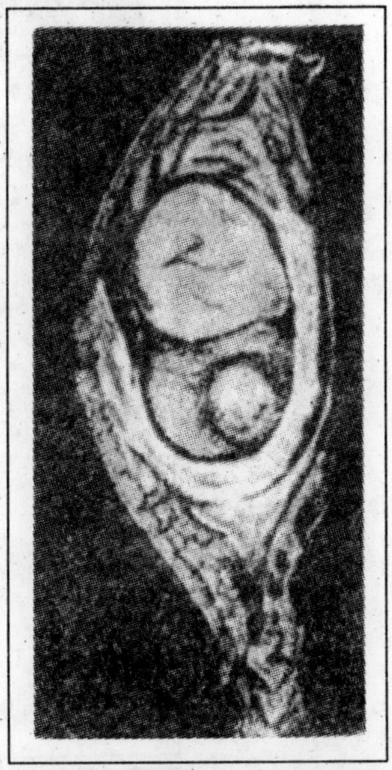

Fig. 17.34: Pericanalicular fibroadenoma of the breast

VIII. BREAST Contd.

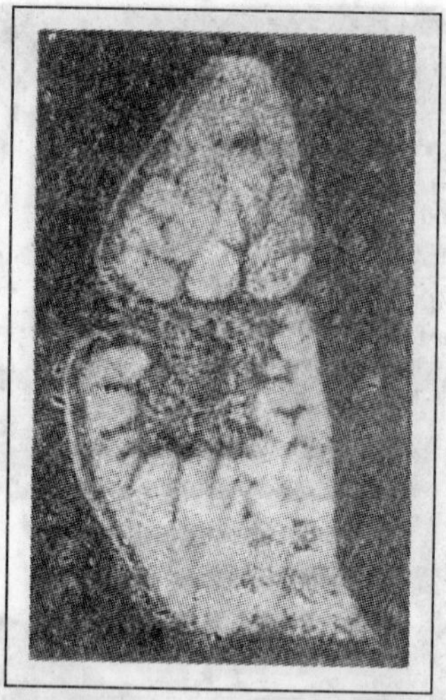

Fig. 17.35: Scirrhous carcinoma of the breast with retraction of the nipple

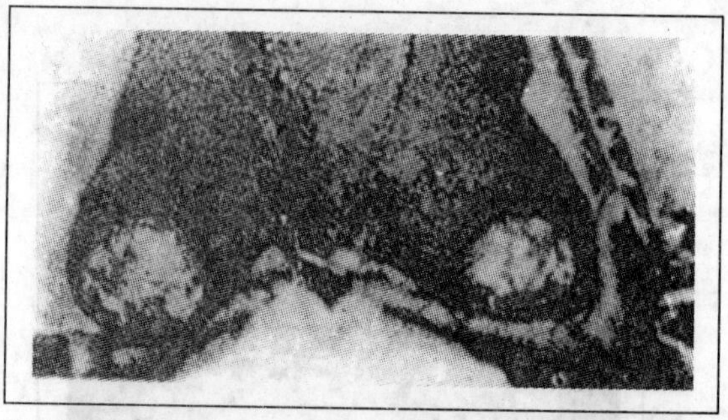

Fig. 17.37: Cancer of the breast (*carcinomatous ulcer in upper and inner quadrant of the breast, bilateral*)

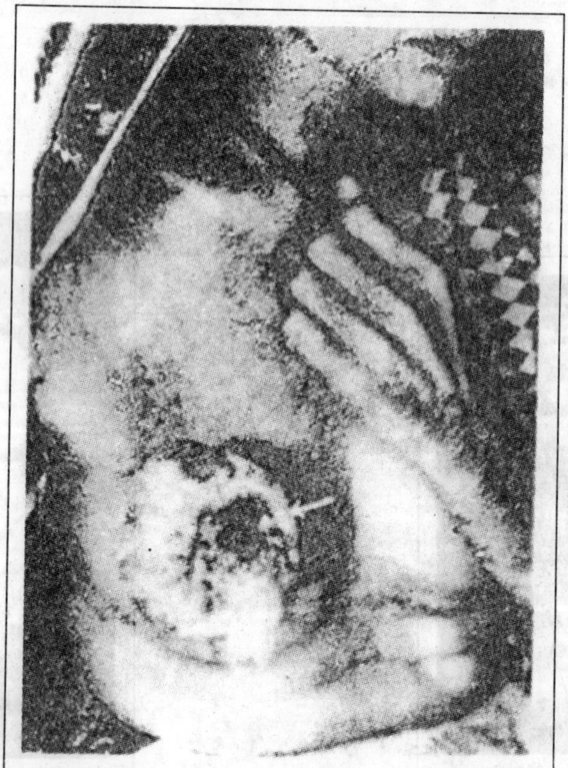

Fig. 17.36: Breast cancer (*fungating with ulceration*)

IX. BONES

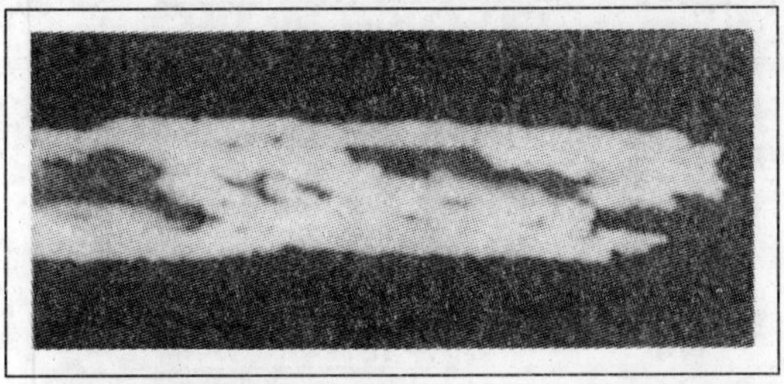

Fig. 17.38: A sequestrum

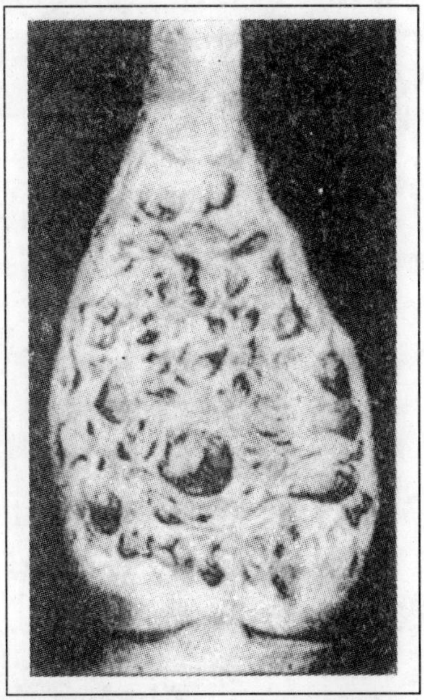

Fig. 17.40: Giant cell tumor of the lower end of the femur with cystic areas of degeneration, which in X-ray shows soap bubble appearance ⇨

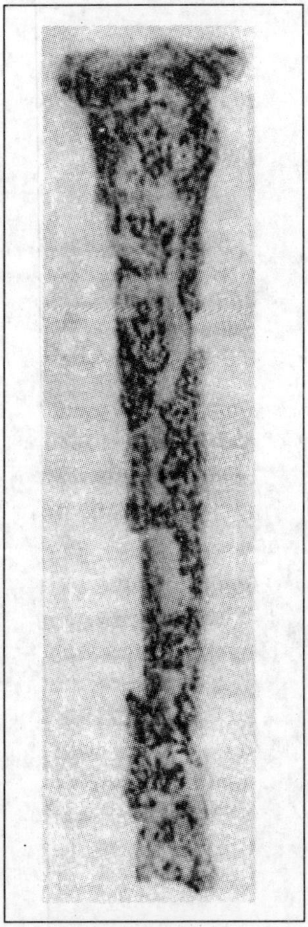

Fig. 17.39: Acute osteomyelitis of the tibia. The whole of diaphysis has undergone necrosis with a shiny, smooth sequestrum (inside) surrounded by involucrum (the necrosed bone shaft)

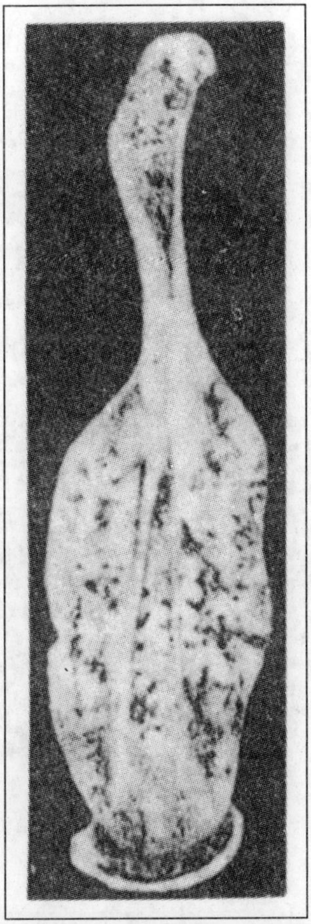

Fig. 17.41: Osteosarcoma involving the lower end of the femur. The epiphyseal cartilage is not involved

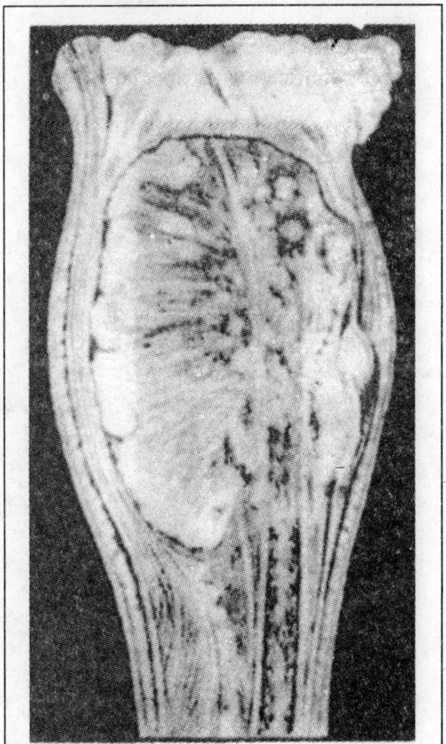

Fig. 17.42: Osteosarcoma arising from the proximal metaphysis of tibia with *sun ray* appearance due to new bone formation and periosteal reaction in an X-ray film (Codman's triangle)

Diagrams/Notes

Appendix

BUFFERS

H-ION INDICATORS

(after N. M. Clark, 1926; The determination of Hydrogen Ions). Baltimore: Williams and Wilkin's

Indicator	Chemical name	Concentration recommended % dye in 95% ethyl alcohol	0.1 N NaOH/0.1 g to make sodium salt	pH range	
				Acidity	Alkalinity
1. Cresol red	Ortho-cresol-sulphonphthalein	0.02	2.62 ml	Red 0.2 –	1.8 yellow
2. Meta-cresol purple (acid range)	M-cresol-sulphonphthalein	0.04	2.62 ml	Red 1.2 –	2.8 yellow
3. Thymol blue (acid range)	Thymol sulphonphthalein	0.04	2.15 ml	Red 1.2 –	2.8 yellow
4. Bromo-phenol blue	Tetra-bromo-phenol sulphonphthalein	0.04	1.49 ml	Yellow 3.0 –	4.6 blue
5. Bromo-chlor phenol blue	Di-bromo-di-chloro-phenol sulphonphthalein	0.04	1.72 ml	Yellow 3.0 –	4.6 blue
6. Bromo-cresol green	Tetra-bromo-meta-cresol sulphonphthalein	0.04	1.43 ml	Yellow 3.8 –	5.4 blue
7. Chloro-cresol green	Tetra-chloro-meta-cresol sulphonphthalein	0.04	1.92 ml	Yellow 4.0 –	5.6 blue
8. Methyl red	Di-methyl-amino azo-benzene-o-carboxylic acid	0.02	3.72 ml	Red 4.4 –	6.0 yellow
9. Chloro-phenol red	Di-chloro-phenol sulphonphthalein	0.04	2.36 ml	Yellow 4.8 –	6.4 red
10. Bromo-phenol red	Di-bromo-phenol sulphonphthalein	0.04	1.95 ml	Yellow 5.2 –	6.8 red
11. Bromo-cresol purple	Di-bromo-orthocresol sulphonphthalein	0.04	1.85 ml	Yellow 5.2 –	6.8 purple
12. Bromo-thymol blue	Di-bromo-thymol sulphonphthalein	0.04	1.60 ml	Yellow 6.0 –	7.6 blue
13. Phenol red	Phenol sulphonphthalein	0.02	2.82 ml	Yellow 6.8 –	8.4 red

Contd.

Contd.

Indicator	Chemical name	Concentration recommended % dye in 95% ethyl alcohol	0.1 N NaOH/0.1 g to make sodium salt	pH range Acidity Alkalinity
14. Cresol red	Ortho-cresol-sulphonphthalein	0.02	2.62 ml	Yellow 7.2 – 8.8 red
15. Meta-cresol purple (alkaline range)	M-cresol-sulphonphthalein	0.04	2.62 ml	Yellow 7.4 – 9.0 purple
16. Thymol blue (alkaline range)	Thymol sulphonphthalein	0.04	2.15 ml	Yellow 8.0 – 9.6 blue
17. Cresolphthalein	Ortho-cresolphthalein	0.04	2.89 ml	Colorless 8.2 – 9.8 red
18. Phenolphthalein	Di-hydroxyphthalophenone	0.05	–	Colorless 8.3–10.0 red

N.B. To make this, dissolve 0.4% aqueous solution of each indicator is prepared by dissolving 0.1 g of each chemical powder in indicates volume of 0.1N NaOH and making up the volume to 250 ml with distilled water (D/w).
Preparation for use: Dissolve indicator powders in alcohol and add sufficient (of the) alkali to produce a green color; label.

UNIVERSAL INDICATORS

A mixed indicator for use in approximate pH determinations.

Methyl red	0.0185 g
Bromo-thymol blue	0.0600 g
Phenolphthalein	0.0640 g
Ethyl alcohol, 50%	100.0 ml
NaOH, 0.1 N	As required

pH	Color	pH	Color
upto 3.0	Red	7.0	Greenish-yellow
4.0	Deeper red	8.0	Green
5.0	Orange red	9.0	Greenish-blue
6.0	Orange yellow	10.0	Violet
		11.0	Reddish-violet

British Drug House "Universal Indicator" (color range)

pH	Color	pH	Color
upto 3.0	Red	8.0	Green
4.0	Deeper red	8.5	Bluish-green
5.0	Orange red	9.0	Greenish-blue
6.0	Orange yellow	10.0	Violet
6.5	Yellow	10.0	Reddish-violet
7.0–7.5	Greenish-yellow	11.0	Deeper reddish-violet

GOMORI'S TRIHYDROXYMETHYLAMINOMETHANE MALEIC ACID BUFFER

pH range 5.08–8.45

pH	Vol. in ml of M/1 maleic acid	Vol. in ml of M/1 trihydroxymethylaminomethane	Vol. in ml of M/2 NaOH	Vol. in ml of distilled water to make 50 ml
5.08	5	5	01	39
5.30	5	5	02	38
5.52	5	5	03	37
5.70	5	5	04	36
5.88	5	5	05	35
6.05	5	5	06	34
6.27	5	5	07	33
6.50	5	5	08	32
6.86	5	5	09	31
7.20	5	5	10	30
7.50	5	5	11	30
7.75	5	5	12	29
7.97	5	5	13	28
8.15	5	5	14	26
8.30	5	5	15	25
8.45	5	5	16	24

MICHAELIS' VERONAL-HYDROCHLORIC ACID BUFFER

pH range 4.95–9.2

Veronal Acetate solution

Sodium acetate	1.943	g
Veronal (**sodium barbiturate**, i.e. barbiton or barbital)	2.943	g
Distilled water	to 100	ml

Mode of preparation

Using a 100 ml volumetric flask dissolve the salts in part of the distilled water, make up to the mark; bottle and label.

pH	Vol. in ml of veronal acetate solution	Vol. in ml of M/10 HCl	Vol. in ml of distilled water to make 25 ml
4.95	5	9.00	11.00
5.30	5	8.00	12.00
6.10	5	7.00	13.00
6.75	5	6.50	13.50
7.00	5	6.00	14.00
7.25	5	5.50	14.50
7.40	5	5.00	15.00

Contd.

Contd.

pH	Vol. in ml of veronal acetate solution	Vol. in ml of M/10 HCl	Vol. in ml of distilled water to make 25 ml
7.66	5	4.00	16.00
7.90	5	3.00	17.00
8.20	5	2.00	18.00
8.60	5	1.00	19.00
8.70	5	0.75	19.25
8.90	5	0.50	19.50
9.20	5	0.25	19.75

HOLMES' BORIC ACID—SODIUM TETRABORATE BUFFER

pH range 7.4–9.0

pH	Vol. in ml of M/1 H_2BO_3	Vol. in ml of M/20 $Na_2B_4O_7$, $10H_2O$
7.4	18	02
7.6	17	03
7.8	16	04
8.0	14	06
8.2	13	07
8.4	11	09
8.7	08	12
9.0	04	16

CLARKE AND LUBS' BORIC ACID—POTASSIUM CHLORIDE—SODIUM HYDROXIDE BUFFER

pH range 7.8–10.0

pH	Vol. in ml of M/1 H_3BO_3 and M/1 KCL mixture	Vol. in ml of M/1 NaOH	Vol. in ml of distilled water to make 200 ml
7.8	50	2.61	147.39
8.0	50	3.97	146.03
8.2	50	5.90	144.10
8.4	50	8.50	141.50
8.6	50	12.00	138.00
8.8	50	16.30	133.70
9.0	50	21.30	128.70
9.2	50	26.70	123.30
9.4	50	32.00	118.00
9.6	50	36.85	113.15
9.8	50	40.80	109.20
10.0	50	43.90	106.10

SORENSEN-WALBUM GLYCINE—SODIUM CHLORIDE—SODIUM HYDROXIDE BUFFER

pH range 8.45–12.77

pH	Vol. in ml of M/10 glycine and M/10 NaCl mixture	Vol. in ml of M/10 NaOH
8.45	95	05
8.79	90	10
9.22	80	20
9.56	70	30
9.98	60	40
10.32	55	45
10.90	51	49
11.14	50	50
11.39	49	51
11.92	45	55
12.21	40	60
12.48	30	70
12.66	20	80
12.77	10	90

SORENSEN'S PHOSPHATE BUFFER

(After Lillie R.D; 1954. Histopathologic Technique and Practical Histochemistry 2nd ed. P. 45, New York, Blakiston)

pH using M/10 solution	pH using M/15 solution	Vol. in ml of M/10 or M/15 KH_2PO_4	Vol. in ml of M/10 or M/15 Na_2HPO_4
4.41	4.47	100	0
5.31	5.42	96	4
5.53	5.60	94	6
5.67	5.74	92	8
5.78	5.83	90	10
5.86	5.91	88	12
5.94	5.99	86	14
6.02	6.07	84	16
6.08	6.14	82	18
6.12	6.19	80	20
6.17	6.24	78	22
6.23	6.28	76	24
6.28	6.32	74	26
6.33	6.37	72	28
6.37	6.41	70	30

Contd.

Contd.

pH using M/10 solution	pH using M/15 solution	Vol. in ml of M/10 or M/15 KH_2PO_4	Vol. in ml of M/10 or M/15 Na_2HPO_4
6.41	6.45	68	32
6.45	6.49	66	34
6.49	6.53	64	36
6.55	6.59	60	40
6.61	6.68	56	44
6.65	6.72	54	46
6.70	6.76	52	48
6.76	6.81	50	50
6.81	6.86	48	52
6.87	6.94	44	56
6.89	6.96	42	58
6.91	6.98	40	60
6.97	7.03	36	64
7.00	7.05	34	66
7.06	7.11	30	70
7.10	7.15	28	72
7.14	7.20	26	74
7.19	7.24	24	76
7.24	7.28	22	78
7.30	7.33	20	80
7.36	7.40	18	82
7.42	7.47	16	84
7.49	7.54	14	86
7.57	7.61	12	88
7.65	7.69	10	90
7.73	7.77	8	92
7.81	7.85	6	94
7.92	7.97	4	96
8.98	8.93	0	100

McILVAINE'S PHOSPHATE—CITRIC ACID BUFFER

pH range 2.2–8.0

pH	Vol. in ml of M/5 Na_2HPO_4	Vol. in ml of M/10 citric acid
2.2	0.40	19.60
2.4	1.24	18.76
2.6	2.18	17.82
2.8	3.17	16.83
3.0	4.11	15.89

Contd.

Contd.

pH	Vol. in ml of M/5 Na_2HPO_4	Vol. in ml of M/10 citric acid
3.2	4.94	15.06
3.4	5.70	14.30
3.6	6.44	13.56
3.8	7.10	12.90
4.0	7.71	12.29
4.2	8.28	11.72
4.4	8.82	11.18
4.6	9.35	10.65
4.8	9.86	10.14
5.0	10.30	9.70
5.2	10.72	9.28
5.4	11.15	8.85
5.6	11.60	8.40
5.8	12.09	7.91
6.0	12.63	7.37
6.2	13.22	6.78
6.4	13.85	6.15
6.6	14.55	5.45
6.8	15.45	4.55
7.0	16.47	3.35
7.2	17.39	2.61
7.4	18.17	1.83
7.6	18.73	1.27
7.8	19.15	0.85
8.0	19.45	0.55

GOMORI'S TRIS (HYDROXYMETHANE) AMINO METHANE—HYDROCHLORIC ACID BUFFER

pH range 7.19–9.10

pH	Vol. in ml of M/5 tris (hydroxymethyl) amino-methane	Vol. in ml of N/10 HCl	Vol. of distilled water to make 100 ml
7.19	25	45.0	30.0
7.36	25	42.5	32.5
7.54	25	40.0	35.0
7.66	25	37.5	37.5
7.77	25	35.0	40.0
7.87	25	32.5	42.5

Contd.

Contd.

pH	Vol. in ml of M/5 tris (hydroxymethyl) amino-methane	Vol. in ml of N/10 HCl	Vol. of distilled water to make 100 ml
7.96	25	30.0	45.0
8.05	25	27.5	47.5
8.14	25	25.0	50.0
8.23	25	22.5	52.5
8.32	25	20.0	55.0
8.41	25	17.5	57.5
8.51	25	15.0	60.0
8.62	25	12.5	62.5
8.74	25	10.0	65.0
8.92	25	7.5	67.5
9.10	25	5.0	70.0

WALPOLE'S SODIUM ACETATE—HYDROCHLORIC ACID BUFFER

pH range 0.65–5.20

pH	Vol. in ml of N/1 $Na_2C_2H_3O_2$	Vol. in ml of N/1 HCl	Vol. in ml of distilled water to make 250 ml
0.65	50	100	100
0.75	50	90	110
0.91	50	80	120
1.09	50	70	130
1.24	50	65	135
1.42	50	60	140
1.71	50	55	145
1.85	50	53.50	146.5
1.99	50	52.50	147.5
2.32	50	51	149
2.64	50	50	150
2.72	50	49.75	150.25
3.09	50	48.50	151.5
3.29	50	47.50	152.5
3.49	50	46.25	153.75
3.61	50	45	155
3.79	50	42.50	157.5
3.95	50	40	160
4.19	50	35	165
4.39	50	30	170
4.58	50	25	175
4.76	50	20	180
4.92	50	15	185
5.20	50	10	190

WALPOLE'S SODIUM ACETATE—ACETIC ACID BUFFER

pH range 2.7–6.52

pH	Vol. in ml of M/5 $NaC_2H_3O_2$	Vol. in ml of M/5 $CH_3 \cdot CO \cdot OH$
2.70	–	20.0
2.80	0.1	19.9
2.91	0.2	19.8
2.99	0.3	19.7
3.08	0.4	19.6
3.15	0.5	19.5
3.20	0.6	19.4
3.32	0.8	19.2
3.42	1.0	19.0
3.56	1.5	18.5
3.72	2.0	18.0
3.90	3.0	17.0
4.05	4.0	16.0
4.16	5.0	15.0
4.27	6.0	14.0
4.36	7.0	13.0
4.45	8.0	12.0
4.53	9.0	11.0
4.62	10.0	10.0
4.71	11.0	9.0
4.80	12.0	8.0
4.90	13.0	7.0
4.99	14.0	6.0
5.11	15.0	5.0
5.23	16.0	4.0
5.38	17.0	3.0
5.58	18.0	2.0
5.90	19.0	1.0
6.21	19.5	0.5
6.52	20.0	–

BARBITAL BUFFER FOR PROTEIN ELECTROPHORESIS

pH 8.6 (Ionic strength 0.1)

Sodium barbital	41.2 g
Barbital	7.0 g
Distilled water	to 2 litres

BARBITAL BUFFER FOR HEMOGLOBIN ELECTROPHORESIS

pH 8.6 (Ionic strength 0.05)

Sodium barbital	20.6 g
Barbital	3.5 g
Distilled water	to 2 litres

Index

A

B

C

I

M

N

T

U

V

W